The Restaurant Diet™

How to Eat Out Every Night and Still Lose Weight

by

Fred Bollaci

Foreword by Dick Smothers

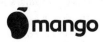

The Restaurant Diet™: How to Eat Out Every Night and Still Lose Weight

Library of Congress Cataloging
ISBN: (p) 978-1-63353-702-6, (e) 978-1-63353-703-3
Library of Congress Control Number: 2017958203
BISAC - HEA017000 HEALTH & FITNESS / Diet & Nutrition / Nutrition
        - HEA010000 HEALTH & FITNESS / Healthy Living

Printed in the United States of America

DISCLAIMER: The author of this book does not dispense medical advice or prescribe the use of any of the techniques in this book as a form of treatment for physical, mental, or emotional problems without the advice of a trained health professional. The information contained herein should be considered as being of a general nature to help you in your quest to lose weight and for emotional well-being, good health, and spiritual growth. Every individual's situation and needs are different. In the event you use any of the information in this book for yourself, the author and publisher assume no responsibility for your actions.

Some of the names, places, and events depicted in this book have been changed to protect the privacy of individuals.

I dedicate *The Restaurant Diet* to my parents: my mother, Marianne Siegal, and my father, the late Dr. Frederick Bollaci, without whom there would be no *Restaurant Diet*.

You both introduced me to the finer things in life—the best food, the best restaurants, and travel to many amazing places. It is all of these experiences that have come together to make me who I am today and form the foundation for *The Restaurant Diet*. You also encouraged me to do things my own way, to make a difference in this world, and to never give up when I believe in something.

I am grateful to own this legacy and build upon it, by learning to enjoy the very best that life has to offer and to be able to appreciate and share all that I've been given.

"You've lost so much weight they need to file a missing person's report."
—Dr. Daniel Galvin, General Surgeon, New York City

Contents

Foreword by Dick Smothers

When my friend Fred Bollaci asked me to write a foreword to his book, I decided to Google the words "forewords for books" before accepting. The search results indicated that, to write a foreword for a book, one generally should be famous, a well-known expert in the field, or maybe a friend to the person writing the book who has had a similar or shared experience with the subject of the book. I believe I qualify in most of those areas, so here goes.

Fred Bollaci is a friend of mine, and I can identify with what he's done to create a healthy life. The old Fred never really had a meaningful life. Due to his unhealthy lifestyle and eating habits, it looked like he was going to have a short, unhappy existence at best. He soon came to realize that he had no future living the destructive way he was living.

Only Fred can tell you—as he does in this book—how and why he came to make the changes that made this transformation possible.

The reason I can identify with my friend Fred is because, for both of us, our lives had become unmanageable and out of control. We had the same problem: ourselves. Our way of thinking had gotten us into serious trouble. Fred medicated his issues by overeating, and I medicated my issues with alcohol. The effects of his overeating and obesity and the effects of my alcohol consumption seriously diminished the quality of our respective lives.

It's been over eighteen years since I had my last drink. Every day since then, I have thanked my higher power for restoring me to sanity and helping me recreate a life that is superior to my old one in every single way. I cannot tell you the joy I feel watching my good friend do the same thing by creating a new life for himself: one full of joy, passion, and adventure.

What Fred has done, and the way he did it, is quite unique. Dining with Fred in gourmet restaurants—the ones he always went to and will continue to enjoy—is a thrilling and fascinating experience to behold.

Bottom line: what did Fred actually accomplish? He reshaped his outside *and* his inside. That is the best way to accomplish everything, isn't it? The two go together—which reminds me of the old Frank Sinatra song "Love and Marriage," by Sammy Cahn and Jimmy Van Heusen. Love and marriage is like a horse and carriage. You can't have one without the other. You also can't change your outside appearance without healing yourself inside, either. That is why has succeeded—and he will teach you how to do so too.

Enjoy the read—and *bon appetit!*

—Dick Smothers, comedian

Letter from Fred's Personal Physician and Cardiologist, Dr. Gene E. Myers, MD, FACC

As a practicing physician and cardiologist for over thirty years, I have had firsthand experience in treating thousands of patients. Having performed over 30,000 invasive cardiac and vascular procedures, I am a strong proponent of preventative medicine. I encourage my patients to adopt healthier lifestyles, including a healthy, balanced diet with daily exercise, so they can live life to the fullest and hopefully prevent heart disease, diabetes, hypertension, and numerous other ailments related to poor diet, inactivity, and unhealthy lifestyle choices.

Weight loss shouldn't be viewed as a short-term means to an end. Rather, reaching and maintaining a healthy weight should be part of a comprehensive healthy lifestyle. This is the best way to ensure permanent success. As a culture, we should start by changing how we feel about diet and exercise. A realistic food and exercise plan must be part of every healthy and active lifestyle.

In my lengthy career, Fred's success story is truly one of the most, if not *the* most, exciting case I have ever been involved with. I am thrilled and honored to have witnessed and been a part of his seemingly miraculous transformation from an unhappy, morbidly obese adult—who risked certain, untimely death from sleep apnea, hypertension, diabetes, and likely related cardiac issues—into a bright, handsome, and vivacious young man who has gotten a new lease on life and plans to make it count.

I cannot emphasize enough the importance of a good doctor-patient relationship. Without the "one-on-one" rapport between Fred and I, the outcome may well have been different. Having a patient with a good attitude, a desire to get well, a willingness to share, and a doctor who was willing to listen and connect the dots, made all the difference. Thirty minutes up-front allowed us to quickly focus on the likely problems and solutions that otherwise may have gone unresolved and made losing weight, and keeping it off, much more difficult.

From a medical standpoint, I oversaw Fred's entire weight loss. We first made sure he was able to exercise, established a baseline with blood tests and a cardiac workup, and helped him establish reasonable guidelines for dietary and exercise plans, which he then tailored to his specific tastes and circumstances. And he has achieved something extraordinary. If there is anything to learn from Fred's story, it is this: weight loss and recovery is an "inside job." You can eat healthy, exercise, reach a healthy weight, and still be miserable, as Fred shares in his story. Until Fred dealt with his emotional issues, the compulsion to give up and go back to overeating and an unhealthy lifestyle was great. In looking for the answers within, establishing a strong support system, and adopting healthy, permanent habits, Fred became poised for a long, happy, healthy, successful life!

—Dr. Gene E. Myers, MD, FACC, Sarasota, Florida
Spring 2017

A Letter from Fred's Nutritionist, Maureen Buchbinder, Nutrition and Health Coach, Educator, and Chef

I am honored and thrilled to be part of Fred Bollaci's book and ongoing success. When Fred walked into my office in December 2009, he was 315 pounds and seemed very enthusiastic and determined to lose the weight. After talking with Fred for a few minutes and witnessing the commitment he had to his goals, and the progress he had already made, I felt he was going to be a success.

To begin, I reviewed Fred's eating and exercise plan and made suggestions. He listened, learned, and came to each meeting eager and determined. I grew very excited by his continued progress; his attitude was fabulous, as he embraced any struggles that came into his path, such as emotional issues from his past and inevitable plateaus. Like anyone trying to lose weight, Fred did not live in a bubble, impervious to stressful situations going on around him. During this time, his dad was battling Stage IV cancer, something that was no doubt very upsetting and difficult for Fred—an only child. This could easily lead someone like Fred, with a history of emotional overeating, to give up. Despite any obstacles, his weight loss was progressive and steady.

As the weight came off, exercise became easier. To adjust to his improvement, he continually modified his exercise regimen by implementing longer and varied physical endurances with intervals.

As for nutrition, his eating plan focused on lean protein, high fiber, and low sugar and carbohydrates. The most unique aspect of his plan was that he made dining out a key component. During his weight loss, Fred shared with me the details of meals he was able to enjoy at many great local restaurants, something that many people would find appealing. Some of his favorite carbs, especially early on, were oatmeal, sweet potato, and barley (vegetable or beef barley soup). When Fred began losing weight, he especially feared carbs such as bread, pasta, and pizza, which represented some of the foods he used to eat to excess, growing up in an Italian-American family with great cooks. After several years in his new healthy lifestyle and at a healthy weight, Fred has made peace with food and is able to enjoy almost anything in moderation.

Fred used to weigh himself daily. Now, he weighs himself several times a week and has established a healthy weight range to stay in. He has become comfortable and confident with the "New Fred" and no longer fears going back to his old ways.

It is now spring 2017, and Fred looks and feels fabulous. His attitude is positive, and he seems happier, more relaxed, and more at peace than ever.

The Restaurant Diet is an inspirational read for anybody who wants to get healthier and reach his or her ideal body weight by making permanent, positive changes to their lifestyle. The menus and recipes are from fabulous restaurants and are a very helpful resource for anyone looking to enjoy gourmet weight-loss, both at home and in some of America's best restaurants.

Fred's story is remarkable, and proof that anyone can totally change for the better. Fred is an amazing young man, and I am hrilled I helped him in his journey to better health.

—Maureen Buchbinder, Palm Beach Gardens, Florida
Spring 2017

Letter from Fred's Therapist, Linda B. Sherr

I feel privileged to contribute this letter to Fred Bollaci's book. Fred is a fine man: intellectually gifted, well educated, thoughtful, and admirably motivated to have made the changes in his life that you will read about in this book.

In my almost forty years of practice as a psychotherapist, I have witnessed the recovery of many eating disordered people. In the recovery process, there is a point at which the negative behaviors—whether bingeing, gluttony, bulimia, or anorexia—abate. The recovering person must then undertake a new relationship with food, as well as with themselves and those around them. Unlike drugs and alcohol, this is not an "all or nothing" experience or abstinence. Rather, the daily need for nourishment requires a complete reestablishment of food as a positive life force.

Fred Bollaci is unique in that he has a gourmet's appreciation of food as healthy nourishment. This allowed him to develop a very creative and positive experience with food. In *The Restaurant Diet*, Fred shares his experience with healthy recipes and healthy, happy eating. I continue to admire Fred's commitment to the recovery process in all aspects of his life. I know his story cannot help but be a benefit and inspiration to all who read it

—Linda B. Sherr, Sarasota, Florida
Spring 2017

Preface

You can't lose weight eating out.

Losing weight in restaurants is impossible!

You especially can't eat in Italian restaurants, French restaurants, Chinese restaurants, Japanese restaurants, Mexican restaurants, Greek restaurants, Indian restaurants, Jewish delis, or steakhouses (insert any kind of restaurant you may like)!

These were just a few of the things people said to me for years, and continued to say countless times when I started to lose weight, by working through what would ultimately become *The Restaurant Diet*. I've since proven them all wrong—and you can, too.

In our culture, eating out is almost as essential to our lives, sense of well-being and normalcy as sunshine, water, and air. As human beings, we need to eat in order to live and, as we are social creatures, it is inevitable we will find ourselves drawn to dining out in restaurants. Restaurants can offer fun, social experiences you just can't get at home. Whether you love food as much as I do or not—and whether you love to dine out as much as I do, or need to dine out for whatever reason—if you are trying to lose weight, the following thoughts may enter your head:

Do I dare go out to eat?

My doctor, or nutritionist, or coworker, or the last diet book I read said to stay out of restaurants if you want to lose weight!

Do I turn down that lunch meeting or dinner invitation?

Do I join my coworkers for lunch, dinner, or—heaven forbid—a snack and a drink?

I'm too tired to go home and cook, can't I just stop at a restaurant on the way home?

If I go, I'll be too tempted!

I'll eat too much, I always do!

If I don't go, I'll be the only one, I won't know what anyone's talking about tomorrow, and I'll feel left out.

If I go, how can I possibly get out of there without blowing my diet?

How am I going to meet anybody if I can't go out to eat?

What about when I'm traveling—if I'm away from home I'll have to eat out!

I don't like to cook. I don't have time to cook. Eating out is so much simpler.

Maybe I shouldn't go on vacation. Maybe I should find a job that doesn't involve travel.

I'm overweight. I'm living proof that I can't be trusted around food. I've never been able to sit down in a restaurant without overeating.

I need to be at home in a controlled environment and eat foods I don't like.

I'm not supposed to enjoy eating. The reason I'm fat is because I "enjoy" eating too much.

A "diet" is the only way I'm going to get control of my weight.

I'm a bad, undisciplined person. I shouldn't reward my bad behavior and lack of willpower by going out to eat.

I should be stuck at home, like a kid in detention.

There's something wrong with me. I'm the problem none of these diets I've tried have worked. I've wasted so much money on pills, shakes, and unpleasant meal plans that were supposed to work, and I'm right back where I started—fat, miserable, and out the money. I'm such a failure!

For people with weight problems and a history of failed attempts at dieting, these and other thoughts swirl around in our heads like a cyclone. Just the mere suggestion of something as simple as a lunch meeting or dinner date can send our minds spinning out of control. Overweight people are stuck on an endless merry-go-round of unpalatable, unrealistic diets and face almost inevitable failure and weight gain.

Allow me to emphasize this point: *People fail at dieting not because they are failures—they fail because the diet plans they follow are flawed.* They are unpalatable and totally unrealistic in the real world. They are designed for quick, gimmicky weight-loss, and fail to offer the desperate dieter a reasonable long-term solution they can sink their teeth into.

As a former morbidly obese person who struggled with these concerns for years, let me be the first to tell you that, like so many other folks, I was fearful that eating out is a surefire way to blow a diet or gain weight.

What should an overweight person do? Go out to eat anyway and hope for the best? Decline any invitation or opportunity to have fun? Lock yourself in your house or apartment for the rest of your life and throw away the key?

The reality is, whether we like to eat out or not, there are going to be times and situations that require us to. For most of us, eating out is a convenient and enjoyable part of life. A 2013 study by Rasmussen revealed that 58 percent of American adults eat out at least once a week. A recent article in *NY Magazine* states that, for the first time ever, Americans are spending more in bars and restaurants than on groceries. Also, due to changing demographics, tastes, and preferences, the largest generation—the millennials—eats out an average of 3.4 times per week, compared to the rest of the population, which eats out an average of 2.8 times per week. If you are part of roughly 50 percent of the population that is overweight and either enjoys eating out or has to eat out, wouldn't you like to know how you can eat out *and* lose weight?

Years ago, I had been conditioned like the rest of our society to believe that essentially everything I enjoyed eating was "off limits" if I hoped to get in shape, lose weight, and keep it off. We are made to believe that food is our enemy, not our friend. We are taught that we should avoid restaurants and limit our food choices to things that look and taste inedible in order to lose weight. In our minds, dieting is supposed to feel like punishment. Remember, this same kind of collective awareness and propaganda led to major misnomers like margarine is better for you than butter, and that eggs are bad for you. Today, the health community has found the exact opposite to be true.

The reality is this: Yes, restaurants can be bad for weight loss. But, by the same token, so can eating at home if you make the wrong choices. The truth is, dining out and weight loss can go together and actually be enjoyable and successful if you learn to do it right.

I believe that dieting in restaurants actually offers a more realistic chance at long-term success than traditional deprivation-based diets. Why? Because dining out is such an integral part of our culture. To be successful at weight loss, we need to learn how to eat better wherever we eat—whether it is at home, or in restaurants. We need to develop a better appreciation for food and make it our friend. I know many people who manage to eat "healthy" at home, who go out to eat one night a week and complain the next day at the gym that they "gained three pounds" from dinner the previous night. Whether they actually gained the weight because of poor food choices—such as too much sodium, alcohol, or other factors—is unknown. The point is, many people who are able to dine at home lose all sensibility when they sit down and are handed a menu. It's the dining equivalent to forgetting how to drive when it starts to rain. We need to train ourselves to make peace with food, regardless of where we are. Just because you're in a restaurant doesn't mean you have to overeat or make poor choices. Most restaurants have tasty choices that are actually good for us!

The only way to be successful at losing weight and at keeping it off is to be able to overcome our issue with food, and to disprove the myth that dining out is bad for our waistlines. Learning how to walk into a restaurant and order a healthy, delicious meal is a very powerful, positive experience—especially for someone who has struggled with overeating for years. What is the point of going on a diet, eating things you can't stand, and avoiding your favorite restaurants for as long as it takes to hopefully lose the weight you want to lose—only to have no clue what to do the next time you set foot in a restaurant?

What happens if you do manage to lose the weight while depriving yourself? You fail to stick to the unrealistic plan you practiced to lose the weight and end up gaining it back. As soon as you return to your favorite restaurant you select the same bad foods you ate before your diet and probably eat more than you did while you were dieting, and likely way more than you need to stay healthy. Most diets don't teach you how to realistically eat in restaurants (or even at home) and hence don't offer a shred of hope for long-term success.

The Restaurant Diet teaches you how to dine out and lose weight. I will show you how to take back some of the control you have been conceding every time you avoided eating out or sat down at a restaurant and struggled or feared the enormous amount of extra calories and fat you were subjecting yourself to, simply because you were not in control of the cooking.

Trying to lose weight in restaurants doesn't need to be a scary experience. In this book, I you will guide you on how to make restaurants a partner in your weight-loss success, not your enemy! Not once will you feel restricted as you learn how to order, eat, and enjoy the restaurant experience—guilt-free—so you can easily lose weight in your favorite restaurants and keep it off. Trust me when I tell you that food shouldn't be bland or boring in order to lose weight. It should be beautiful and delicious, and you shouldn't be stuck at home eating things you despise on your journey to shedding pounds.

There are a number of restaurants today that actually specialize in healthy gourmet cuisine. Seasons 52 is a top nationwide chain that does just that. Surprisingly, I know many people who don't want to eat there, despite the fact that I tell them the food is good, there is a lot of variety, and nothing tastes "dietetic." Seasons 52 utilizes a fresh, seasonal approach to dining; they offer slimmed-down cocktails and shot glass-sized mini desserts in an upscale, lively atmosphere. They also take the guesswork out of counting calories—they provide them for you! What's not to like about that? I hear things like, "I'm not going to eat at that diet place!" All I can say is these people are missing out on a lot of great food that truly doesn't taste like "diet" food.

Many people are convinced that food must be unappealing in order to be considered healthy or appropriate for weight loss. Those of us who have ever tried to diet would probably agree. This is exactly why my message in *The Restaurant Diet* is so timely and a big part of why it works.

The problem begins when we eat too much, eat the wrong foods, or eat for the wrong reasons. These are all things we can learn to manage in order to make eating a pleasurable activity that we need in order to sustain life, rather than something we do in excess or fear.

One thing that surprised me when I began my quest to lose weight eating out was how many chefs, restaurant owners, and staff actually do care about their customers and are happy to work with you by doing things like reducing the amount of butter or oil, or serving the sauce on the side. It's all about how you approach it. Later in this book I will show you how to make your favorite restaurants your friends. One chef summed it up well to me: "I was delighted to accommodate you and be a partner in your successful weight loss. I am glad that you were able to lose weight eating in my restaurant and delighted you will be eating in my restaurant for many years to come."

As you will discover, I love eating out in great restaurants more than just about anything else. You can call me a foodie, and one might go as far as saying that good food is my passion—or perhaps even an obsession. Dining out in great restaurants for me is about more than just the great food. It is an experience I liken to art and theater. It is a performance or a show that I become part of. Every day I am romanced by delicious food and think it like a love affair. Every morsel I consume is not only for pure pleasure but also for my body to create energy, replenish muscles, and build new cells.

The art is in the execution and presentation of a beautiful plate of scrumptious, perfectly cooked food. The theater is the background—the ambience, the service, the décor, and atmosphere. A good restaurant is like a Broadway show: the lighting, the props, the actors, actresses, music—everything has to be choreographed just so. Then you bring in the food. Great food can either be significantly enhanced by an engaging restaurant environment, or substantially diminished by its surroundings. You've no doubt heard the expression "dinner and a movie." In fact, many movie theaters today have raised the bar, offering a full service fine dining and bar experience, complete with cushy leather chairs for their patrons. In trying to figure out how to combat dwindling attendance at movie theaters, savvy operators have zeroed in on exactly what *The Restaurant Diet* is telling you: people want to go out and have a memorable experience. We want to be pampered, served, indulged, treated well, and made to feel special. This is part of why the spa industry is so successful. Dining out is a convenience and can be called a "feel good" experience. Someone else does the shopping, the prep work, sweats over a stove, serves us, and does the dishes. Especially after a long day, who really feels like going home and throwing dinner together, then doing dishes—and worrying about being healthy?

One of the biggest complaints I've heard from people I've counseled is that, while on previous diets, they either couldn't go out to eat or they were afraid to eat out. Dieters are adjusting to a completely new lifestyle. They are grieving the loss of gluttony, dealing with eating a lot less food, and having to face their raw emotions—which is very difficult. Doing this at home, alone, and eating foods we don't like is even tougher. Dieters miss socializing and they miss eating foods that taste good—and not every dieter wants to spend their free time in a group talking to other people who are also struggling to diet. Dieters want freedom, they want flexibility, they want options. They want to be able to eat out and not feel fearful or guilty. *The Restaurant Diet* gives you the freedom and permission to do just that!

People don't necessarily need to go out to eat, but they choose to spend some of their income on exactly this sort of convenience and enjoyment. If you build or offer something great, people will want to leave their homes to go out and enjoy it. Why should you miss out on these kinds of experiences just because you need to lose weight?

Having enjoyed meals at countless excellent restaurants—from cozy "mom and pop" establishments, where the owners know your name and treat you like you are a guest in their home—to world famous "bucket list" destinations, like Thomas Keller's The French Laundry in Napa—the experience of dining out has become an inextricable part of who I am. As you will learn, I also enjoy cooking at home, but find something especially magical about a wonderful restaurant experience. Great chefs and restaurants inspire me with their creations, to try new things when I cook at home.

As an only child, my parents taught me how to appreciate and enjoy the very best that life had to offer. We traveled internationally, had many great cooks, and appreciated gourmet food and wine; my aunt owned a spectacular Italian restaurant. However, I also witnessed family members using food as an emotional crutch and, when my parents divorced, I began to use food as a way to deal with my emotions. When I wasn't eating, I felt empty. Weighing over 200 pounds by age 13, I was determined to change my life. I lost weight then, but my success was only temporary. Shortly after finishing law school, my weight ballooned to 329 pounds. I had a body mass index (BMI) of 46, practically double that of a person at a healthy weight.

I embarked on a successful career as a trusts and estates attorney but, despite earning a law degree and an MBA, I felt empty and unfulfilled without being able to enjoy food. The problem wasn't so much the food; rather the problem was *so much* food, and my inability to disconnect food from my emotions. Every diet I tried seemed like torture. I loved to cook gourmet meals and entertain, and loved to eat out in great restaurants even more. But nothing gave me as much pleasure as enjoying a delicious dish in a gourmet restaurant; I was always looking for the next great restaurant and meal.

Unfortunately, my love of good food was standing in the way of my health and happiness. My health and very life were at stake. Eating wherever, whenever, and whatever I wanted had made me overweight and miserable. Overeating in response to some kind of stressor was not a recipe for health or happiness. A great meal out and eating too much were temporary distractions from something

I didn't want to deal with: my emotions. For instance, I would have a stressful day and I would then go overeat. I made excuses for overeating. I punished myself for overeating. I felt ashamed of myself for overeating. I would then "diet" and lose some weight, feel worse, and gain it back—only to feel even worse. This was my lifestyle for years.

Weighing over 300 pounds came with a hefty price tag. I couldn't shop where regular people shopped. Nobody wanted to date me. Exercise was difficult and painful. Simply trying to perform routine daily tasks like grocery shopping, light housework, or getting the mail were difficult. My back, bones, and joints ached. Sitting, standing, and even sleeping were painful. My doctors warned me that if I didn't change my lifestyle and eating habits, I would likely die of a heart attack, stroke, or diabetes before I reached the age of forty. As you will read, I almost died from sleep apnea, a condition related to my obesity.

Despite the cold hard facts staring at me in the face, I couldn't imagine a lifetime avoiding eating in my favorite restaurants or living on foods I found inedible. I envisioned what I needed to do in order to lose weight and keep it off as being some permanent form of torture I was unwilling to try. Still, I was determined to keep trying every diet, pill, shake, and gimmick under the sun to find a quick or easy solution to my problems. I even went away to two top residential weight-loss facilities. Yet none of the traditional diets worked—I couldn't stick with anything long enough to make a lasting impact. I felt deprived and miserable. I couldn't stand being "forced" to exercise for the sole purpose of losing weight. I felt empty and vanquished to be blessed with the very best in taste—and cursed by what this did to me.

My love affair with food was killing me, and I desperately needed to lose a ton of weight and somehow keep it off. It seemed totally unfair for someone who enjoyed great food to suddenly face eating diet food they didn't like.

For years, I had fallen hook, line, and sinker for the myth that it is impossible and certainly unwise eat in restaurants while dieting. I found myself struggling for years to diet the traditional way: eating foods I didn't like and avoiding my favorite restaurants. I tried nearly every diet out there, thinking that these so-called "experts" knew something I didn't. I eventually got fed up. I realized I was part of the problem—and so were the diets. My problem was emotional, and my unwillingness to deal with it. The problem with every diet I had tried was they offered no realistic approach to dieting in the real world, which is where all of us live—a world in which people like, and often need, to eat out. Typical diets take our money and offer no secret shortcuts or realistic advice that enable us to succeed at losing weight and keeping it off long-term. These diets simply feed us misinformation, that we need to eat things we don't enjoy and that we are bad, undisciplined people who need to keep coming back for more.

Most diet programs and supplements are good at keeping me and millions of other dieters stuck in a pattern of deprivation and despair. Diet meant eating things I didn't like to lose weight. After the diet either succeeded or went bust, there was no chance of sticking to the routine, so it meant go back to eating "normally" and gaining the weight back. Most diets teach us how to deprive ourselves for a short-term objective, they don't teach us how to be successful long-term. We are led to believe that food is our enemy, and we are failures, when neither is true. I had grown sick and tired of trying to stick to a routine I didn't enjoy and eating foods I couldn't stand, like a plain broiled piece of chicken with no flavor. I felt like I was being punished and I struggled with accepting I either had to give up my love of food, or I was going to be fat, unhappy, sick, and likely dead in a few years. No matter how I sliced it, neither option seemed acceptable.

The bottom line: I loved to eat out, I loved gourmet food *and* I needed to lose weight. And keep it off. Period.

Being told "no" over and over again just made me more determined to prove everybody wrong and show that there is a way to eat at great restaurants and lose weight. But it had to be easy, tasty, and had to allow me the ability to eat out and enjoy a variety of foods. I figured if anyone could figure it out, I could. Just like Thomas Edison must have known 1,000 ways *not* to make a light bulb, it was the 1,001st attempt that worked. In my case, it was trying to lose weight so many *ineffective ways* that enabled me to come up with a way that worked.

Whether you are a foodie like me, or just someone looking to lose weight who enjoys eating out, finds restaurant dining convenient, or perhaps doesn't like to cook, you shouldn't have to forego the restaurant experience just because you want to lose weight and get healthy. I will show you how to eat out in great restaurants and lose the weight you need to, even if you've gone through a lifetime of unsuccessful dieting. I will also teach you how to shop and cook better at home, and to prepare healthy gourmet meals like a top chef, by sharing recipes from some of my favorite restaurants!

While in my early thirties, I developed a diet I could live with—my revolutionary approach to healthy, gourmet, *"La Dolce Vita"* living. People were amazed; I even amazed myself. Over a one-year period, I lost 150 pounds following a comprehensive diet and lifestyle plan that I had carefully designed and developed while working with my doctor, nutritionist, and psychologist.

Using my unique approach, I've kept the weight off for over seven years. Along the way, I developed mouth-wateringly delicious recipes and a lifestyle plan for people wishing to achieve the same successful outcome—no matter how many pounds they want to lose. In addition to making healthier choices when dining out, without scrimping on taste, satisfaction, or the foods I love, I learned how to choose the most nutritious, delicious, and clean foods to make at home. I will show you how to walk into your favorite restaurant, enjoy a delicious meal, drink a glass of wine if you like, and still lose weight!

The Restaurant Diet is unlike any other diet out there. It teaches us to love and respect food again, and helps us address why we overeat in the first place. Rather than simply eat less and be miserable, *The Restaurant Diet* shows us not only how to enjoy eating out, but also encourages us to look within for the answers on how to love ourselves and want to give ourselves the very best—enough delicious food for us to enjoy and be healthy, not excess food to compensate for any deficiency elsewhere. Looking within and getting help understanding why we overeat are critical to our success. Without this understanding, we are susceptible to go back to overeating, or even replace one addictive behavior, such as compulsive overeating coupled with alcohol, tobacco, or even drugs. Why do many people who quit smoking gain weight—they replace one oral dependency (smoking) with another (eating). Without dealing with the emotional root, we run the risk of adopting other harmful compulsive behaviors, even if we do succeed at dieting.

My goal is to give you permission to empower yourself—to take back your life and embrace food as a gift we give to ourselves to help sustain life. In fact, I liken *The Restaurant Diet* to a gourmet weight-loss spa for the mind and body.

Doesn't that sound a lot better than "I'm going on a diet?"

Introduction

It was a beautiful evening in the spring of 2017 in Delray Beach, Florida. I was meeting Catherine for dinner, a good friend who was down visiting from New York, whom I had not seen since I had lost the weight. Although we spoke often and she had seen pictures of the "new me" online, she was shocked by what she saw when she approached the table: I was relaxing and sipping a glass of wine in the lovely *al fresco* seating area of a stylish new restaurant, dressed in a slim pair of AG jeans and a colorful Tommy Bahama linen shirt with the sleeves rolled up.

"Fred, you look like you just stepped off the cover of GQ!" she exclaimed. I couldn't believe it, but my friend was in tears. "You look so amazing, I'm so proud of you," she said as she hugged me and sobbed.

My friend and I spent a lovely evening catching up and enjoying a gourmet meal with wine at a nice restaurant, without overdoing it—something that, a few years before, I didn't think could be possible—something Catherine wasn't so sure we could do either. Catherine brought some photos of the last time we had seen each other in New York, back in 2008. I looked at them and couldn't believe I was seeing my old self. I was huge, round, and clearly unhappy at almost twice my current size. My friend was a little concerned about how to behave around me, what to drink, and what to order—for fear she might trigger me to do something I would later regret. So, she said she was leaving the ordering entirely up to me, with the proviso: "I'm picking up the check to celebrate the new you, and I'm really into seafood."

The reality was—after losing an enormous amount of weight my way, by learning to enjoy eating out, by making better choices restaurants, and continuing to practice and build upon what I had learned for a number of years—I was totally comfortable in practically any situation, and assured Catherine that she could eat whatever she wanted and I wouldn't be offended. "No-no," she said, "I want to see firsthand how it's done—how someone who loved to eat like you did can sit down in a great restaurant and do what you have done." "With pleasure," I said. It was like I had won the lottery. I finally found a way to lose a ton of weight and keep it off—while eating at great restaurants.

The truth is, I had lost a lot of weight before—about fifty pounds when I was in middle school. I was tired of being picked on, and took advantage of the opportunity of relocating from Long Island, NY to Florida to feverishly work to lose weight before we moved. For several months, I ate very little, exercised a lot, and hated the experience even more than I hated being fat. I was hoping to leave "Fat Fred" behind, as was my nickname in school, in the hope that a great new life would unfold when I got to Florida. Unfortunately, losing weight, looking normal, and moving to another state didn't do it. I lost the weight, but the baggage came with me, and I was just as unhappy and unsure of myself as when I was fat. I went back to eating what I wanted and not exercising, eventually putting the weight back on. During the course of college, law school, and my legal career, my weight exploded. I tried dieting many times but each time I threw in the towel because I hated the experience so much. Each diet looked something like this: no going out to eat, eat bland, boring foods, exercise, and try to lose x number of pounds by a certain date. This unpleasant, short-term perspective is a large part of what's wrong with most diets. I hated that I couldn't go out to eat in my favorite restaurants. I hated every minute of every day I couldn't go out to eat, or eat whatever I wanted, and I became depressed and obsessed over the numbers on the scale that never seemed to drop as much as I thought they should, given the enormous sacrifice I was making. I hated myself for loving food so much and being convinced I had to either stop loving food, or remain fat and unhappy.

The Restaurant Diet is my love letter to food, and my recipe for successful, flavorful weight loss. It puts us in touch with the best version of ourselves as we learn to eat better, respect and appreciate food, and love and take better care of ourselves. It can also be called "the food lover's diet" since, although it involved losing a lot of weight and learning to treat food differently, it really isn't like any other diet out there.

I've divided *The Restaurant Diet* into four easy-to-follow Phases that can be easily tailored to your specific situation.

Phase One, *Beginning*, is the shortest phase. It is designed to literally jump-start your weight loss, while exercise is difficult. In this phase, calories are the most restricted, as are sugar and carbohydrates. However, you will still be able to enjoy foods like steak, shrimp, lobster, fish, chicken, turkey, lamb, veal, pork, eggs, salads, grains, fruits, vegetables, yogurt, and gourmet meals in the best restaurants and at home. You will even be able to enjoy a glass of wine with dinner.

Phase Two, Opportunity, allows for greater opportunities food-wise, in exchange for more challenging exercise, after a successful jump-start.

By *Phase Three, Challenge,* you will be in much better physical shape and will want, and need, to challenge your body with a wider range of activities, to take more weight off, and replace the fat with muscle. This is the final phase of losing the weight, and by now exercise is easier and more enjoyable, and you are able to enjoy more foods than before. By this point you, will have lost a considerable amount of weight and your new way of eating will become second nature. You are well on your way to a healthy and permanent new lifestyle.

Phase Four, Achievement, is for maintenance. By the time you have reached a healthy weight range, you will have developed many good eating and exercise habits. You will not only be rewarded with a new life and an attractive, fit new body—you will have the benefit of a healthier, balanced lifestyle and most likely have many more years to enjoy the new you. You will continue to exercise and eat the foods you enjoyed in Phase Three, but with reasonable additions and occasional treats. You will be able to continue this for life and enjoy many delicious foods in moderation, as long as you create a healthy balance, keep up with reasonable daily exercise, and continue to look after your emotional and spiritual well-being. You will establish a healthy "weight range" that you wish to remain in for the rest of your life. And, in the event some pounds return and you get near the top of the range, you will temporarily go back to an earlier phase until you are comfortably within your range once again. While losing the weight, you will need to address the emotional issues that come up and learn healthier ways of living. By building a solid foundation, and having a good set of tools and support system at your disposal, you are much more likely to experience lasting success.

The concepts in *The Restaurant Diet* are easy to follow and incorporate into your life. You will learn to enjoy food again, and learn that it is entirely possible to eat in great restaurants and lose weight. It's all about attitude. You will learn to love and accept yourself, even if you failed at dieting many times. Instead of reminding yourself how undisciplined or unsuccessful you've been in the past, or how much you hate dieting and exercise, go enjoy your favorite restaurant and tell yourself: "You deserve the best!"

The Restaurant Diet's approach to eating better, cooking better, and treating ourselves better can be of benefit to everyone—not just the millions of overweight folks who have struggled with dieting and are looking for a better way. Anyone who is interested in a long-term, realistic, healthy, gourmet approach to dining and living will likely find something beneficial in *The Restaurant Diet*, even if it is just some great recipes and places to eat.

If you learn to diet and eat out the right way, you can achieve your weight-loss goals, transform your life, and enjoy yourself on the journey!

PART ONE

Taking It Off! The Four-Phase Gourmet Weight-Loss Plan

Chapter One
Solving the Restaurant Problem

Successful dieting in a restaurant is a lot more than a matter of willpower, planning, choices, and self-control. It is all of these things, plus the added requirement of learning how to embrace losing weight by going out in public and dealing with people who will be preparing and serving you a substance you've likely had major problems with—food. You have to train them to help you, not tempt you. This can be done in a nice, but firm way. You don't want to come across as a jerk, but you don't want to be afraid to speak up, either. For years, I was afraid of what other people thought of me, so I often wouldn't say anything—even if keeping quiet had been against my best interests. To succeed, I needed to change how I conducted myself.

Learning to lose weight in restaurants is partly a social skill that can be learned and practiced. I liken this to how our parents teach us etiquette or enroll us in classes when we are kids—so we know how to go out into the world and behave like ladies and gentlemen, rather than barbarians. People who work in restaurants will be far more responsive and cooperative to someone who is civilized and well-mannered than not.

The first time I sat down in a gourmet restaurant with my mom as a little kid, I saw at least five forks in front of me and started to cry. My mother had to teach me how to use these utensils. There is a proper etiquette to dining out: saying please and thank you; knowing which fork to use and where to rest your knife; and things like chewing with your mouth closed, using your napkin, etc.

It is important to have good social skills and physical presentation for a variety of reasons. Mainly, though, if you are overweight there might be some stereotypical perceptions from the restaurant staff that work against your favor. As an obese person, I was frequently ridiculed in both my personal and professional lives. I can attest that fat people are often treated worse than thin people. We need to work harder to overcome perceptions and act comfortable in our skin. In business or anything in life, you need to play the part in order to gain respect. If you are well dressed, polished, and presentable, you are already halfway there.

Your goal is to win over the restaurant folks by being as engaging, open, polite, and respectful as possible. You want them to *want* to help you. You want to be welcomed with open arms, not shunned. As a formerly overweight diner, I used to think I was expected to order a lot; first, because I wanted to eat it; second, because I thought the folks in the restaurant would find it odd that someone fat would not want to eat; and third, because I had done it for so long at many of the same restaurants, I thought it was expected. I used to think the owners, chefs, or staff who I tipped based upon the large amount I ordered (and large check) would be offended if I started ordering less. In my family growing up, some of my older Italian relatives were truly offended if we didn't clean our plates! Combine the fear of offending your grandparents, aunts, uncles, or whomever with mind-blowingly delicious food, and we have a problem. I thought this was the way the world worked. For many years, I ate out many times a week, and frequently ordered and ate too much. I was a regular at many restaurants where the staff knew me and treated me well, serving me everything I ordered and telling me about fattening specials, since they knew I would likely try them. Many places made a lot of money having me as their guest, and the staff members were well tipped based upon how much I ordered and ate. Changing my mindset and attitude was the first step towards changing my entire restaurant experience, which would enable me to be comfortable in restaurants—both the old and familiar as well as the new and make these places part of my successful weight loss.

I was at my heaviest weight ever. I wanted to lose weight. How was I going to do it? I decided from day one that I needed to walk in with a positive and determined attitude and share with the folks at the restaurant that I was seriously trying to lose weight and wanted them to work with me so I could continue to enjoy dining there. A hallmark of great service is knowing your customer. People used to assume I wanted to eat a lot when I was fat—especially at many of the restaurants I frequented, where I often ordered and ate way too much food. Whether I was going to eat someplace where I was known as an overeater, or someplace new, I needed to change that perception and broadcast loud and clear what I was doing. I needed to introduce people to the "new me" and, in many cases, reintroduce myself to people who knew the old me. I had to let the world know I was now the guy who was getting healthier, changing his life, and developing a more positive relationship with food. Anybody who didn't understand or like it—that was their problem. I was determined to keep eating out but I was going to eat better, and eat less. I was going on a diet unlike any other. I was finally doing it my way!

As the customer, it is your prerogative to tell the folks at any restaurant what you need and want, and how you need them to work with you. For example, in a nice way you will want to ask them not to bring bread to your table or to stop them from telling you about the twelve-layer chocolate cake for dessert.

If you are among the many people who have a long history of overeating and failed attempts at dieting, you are extremely vulnerable to mistreatment and neglect at a restaurant—even if the folks working there don't realize it. I know firsthand how one little comment can throw off an otherwise successful day and send you into a tailspin. It will take practice to become partners with restaurants, but it is well worth it. The majority of your experiences are likely to be wonderful, and you will find pleasure in the food and the camaraderie. However, if the people in the restaurant have a negative attitude towards you, then move on. If you are uncomfortable in any restaurant for any reason, or have difficulty controlling yourself, or you come across an owner, manager, or staff member who is less than accommodating, go somewhere else. No matter how good the food might be, it's not worth the aggravation or temptation—there are many other fine establishments with food just as good that would warmly receive you.

Especially early on, be cautious when dining with others. You'll want to eat with people who respect your goal and your need not to have food pushed on you. Preferably, you'll find friends, colleagues, or family members who will be glad to join you, and respect your request that they work with you. If you are uncomfortable dining with anyone or in any situation, it is perfectly alright to politely excuse yourself. Lastly, avoid dining with anyone who is an overeater, that you may have overeaten with in the past, and who is not interested in changing their habits. Why subject yourself to the added pressure? You need to maintain as much control over your environment as possible in order to succeed.

What about fast food establishments? The strategy of making the staff, chefs, and owners partners in your weight-loss success story is of course better suited to fine dining establishments and family-run operations, than it is to fast food restaurants. While I am not a big fan of fast food, there are times when fast food is the only convenient option. Yes, you can occasionally eat fast food, but you need to choose selectively. Fast food restaurants frequently offer many unhealthy choices and the staff isn't interested in your desire to lose weight.

Here, especially, we are responsible for making the right choices, often in a hurry, and from a large menu board filled with many unhealthy choices. Still, most fast food restaurants offer some healthy options, and many also have nutritional information available which will soon be required to be conspicuously posted in chains nationwide, making your life much easier. It takes a little effort, but you can navigate even a fast food establishment by taking a little extra time to review the nutritional information and make healthy choices. In fact, before going to any restaurant, you should get into the habit of doing a little research and making your choices before you get to the restaurant. I will show you how in the coming chapters.

For success at a fast food establishment, I suggest always having a few "go-to" items that you can eat in a pinch, like a salad with low-fat dressing, a healthy wrap, or grilled chicken sandwich, for times like when you are rushing between business meetings or running through an airport to catch a plane and haven't had time for a proper meal. Although my focus and passion is on eating in gourmet restaurants, we all find ourselves from time to time in a situation where fast food is the only option available. I know, the above options may not sound as enticing as a burger with fries, but at least you will have put something healthy and nutritious in your stomach rather than blow it on a meal that contains as many calories as you wish to consume in an entire day. If you think smartly ahead on this, and can hold off while traveling, then you will have a gourmet meal awaiting you when you arrive at your destination.

TOP DIETING TIPS

For your convenience, I've provided a list of my Top Dining Out Tips—your very own starter's guide to eating out and losing weight. It arms you with a strategic plan to help make losing weight in restaurants easier. Fortunately, in today's world we can let our fingers, web browsers, and apps do most of the work for us. Gone are the days when dieters had to awkwardly carry around a book and look up calories or point values, make often inaccurate guesses, or blindly worry about whether we are "being good." Today, we can map out our entire meal in just a couple minutes before we leave our home or office.

1. Review the menu and plan in advance whenever possible. Many restaurants post their menus online, others may e-mail or fax you a copy of the menu at your request. If you want to know the daily specials, or have any special requests as far as a specific item or special preparation, a phone call in advance is a good idea. I always try to do my "due diligence" by looking over the menu and figuring out what I am going to eat before leaving for

the restaurant. Make realistic selections for your proposed meal, and then plug the foods you are planning to eat into a calorie counting program or app, such as Livestrong.com; you can determine if your choices are within the calorie budget you will adopt in Phase One with the help of your medical practitioner. If the restaurant has "heart-healthy" or reduced calorie menu items with the calories listed, take advantage of them. Some restaurants publicize their calorie counts, but if your restaurant or the exact dish is not listed, make well-reasoned estimates. Taking a little time and thinking before you go out, order, and eat will save you in the long run. Know before you leave the house what you are going to have, and stick with your plan. Print or take home a "to-go" copy of the menu with your selections circled and calorie estimates written down and save them in a folder at home for easy future reference. In the rare exception that you are unable to view the menu in advance, ask for a menu when you arrive at the restaurant. Take it outside and look over it. If you don't have the luxury of pre-planning for a particular meal, have your smartphone handy with your calorie counting app and see if what you are planning to eat is within your budget before you decide to order. Walking in knowing what you're going to have and then vetting those choices is your best bet.

2. Further to number one, after you eat, be sure to log everything you consumed in your calorie counting app (such as Livestrong.com). Be sure to plug the food/calories you consumed into your app after each meal. (In many cases, I did it before I even went to the restaurant, and I would simply follow along, so my meal was a well-planned roadmap.) This is helpful especially early on when you are new to this. I mention Livestrong specifically because it is the primary program I used throughout my weight loss, in addition to several other calorie analyzing software I used to calculate calories in recipes I made at home, which I will share later. There are other programs and apps available; my advice is to try using several for a few days and see which one works best for you.

3. Look for things that are baked, broiled, grilled, pan-seared, poached, or roasted, as opposed to fried or sautéed.

4. Look for sauces, soups, and preparations without butter or heavy cream.

5. Don't be afraid to ask questions about how a food is prepared or what ingredients are in it. Not everything is obvious. For example, "Seafood Chowder" doesn't clarify whether or not there is butter or cream.

6. Avoid dishes with sugar (especially Phase One) and fattening desserts.

7. Pairings are important: If you are trying to be healthy, choose a light pasta *or* a fish or meat dish, not both.

8. Order colorful foods: Foods that are "colorful" often have more vitamins and are healthier than their less colorful counterparts. For example, a sweet potato is much better for you than a white potato. Sweet potatoes are loaded with vitamins A and C and beta-carotene. Vegetables like multi-colored peppers are great roasted and are full of vitamins; Swiss and rainbow chard are also great options.

9. Don't go out to eat while starving. It's best to have a couple of light, healthy snacks during the day in addition to your main meals. Never allow yourself to get to the point of being famished. If you are really hungry, have a handful of grapes, cherries, or strawberries a few minutes before you go out, or drink a glass of water. This will take the edge off so you don't arrive at the restaurant famished.

10. Stop eating before you are stuffed. (This goes for eating out and at home.)

11. Timing is important. Don't go out to eat late in the evening, unless you plan to be up to take a walk and digest before bed. Plan to finish dinner two hours before bed and be sure to leave enough time to take a leisurely walk after you eat. If you are traveling or have to eat late, make a point to walk afterwards. People who work late hours often fit a workout into their day, before dinner. Another timing tip is to go when the restaurant is less crowded, if possible; try to avoid the ever-popular 7:30 p.m. dinner reservation. Going a bit earlier or later will likely result in a more relaxed experience, where the restaurant's staff is more likely to "get it right" the first time. In the event anything gets lost in translation (like a sauce ends up on the meat or fish instead of on the side), politely send it back; you are the customer and you are entitled to get your food the way you ordered it.

12. When you arrive at the restaurant, start by introducing yourself to your server and staff. Politely them that you are trying to lose weight and you would appreciate their help and assistance—before anyone starts describing the decadent chocolate cake. Meet the manager, chef, and owner. If you are already a regular customer, tell them why you would like to continue patronizing their restaurant (the food, the atmosphere, you have been dining there for

years, etc.). If you are trying the restaurant for the first time, tell them that and let them know you will be happy to return if the experience is good.

13. Be polite and friendly to everyone—smile. Most restaurant owners, chefs, and staff will be glad to work with a customer who has a good attitude and is looking to get well. People also like a comeback story. Smart restaurant owners would prefer to help a customer than lose a customer.

14. Eat either in the bar area or in the restaurant—not both. Starting at the bar with a drink (and possibly snacks or tapas) and then sitting down in the dining room is a temptation to drink and eat more than you need to. It's easy to lose track of what you've eaten or continue to pile on. Occasionally, I would just eat tapas, or small plates, in the bar area with a glass of wine. (Refer to the discussion about the pros and cons of Happy Hour dining in the next chapter.) Some Happy Hour menus offer great values and healthy choices.

15. Avoid salty nuts and chips. The salt causes thirst and makes you retain water; salt may also lead to hypertension. Nuts and chips are a favorite "freebie" at bars, which encourages you to eat continuously as bowls are refilled—and also order more high-calorie drinks. Nuts aren't bad *per se*, in moderation. Chips, however, are essentially high in fat and calories and are lacking in nutritional value. If you are considering guacamole, many restaurants serve it with fresh vegetable crudités as a healthy alternative to nachos.

16. Consider choosing restaurants you are familiar with—at least in the beginning. You will have a comfort level and idea about the kinds of foods they offer, and people may know you. If this is the case and they view you as an overeater, it is important that you change this perception immediately by telling them that you are in the process of losing weight and want to continue to eat there—only you need to eat healthier. However, you should avoid any restaurants that have been particularly problematic in terms of overeating or too much temptation with high-calorie foods, especially in the beginning. Some people prefer trying places they have never been and hence where they have no history of overeating. I first went to familiar restaurants and then tried new ones. I found it much easier because I felt comfortable at these restaurants and knew the staff, chefs, and owners at many of them quite well. In fact, the very first night of my weight loss I dined at Morton's of Chicago (see the next chapter for an illustration of how I dined there). Each of us is different. You'll have to go out, try it, and decide what works best for you.

17. In the unlikely event the staff is not agreeable to making reasonable accommodations, or you simply can't find anything remotely healthy on the menu, leave and go somewhere else. There is no shame in this at all. I recently went to a restaurant whose 300-pound manager informed me they never do half portions or make any sort of adjustments in the preparation of anything for anyone. They may have good food at these restaurants, but they will not be partners for you in your quest to lose weight—and therefore don't deserve your business.

18. Politely decline the bread and butter or anything else fattening the kitchen may send out. If you are dining with others who insist on having bread, politely decline or keep passing the basket and ask that they keep it out of your reach. Why do people tend to eat several pieces of bread and butter when they go out before eating anything else? Because it's there? It's good? It's free? If you don't normally eat a loaf of bread at home before a meal, why do it in a restaurant? Take it out of the equation completely; you don't need the calories. If you are dining with people who want bread, let them have their bread and then ask them to remove the basket or keep it out of your reach.

19. Consider asking for a pitcher of water (or several refills of water) if it doesn't come automatically to your table. Order it with lemon or lime, if you prefer. Consider mineral water, which Europeans swear by for digestive benefits. I also recommend unsweetened iced tea. Water and unsweetened tea are excellent options for filling you up to avoid overeating. Sip as soon as you sit down, before eating anything. Do the same in between bites and courses. This will help you feel full faster.

20. Politely ask not to hear about fattening specials, desserts, etc. You can say you've researched the menu in advance and know what you'd like to order.

21. Ask for sauces and dressings on the side. This doesn't mean you can't have any. If you dip your food in the sauce, you will consume a lot less calories than if the food were covered with it. Avoid high-calorie side sauces like béarnaise, Hollandaise, and drawn butter. Be careful about condiments: Ketchup contains a lot of sugar (high fructose corn syrup, which should be avoided). Mayonnaise is high in fat and calories (opt for light mayo or skip it). Mustard is very low in calories.

22. If you would like, order a glass of wine with your meal. I enjoyed a glass of wine with dinner on most days, starting in Phase One! Refrain, however, from cocktails/sugary beverages/soda/diet soft drinks. Be sure to count the calories. A typical 5-ounce glass of wine is 125 calories, and a flute glass of champagne is approximately 95 calories. (Cocktails are permitted in lieu of the glass of wine in Phase Three and Four.) If you are not a wine drinker, consider opting for light beer, such as Michelob Ultra or Beck's Light. Also, many restaurants offer slimmed-down versions of classic cocktails on their drink menus. A restaurant I recently visited featured slimmed-down Cosmopolitans made with light cranberry juice, which contains 50 calories per 8 ounces compared to regular cranberry juice, which has 110 calories. You can slim down your cocktails at home as well.

●

Where to Drink in the Hamptons

If you enjoy mixed drinks, such as margaritas, you might want to check out Keith's Nervous Breakdown Ultra Premium Cocktail Mixes. Developed by Keith Davis of The Golden Pear Café's in the Hamptons (featured in the Recipes section), they are all-natural and, unlike most, are sweetened with organic agave nectar, rather than high fructose corn syrup. They are currently available in the New York area at fine restaurants and retailers, and may be ordered online: www.nervousbreakdown.com.

●

A word of caution: Alcohol impairs your ability to think, judge, and remember. You want to enjoy and relax, but if you drink, you may slacken the rules, forget that you ate something you shouldn't have, or revert to the old, familiar habits that got you in trouble in the first place.

●

The Low-Cal Sparkling Wine

One of my favorite sparkling wines is Syltbar Prosecco from Italy. Due to a natural double fermentation process, it contains less than half the number of calories in Syltbar's Prosecco than in ther brands of Prosecco, champagne, or sparkling wines, and tastes as good as, if not better than, other brands of Prosecco. It's a "light" beverage, if you will, that wasn't even designed to be a light beverage. They make a regular brut variety, as well as a rosé, which are currently available at fine restaurants and retailers in a handful of states, including Florida, Massachusetts, Illinois, Nevada, and New York and may also be ordered online. If you enjoy bubbles, minus the guilt, it is worth looking for (www.syltbar.com). Whether you choose to enjoy a glass of wine, or prefer a different kind of cocktail, limit it to one drink per day with dinner in Phase One.

●

23. You don't have to order everything at once. One strategy is to pace yourself; start with a soup and/or salad and/or appetizer that is within your calorie budget. Then order one course at a time. We've all heard the expression, "Your eyes are bigger than your stomach." Ordering everything when you sit down, and are hungry, is not a good idea; chances are, you will end up with more food than you need. You may find you are full with just a soup and salad (or an appetizer) and stop the meal there. Alternately, you can start by just ordering a salad and entrée with vegetables and avoid any starters. Once you start to eat, you will find you are less hungry and therefore not as inclined to order nearly as much food. This saves you money and helps you avoid the temptation to overeat.

24. Be careful with appetizers. These are made to taste good, but are often high in fat and calories. Opt for items like shrimp cocktail, seared ahi tuna, tuna tartare, carpaccio, grilled vegetables, hummus, or baba ganoush. Skip things like loaded nachos, chicken wings, and fried calamari. A good idea for your waistline and budget is to order small plates—especially if you are dining

with friends. Tapas have never been more popular. Just be sure to look for things that are light and healthy, such as grilled octopus, ceviche, or grilled artichokes. You can also order things like sliders without buns. I've never heard restaurant staff complaining if they don't have to bring you a bun you're paying for. Don't be afraid to ask—you might be pleasantly surprised and you might even find a new favorite dish or restaurant, or discover a healthier way to enjoy a restaurant favorite. For example, I've always enjoyed the Spinach and Artichoke Dip at Houston's/Hillstone. I have eaten there for years and was not aware that they offer crudité in place of the tortilla chips—all you have to do is ask!

25. In the event that the portion size is considerably more than your caloric budget, ask for a box in advance and have it ready. American restaurants, in particular, are known to serve gigantic portions of food and you need to protect yourself from such temptation. When the food comes, automatically portion out the amount you aren't going to eat and take it home for another meal. This way, you won't be tempted to overeat.

26. An appropriate portion of protein (i.e., steak) is four to six ounces. A four-ounce size is equivalent in size to a deck of cards—what most people consider to be "small" portions are actually *appropriate* portions. One person doesn't need a sixteen-ounce steak; when dining out, I encourage people to share their entrée with a dining companion. Even if a restaurant charges you extra to share, most will provide each diner with whatever comes with the meal (such as soup or salad). You can also box up the steak when it arrives at your table. If having half of your dinner in a to-go container in your refrigerator is too much temptation, write down the date and contents, wrap it up, and immediately freeze it for later enjoyment. If this is not an issue, leftover meat, seafood, and poultry make excellent additions to a salad the following day.

27. Focus on lean proteins and vegetables. When we start losing weight, we quickly learn to balance our need to satisfy our large tummies and stick to a realistic calorie budget. I've found the best way to do this is to include a lot of fresh fruits and vegetables that are low in calories and high in satisfaction (they contain a lot of water) along with protein, which is nutrient-dense and satisfying.

28. Go-to proteins: Lean cuts of beef (Filet Mignon or New York Strip). Seafood, such as flounder, grouper, halibut, salmon, snapper, sole, and swordfish are excellent when grilled, baked, poached, or pan-seared. Roasted or grilled

chicken, as well as dishes like Chicken Cacciatore, are great choices. Lamb is fine and even burgers are okay, as long as you use quality meat, skip the bun, and don't overdo the toppings. One of my favorite burger places, Zinburger (locations nationwide), offers quality beef, cooked to order, and they will give you a "lettuce" bun if you ask.

29. Beware of restaurant psychology. For example, a restaurant may offer an 8-ounce filet at $40 and a 12-ounce at $44. Any value-conscious consumer would likely order the 12-ounce, since you are essentially getting the extra 4 ounces for the price of 1 ounce. It is foolish to buy something you don't need just because it is a better value—especially if the temptation is too great to overeat either at the restaurant or when you get home. The other option is to order the larger steak, ask for a take-home container right away, divide the steak, and pack up a portion for lunch or dinner the next day. A salad with sliced leftover Filet Mignon is a wonderful meal. If you're concerned about it being in your refrigerator overnight (temptation), consider wrapping it as soon as you get home and freezing it to enjoy on another day. This is a good strategy for any kind of leftovers that can be frozen.

30. Ask about half portions. Many restaurants offer them especially for certain pasta dishes. Make sure to avoid restaurants and dishes that are served "family-style," which makes portion control much more difficult.

31. A portion of pasta should only be 3–4 ounces, as is typical in Italy. Pasta is a personal favorite of many people, including me, but it is also high in calories—even without any sauce or cheese. Each ounce of pasta is 100 calories and, unfortunately, it does not offer the same nutritional value that can be found in 100 calories worth of meat, fish, poultry, or vegetables. Many restaurants serve pasta portions that are as many as 12 or even 16 ounces! Topped with whatever sauce and cheese, you could easily be looking at *2,000 or more calories*. The key to pasta (like everything else) is quality, not quantity. Prepare a 4-ounce serving at home, so you can see what it looks like. Opt for tomato-based sauces, as opposed to anything containing butter or cream. If you order pasta in a restaurant, order a half serving *al dente* (still slightly firm when bitten) and eat it with vegetables and protein. A never-ending bowl of pasta is a very bad idea. You can sprinkle a few flakes of grated Parmesan cheese, but be careful, as it contains a lot of calories.

32. Avoid fried foods—especially those with trans fats, which the body has a hard time processing. These are not always easy to identify; trans fats are

found in foods that are fried in partially hydrogenated oil. The best thing is to avoid fried foods in restaurants altogether. Other foods that contain trans fats include pie crusts, margarine, Crisco, cake mixes and frostings, many pancake and waffle mixes, non-dairy creamers, and flavored popcorn. Ask for less oil and butter in all food preparation. Eliminating one tablespoon. of grease removes one-hundred calories.

33. At the deli, ask for half-sour pickles as regular pickles are loaded with sodium. One day I ate pickles and chicken soup for lunch at a deli and gained eight pounds in water weight the next day. Fortunately, it was gone the following day, but your body doesn't need the stress; sodium can contribute to hypertension, or high blood pressure, which can be dangerous. Fatty cuts of meat like brisket, corned beef, pastrami, and tongue, should be avoided in Phase One. When you order a sandwich, skip the bread or make it an "open faced" sandwich in later Phases. Avoid eating Reuben sandwiches, as the bread is sautéed and it contains unhealthy Russian dressing and melted cheese. If you like the Reuben's flavor and must have it, order some cooked meat, a small side of dressing, and some sauerkraut and you'll save hundreds of calories. At a sandwich shop type of deli, the sandwiches are often loaded with cold cuts and cheese. You are better off bringing a sandwich from home and putting more vegetables than meat or cheese, and limiting the dressing (slathered with mayonnaise is always a bad idea, opt for mustard instead). At bagel shops, take the bagels home and serve them yourself. A half of a bagel with low-fat cream cheese and some smoked salmon can be satisfying. If you order a "Nova Sandwich" made there, odds are there will be a lot more cream cheese than you need.

34. Avoid pizza, pasta, and bread in Phase One. Limit cheese. Opt for cheddar or Swiss over American cheese, which is processed. Skip the ketchup and mayonnaise.

35. Consider making salad your meal. Add grilled chicken, steak, turkey, salmon, tuna, or shrimp. Many restaurants offer exciting chopped salads. Ask for things like crumbled blue cheese on the side. A little goes a long way in a chopped salad. Skip fatty things like bacon and beware of fattening dressings.

36. Avoid all-you-can eat buffets. (Refer to the strategies in Phase One about how to handle a buffet if that is your only option.)

37. As previously mentioned, avoid fast food. If you must have it, choose an establishment that has published calorie counts, and make healthy choices. Never "supersize" anything.

38. Avoid restaurants or situations that have triggered your worst binges—or anywhere you feel uncomfortable or fear you may have difficulty controlling yourself. Self-service restaurants and those that offer unlimited quantities of food tend to be problematic for many people.

39. Spicy foods rev the metabolism and can help burn calories. Categorically "Hot" spices are a low-calorie way to enhance flavor. A pinch of chili flakes or some hot peppers are good in many dishes. You may especially enjoy Cholula and Sriracha sauces as accompaniments to food.

40. Avoid white potatoes in Phases One–Three. If you have a baked potato in Phase Four, limit the toppings—skip any butter, bacon, cheese, and sour cream. If you really want sour cream, however, choose low-fat and use just a dollop. Watch out for side dishes, as many of these are loaded with fat and calories and may have more of both than your entrée—avoid creamed, fried, or "loaded" anything. I've seen "mac and cheese" dishes that are as high as 1,600 calories for a side dish! Try ordering steamed, grilled, or lightly sautéed vegetables and pass on things like Lyonnaise or au gratin potatoes, fries, hash browns, onion rings, and mac and cheese.

41. Choose brown rice over white rice. White rice starts as brown rice, which undergoes a refining process, where it is stripped of its fiber and nutrients. If you are into sushi, consider sashimi (without the rice). Also, some sushi restaurants make their sushi rolls with brown rice upon request.

42. If you order a hamburger, opt for burgers made with freshly ground beef rather than a pre-made patty, try it without a bun, and with veggies instead of French fries. Choose a light dressing. Oil and vinegar (including balsamic) or oil and lemon are often the healthiest salad dressings.

43. Eat when you are hungry—not starving—and stop before you are full. Remember, it takes twenty minutes for your brain to tell you that you have eaten enough to be full. If you eat too quickly, you will likely continue eating until suddenly you feel you are ready to burst, which is not good. Slow down, put the fork down, chew slowly, take a sip of your beverage, converse, and then take another bite. If this is difficult, it could be a sign that the food

is a problem substance to be avoided. We will get into how to deal with problematic foods later on.

44. Be sure to allow an adequate amount of time for the kind of meal you are planning. A fast, casual restaurant is best if you only have a short amount of time. In a fast, casual environment, look for published nutritional information and have some ideas of healthy items that should be your "go-to" choices, in the event you don't have time to sit down and be served a meal. When you are planning to dine in a sit-down restaurant, allow adequate time. You don't want to have to rush or eat in a hurry. *The Restaurant Diet* is all about enjoyment!

45. Pick a nutritious, refreshing dessert. Instead of ordering fattening cake, pie, or ice cream, have fresh fruit or berries for a satisfying and healthy dessert.

46. If someone at your table orders a fattening dessert, decline it completely or try only a taste. Look for "mini" personalized desserts, and avoid all sugar in Phase One. In Phases Two–Four, you may treat yourself occasionally—once a week. Be aware that, even if you are eating small or "healthier" desserts, they tend to increase cravings. Over time, you will train yourself to become used to smaller desserts on occasion, rather than simply avoiding dessert altogether. Often, restaurant sized dessert portions are very large, and should be shared. I appreciate being able to enjoy a taste or small serving of dessert on occasion, so long as I don't overdo it. Alternatively, instead of having dessert at the restaurant, walk elsewhere for dessert, such as frozen yogurt, or gelato, which is known for being less fattening than ice cream.

If you enjoyed your restaurant experience, go back and enjoy it again. Make that restaurant and chef a partner in your success. The nice thing is that you can go back and have the same meal again, and not have to explain everything to them from the beginning. You also don't need to search and estimate calories all over again. Share your positive experiences with others! If there is a restaurant or staff member that is particularly accommodating, tell people about it. Write a positive review online, or consider blogging about your own journey. If there are other people in your life looking to lose weight, consider going out together. Make it fun. Just like a workout buddy, having a like-minded dining partner or group of friends all looking to shed a few pounds can be very helpful, just as dining with someone who isn't trying to lose weight and is insensitive to your needs can be harmful. You shouldn't have to go it alone if you have friends or family that are of the same mindset, but you should avoid eating with people who are not of the same mindset and are not considerate of your needs (no breadbasket, don't mention the dessert, etc.), especially at first. Eventually, with practice you may reach a point that you can dine practically anywhere with anyone, and be comfortable in your routine, and not be tempted or derailed by other people's actions.

It is my hope that, if you take away nothing else from *The Restaurant Diet*, you will at least put into practice the above tips and strategies for dining out, as they will help you advance considerably in your weight-loss goals and help you overcome many common pitfalls related to restaurant dieting. Dining out and losing weight isn't rocket science, it just takes some practice getting used to an entirely new way of dining, thinking, and acting. Learning how to lose weight while dining at restaurants takes a form of strategic planning you do in advance and a formula you follow once you sit down at the table. In no time, all of this will become second nature. You will become increasingly comfortable walking into any restaurant, making better choices, enjoying yourself, and losing weight. As a result, you will be a smarter and happier dieter. You will walk confidently into your restaurant of choice armed with knowledge of healthy food choices, calorie counts, nutrition, how to order, eat, and what to avoid. You will start to find it easy and fun to devise a delicious meal plan for each and every meal and stick to it. As the pounds start to come off by dining in your favorite restaurants, you might even have to remind yourself that you're actually on a diet!

As long as you are polite, restaurants should be willing to serve and accommodate you. The nicer and firmer you are, the better off you will be. If you encounter someone who insists on leaving a bread basket or bringing you a fattening *amuse bouche* (bite-sized hors d'oeuvre) or gift from the kitchen, politely, but firmly decline saying, "No thank you" or "I'm sorry, I can't eat that." Be sure to talk to the chef or owner if available and to thank everyone who accommodates you. The more you employ your *Restaurant Diet* way of thinking, the healthier you will become, and better equipped to deal with any obstacles you may encounter, such as a restaurant running out of the item(s) you want.

If you continue to go back to a restaurant, share your success story with others. Most restaurant owners and staff will appreciate and applaud your effort and want to continue to help you. Many times, I have walked into one of my favorite restaurants and announced: "I've lost five pounds so far this month! You were part of my success, I am glad to be able to come back!" I received congratulations from everyone and even more support afterwards, as they felt like they were a part of my success.

A couple of final tips to reiterate: we all have foods and restaurants that may have been a particular problem for us in the past with regard to bingeing. If you are not comfortable going to any restaurant, for any reason, simply don't go there!

If you are part-way through a meal and are having anxiety or self-control issues with overeating: excuse yourself, take a walk, call a friend or sponsor, or possibly get the rest of your meal to-go. Food is meant to be savored and should never cause undue stress, which almost always leads to bad eating choices. You'll find that simply removing yourself from the situation will reduce your stress and prevent bingeing before it goes too far.

Chapter Two
Phase One—Beginning

"All glory comes from daring to begin."
—Eugene F. Ware (1841–1911), soldier, lawyer, politician, and author

---

In designing the four phases of *The Restaurant Diet*, I worked closely with my family doctor (who also happens to be a cardiologist) to help determine a realistic calorie budget to begin with, make sure there were no other underlying medical issues aside from being overweight, and to get medically cleared for an appropriate amount of exercise so I could start my new life.

Once I established and practiced my new routine for two months, I lost 10 percent of my body weight and exercise gradually became easier for me. I had become well versed at walking into practically any restaurant and successfully enjoying a healthy, gourmet meal. Soon I was able to enjoy a few more calories each day in exchange for more exercise. As you will read, the theme of *The Restaurant Diet* is a gradual, lasting progress one phase at a time, until you reach your desired weight.

When beginning any weight-loss program, it is important to establish a realistic, long-term goal or desired weight. You should have some idea where you want to go, but don't impose an unrealistic timeframe (i.e., tell yourself you need to lose twenty pounds by Memorial Day). My best advice is to establish a realistic weight goal, then a weight range to remain in once you have reached Phase Four, to work on developing better habits related to food and exercise, and to work on your emotions. If you do these things, you will succeed in good time.

METHODS FOR DETERMINING IDEAL WEIGHT

In consulting with your doctor, you may wish to utilize a combination of the following methods to establish a realistic weight-loss goal and range to stay in. I have included my personal statistics for illustrative purposes.

METHOD 1:

Below is a simple, easy-to-use method to help determine ideal weight.

Women: 100 pounds for the first 5 feet of height plus 5 pounds for each additional inch. For example, if you're 5 feet 6 inches, your ideal weight is 130 pounds. (100 + 30).

Men: 106 pounds of body weight for the first 5 feet of height plus 6 pounds for each additional inch. For example, if you're 5 feet 11 inches, your ideal weight is 172 pounds. (106 + 66).

You may adjust this for large or small body with. For a small body frame, subtract 10 percent. For a large frame, add 10 percent.

In my case, I have a large or broad frame, so based upon this formula, a reasonable weight would be 172 + 17 = 189 pounds.

METHOD 2: BODY MASS INDEX (BMI)

Body mass index estimates how much you should weigh based on your height and age. Ideally, a BMI should be under 25. To calculate your BMI: multiply your weight in pounds by 703, divide that number by your height in inches, and then divide that number by your height in inches again. For example, my BMI at my maximum weight of 329 (I am 71 inches tall) was 45.9 (46), which is morbidly obese (over 40). Using the BMI method as a guideline, my weight should be 179 or less. Use the chart below to see what category your BMI falls into and whether you need to be concerned about your weight.

BMI	Category
Below 18.5	Underweight
18.5–24.9	Healthy
25.0–29.9	Overweight
30.0–39.9	Obese
Over 40	Morbidly obese

The BMI formula is somewhat controversial, as it does not take into consideration different body types, nor does it consider the fact that muscle weighs more than fat; meaning that a person could have a higher than recommended BMI, yet have very little body fat and be perfectly healthy. My advice is not to be obsessed with a specific number, and to use a combination of the two simply as references. Most importantly, you should consult with your doctor to determine what weight range is appropriate for you.

To convert pounds to kilograms, divide your weight in pounds by 2.2. Example: 130 pounds = 59 kilograms

To convert kilograms to pounds: Multiply your weight in kilograms by 2.2. Example: 80 kilograms = 176 pounds

MONITORING WEIGHT AND STICKING TO A WEIGHT RANGE

Once you reach a desirable weight, your goal, of course, is to stay there. A person's desired weight shouldn't be a single magic number (like "180"). Talk to your doctor and consider establishing a healthy range.

As an example of a healthy weight range, according to the three methods discussed earlier, my ideal weight is 172 with a high of 189 (with the 10 percent allowance for a larger frame, based on the simple formula method), or 179 or less using the BMI formula (for a BMI of under 25). Therefore, my doctor, nutritionist, and I agreed that my ideal weight range would be 180–190 pounds.

My advice is to work towards a realistic and reasonable goal that you and your doctor or team establish, based upon things like your age, sex, mobility, and current weight, and to monitor and evaluate your progress along the way, making any adjustments your team may suggest. I've spoken with both my doctor and nutritionist who have advised that everyone's circumstances are different, so there is no "one size fits all" approach. For some people, simply losing a "good deal of weight" as opposed to reaching what the above methods or any other method suggests one should weigh, is far better than doing nothing.

Each of us was born with certain metabolic and genetic tendencies, and our metabolism changes as we age, regardless of whether we were ever overweight or lost a lot of weight. Therefore, it is important to continue to be mindful and realistic with our weight-loss and maintenance goals, and is important to consult with your doctor on an ongoing basis to determine what is best for you.

PHASE ONE IN MOTION

We all begin in Phase One, when we are at our heaviest, and least fit or able to exercise. Phase One marks the beginning of a new life and new, healthier, more disciplined approach to dining and to living. Twenty-four hours ago, you may have been eating whatever you wanted, and exercise was likely not a priority. Your body may be out of shape, but if you've been overweight for any amount of time like I was, your body will actually be accustomed to being overweight and inactive. Phase One, the shortest and strictest phase of *The Restaurant Diet*, is all about shocking the system. Here you'll greatly reduce, if not eliminate, unhealthy fats, carbohydrates, sugar, processed foods, fried foods, and anything artificial. You will do this in restaurants and at home as you learn to count and estimate calories and stay within your calorie budget, while beginning to incorporate exercise into your daily life based upon what your doctor deems appropriate. If your calorie budget is anything like mine was in the beginning, you'll need to cut back on calories and start to exercise by literally putting one foot in front of the other, literally. Be careful about cutting calories too drastically, however, as the body goes into "starvation" or "save and store fat mode"—which is why most "diets" require at least 1,200 calories per day.

Though it may sound counter-intuitive, shocking the system doesn't happen overnight; it takes the body some time to adjust. In fact, initially, your body will want to hold on to the weight—a primitive survival instinct all humans and animals have to protect us in the event of famine or crisis. Our bodies do not understand that we are deliberately trying to lose weight by eating less and beginning to exercise. Our metabolisms don't instinctively understand that being overweight is harmful. This is one reason people who expect quick results from dieting are often disappointed. We have to stick with a healthier regimen of diet and exercise long enough to overcome our body's tendency to want to resist changing. Therefore, Phase One is designed to be strict, but not so strict as to work against you. You want to give your body a gradual jolt as you reduce calories to a realistic amount, make better food choices, and gradually increase your physical activity.

Phase One is not about forcing you to "hurry up and lose weight fast"; rather, it's about making permanent changes and moving in the right direction, however long it takes for the weight to drop. It's okay to let go of all that pressure. This time losing weight is not about taking off a certain number of pounds in a specific amount of time.

Although the strictest part of Phase One is temporary, the changes you will be making and your overall direction will become permanent. Try not to get impatient or frustrated, even though it won't always be easy. The best advice is to simply start and not give up! I lost very little the first couple of weeks while my body was in shock trying to fight what I was doing. I knew this would be temporary. I got through it, and my weight began to drop.

It's important to recognize that weight loss is about being "well fed" in all areas of our lives—what we eat, how we exercise, and how we deal with our emotions. After using food for years as a way of coping with things such as anger, depression, and anxiety, developing healthier coping skills is a must. We will discuss the importance of therapy as part of a comprehensive path towards wellness in depth in later chapters. Once you start to eat right, exercise, and handle your emotions, you will feel "well fed" and will start to see results. I like to think of the acronym "FED" when addressing weight loss: Food, Exercise, and Deal (with your emotions).

IMPORTANT CAUTIONS

Always consult with your primary care physician before beginning any major weight-loss or exercise program. The first thing you need to do is to have a complete physical. Then you should determine—with the help of your doctor—a realistic calorie goal. This will likely be based upon your age, sex, current weight, level of activity, and realistic weight goal you have established. Also, I recommend continuing to follow up with your doctor during the course of your weight loss and thereafter—especially if any medical issues arise, or if you are looking to increase your level of activity and progress to a new phase of your diet.

After I consulted with my doctor and did some research, we established 1,500 calories per day as a practical budget to start with, given that my level of activity would be low in the beginning due to my overweight condition. Your doctor may run a series of blood tests to check for things like high cholesterol, the results of which could impact your food choices. You and your doctor may also want to enlist the guidance of a nutritionist to help develop your dining plan.

As someone who is likely used to eating more than you should, when you reduce calories, you are going to have to find ways to satiate yourself. You should enjoy a variety of lightly dressed salads and small portions (approximately 4–6 ounces) of lean protein, like beef, chicken, turkey, lamb, veal, pork, and seafood, such as lobster, shrimp, salmon, tuna, flounder, sole, halibut, snapper, and sashimi for lunch or dinner, and items that are low in fat and carbohydrates for breakfast, such as eggs, egg whites, fresh fruit, and yogurt. Snacks should be low-calorie, easy to eat, and take-with-you items like fresh fruit or yogurt. For your main meals, choose items that are grilled, baked, broiled, pan-seared, or poached, and avoid fattening sauces (or ask for them on the side). With a little planning, you too can enjoy many excellent restaurants and delicious meals out and at home without the guilt.

MAKE CALORIES YOUR FRIEND

We need calories to live on, just the way a car needs fuel to run. Knowing just how much we need, and making sure we get it—and in the very best way possible—is key, by eating a balance of quality foods that give us the nutrition and satisfaction, as well as the energy to go about our day. Many diets make the calorie our enemy, or encourage us to avoid dealing with them altogether (eating whatever you want of certain foods). Learning to count calories and keeping track of everything I ate made me accountable, and made it less likely for me to go over budget.

I believe it will do that for you as well. Start fresh each day. If you are under budget one day, do not go over the following day. Stay consistent, and try to consume the entire permitted amount. Going too low does not help. Establish a calorie budget, count calories, and monitor your progress. Remember, everything counts. The only way an overeater can successfully manage losing weight and keeping it off is to keep track of everything and remain accountable.

The Restaurant Diet illustrates how to make better choices in restaurants, to ask your servers questions, to review menus in advance online, and to be specific about requests, like going light on butter or oil. It will take practice and patience to review a menu before going out to eat, make selections, and plug foods into a calorie counter or app, to determine whether your choices are suitable. Before long, you will become a weight-loss wizard, and you will find yourself able to enjoy eating out and losing weight. If you like to eat out as much as I did, you will find it worth the effort to do it right. It actually became fun, a game to eat in great restaurants and lose weight. It made me feel good about myself to be empowered to make my own healthier choices, and to be able to still enjoy dining at my favorite restaurants—something I could never do on other diets.

WRITE AN "AVOID LIST"

While dieting should not be about deprivation, let's face it—we all have problem foods that we need to avoid. There are other foods that are simply not good for you, no matter how you slice it; essentially, these are "empty calories" that do nothing to fill you up and will quickly blow your calorie budget and leave you hungry. These "diet busters" should be avoided. Especially in the beginning, start by replacing these foods with those that are satisfying and lower in calories—foods that are in one of two camps: 1) nutrient dense or 2) high water content. Nutrient dense foods include lean proteins (meat, fish, and poultry). Foods with high water content include fruits and vegetables, which provide nutrition and fill you up for very few calories.

In Phase One, avoid pizza and pasta completely, as well as white rice, white potatoes, white bread, fried foods, butter, cream, whole milk dairy products, sugar, and sugar substitutes. Pizza, pasta, and bread are foods many people tend to overeat the most. White potatoes, white rice, and white bread—which offer little nutritional value—should be replaced with sweet potatoes, brown rice, and either whole-wheat, multi-grain, or sprouted bread. An easy tip is to simply avoid refined for processed foods, such as white flour.

If you enjoy wine as I do, I have good news! A glass of wine is okay in *The Restaurant Diet*, even in Phase One! Just stick to one 5-ounce glass (125 calories) of white or red of your liking, and have it with dinner. As I said earlier, I enjoyed wine, but if you prefer another type of beverage, you may consider having it instead of the glass of wine, as long as the calories are roughly the same.

FOODS TO LIMIT OR AVOID—ALL PHASES

To be successful at losing weight in a restaurant or at home, you need to establish some ground rules of what is good for you and what isn't. I am a visual person and a fan of writing out lists to help me remember. I believe that if you write it down, it has extra impact, and putting it on paper gives it a permanence and credibility. Certain foods like candy, chips, cookies, soda (regular and diet), sugary sports drinks, and other beverages should be avoided by everyone, period. They simply are not worth the amount of calories they contain for the lack of nutrition they offer.

Everyone attempting to lose weight and get healthier should have a written list of foods they need to limit. This doesn't mean you can never eat them again. What it means is you need to pay careful attention to the calories and fat content and may want to reconsider eating them. Copy my personal list below and adapt it as you like, especially early on, when you are getting used to a new way of thinking when it comes to food.

You also need to write a separate "Avoid List" of foods that have caused you significant problems. By this I mean anything you have ever binged on or are unable to eat like a civilized person (i.e., eating uncontrollably, not putting utensils down, or not coming up for air). It could also be any food you obsess about or can't leave alone if it is around you. If at any time you run into a food that is problematic, you should add it to your Avoid List. These foods should not be allowed in the house and certainly not ordered when dining out.

Start by writing your own AVOID LIST. Be sure to include any foods that you know pose a problem and place the paper on your refrigerator or somewhere conspicuous at home. If needed, take it with you when you go out to eat. My Avoid List included things like hot dogs, grilled cheese sandwiches, cookies, chips, soda, candy, sports beverages, and cake. These were foods I either had a problem with, or were high in fat and/or calories and simply not worth it. As a visual, imagine the Avoid List should be regarded as a red light, a stop sign, a DO NOT ENTER sign, or a HAZMAT sign, meaning it is literally poison to you! This is the time to be completely honest. If you are reluctant to put cheesecake on the list because you're afraid of missing it (after you ate three pieces in one sitting last week), add cheesecake to your Avoid List.

Below is what I call my LIMIT LIST. This is a list of foods you should LIMIT forever, and AVOID COMPLETELY in Phase One, along with any foods that fit the HAZMAT description above, which is your permanent AVOID LIST. As a visual, look at this list of foods as a yellow light, requiring you to proceed with caution. Again, if any of these foods pose a particular problem, they should be on your permanent Avoid List.

- Deep fried foods—either savory, or sweet (including but not limited to: fried chicken, chicken wings, egg rolls, French fries, hash browns, Lyonnaise potatoes, onion rings, doughnuts, zeppoles, etc.) as well as fried on the stove
- Brisket/fatty cuts of meat like brisket, corned beef, pastrami, and tongue
- Butter (and sauces made with butter, such as Hollandaise)
- Baked goods—breads, cakes, pies, doughnuts, cookies

- Bacon
- Chips, pork rinds, jerky, etc.
- Chocolate and candy
- Cream sauces made with butter or heavy cream (Alfredo)
- Whole milk or heavy cream
- Cream-based cheeses
- Ice Cream
- Alcohol (with the exception of a glass of wine with dinner in Phase One and Two)
- Soda and sugary beverages, including natural sugars, like fruit juices, as well as sports beverages
- Sugar and artificial sugar substitutes (see sidebar); in Phase One, eliminate all sugar (except that found naturally in fruits)
- Duck and goose (high in fat)
- Hot dogs
- Liver, *pâté, foie gras*
- Pre-made hamburger patties (often high in fat); it is better to buy fresh ground beef
- Sausage, bratwurst, etc.
- Processed deli meats
- Regular mayonnaise and sour cream
- Pasta and rice
- Ribs, short ribs
- White bread, anything made from white flour, pizza, sandwiches, pancakes, waffles, French toast, etc. (opt for multi-grain)
- White potatoes, especially those with toppings
- White Rice (opt for brown rice instead)
- Blintzes
- Shortening or lard
- Cheese (limit portion, opt for part-skim). Feta cheese is a good option, it has fewer calories than most cheeses.

ONE DAY PER WEEK CLEANSE DAY IN PHASE ONE

During Phase One, make one day a week a "cleanse day." On these days you should avoid any carbs, protein, and alcohol (including the glass of wine), sticking with an abundance of fruits and vegetables. Try making salads, and dressing them with a touch of olive oil and either white or traditional balsamic, cider vinegar, home-made raspberry vinaigrette, or home-made honey Dijon dressing, among others. It is important to flush out and cleanse your body.

As an illustration, I have included an example of how *The Restaurant Diet* works at Morton's of Chicago, a top steakhouse with nationwide locations, and a restaurant I enjoyed several times a month during my weight loss.

SLIMMED-DOWN GOURMET DINING: MORTON'S OF CHICAGO

Morton's of Chicago is a prime steakhouse with locations nationwide. The restaurant serves beautiful steaks, cooked to perfection, as well as many excellent (and some fattening) side dishes and decadent desserts. The service is top-notch.

If you enjoy steak, beef can be a good choice for weight loss. In fact, an entire meal at a steakhouse can be a good option—if you know how to approach it. Unfortunately, steakhouses often serve enormous portions and it takes careful monitoring to ensure success. The secret to successful dining out at a steakhouse—or any restaurant, for that matter—begins with counting calories. It means tracking the foods you plan to eat on a reliable website or app. It requires making healthier choices even before heading out to the restaurant—and then you must stick to them. This takes some time and practice, but it is a lot better than avoiding your favorite restaurants or going out to eat with no plan and getting sidetracked.

Start off by reviewing Morton's menu before even making the reservation. Check calorie counts and portion sizes online. If you'd like a glass of wine, that's perfectly fine, but recognize that you would need to sacrifice 125 calories somewhere else.

Once you arrive at Morton's and are seated, engage your server. Introduce yourself to staff who don't know you. Tell them that you are in the process of losing weight, and that you would appreciate them not mentioning any fattening specials that could possibly be a temptation. Tell them no bread and butter. Be as polite and pleasant as possible, but be firm if necessary. If the bus boy tries to insist on leaving you some bread and butter anyway, hand it back to him and say, "no thank you." Don't allow them to tell you about their decadent dessert special. Again, just say, "no thank you." Ask for sauce on the side and that they reduce the amount of butter and/or oil in dishes.

At Morton's, *Prix Fixe* (or all-inclusive) several course meals are a good bet in terms of variety, portion size, and value. The steakhouse occasionally runs a special Steak and Seafood set menu that includes salad, a six-ounce Filet Mignon, three baked shrimp (or scallops or a crab cake), a vegetable or side (my favorite became the grilled asparagus with lemon), and dessert (I would order the mixed berries).

Begin by skipping the bread and appetizers to make room for a full meal. Order a house salad with oil and vinegar or a lettuce, tomato, and red onion salad with olive oil and balsamic vinegar on the side. For taste, you can order a small portion of crumbled blue cheese on the side. For the Steak and Seafood main course, ask for the sauces on the side. Instead of selecting a sugary dessert, order a bowl of rich mixed berries.

Another option is to substitute a soup in place of the salad. Alternately, you can enjoy a Jumbo Shrimp Cocktail, a soup such as a vegetable barley, seafood chowder (tomato base, rather than cream), or Onion Soup (without the bread and cheese), and a salad, which is a completely satisfying and relatively inexpensive, gourmet meal at a nice restaurant.

Morton's lounge offers a "Power Hour" selection consisting of excellent-quality tapas-sized portions of foods like prime sliders (leave off the bun), Jumbo Shrimp Cocktail, oysters on the half shell, tuna tartare, and more for a discounted price in the lounge.

When you go to a steakhouse like Morton's, see if they also offer special *Prix Fixe* meals or discounted bar bites—some of which are healthy. Another thing about Morton's, and many steakhouses, is they also happen to have excellent seafood selections, and many even feature vegetarian and vegan options. Many restaurants now feature heart-healthy options and low-calorie items, and some even post calorie counts on their menus, which is very convenient for people who are trying to lose weight or maintain a healthy lifestyle. Chains with twenty or more locations will soon be required to post calories on their menus.

In the event you are asked to eat out at a steakhouse with little or no advance warning, always opt for foods that are grilled, baked, or poached. Limit your portion size to a maximum of 4–6 ounces for protein (a deck of cards) and 3–4 ounces for pasta (typically a half portion). Always ask for sauces and dressings on the side. Once you have eaten a certain dish at a certain restaurant and estimated and logged your calorie count, you will be able to replicate the meal without doing the research. If you frequent a restaurant, it won't be long before you have a dozen or so "go-to" meals already logged in your tracker and can then easily replicate the meal at any time, and perhaps even translate it to calorie counts at similar restaurants.

ETHNIC RESTAURANTS

One of the things I hated about every other diet I tried—aside from the fact that dining out was either discouraged or forbidden—was that I quickly became bored with the very limited selection of foods I could eat. Frozen meals and "slimmed-down" commercial products, which sought to mimic the tastes of authentic Italian, Chinese, Mexican, or other cuisines, simply didn't cut it. The flavors were not right, and many times they would end up in the garbage. I'd find myself calling a restaurant to deliver, or getting in the car and going out to eat.

We are fortunate to live in a multicultural nation, with so many wonderful examples of cuisines from all over the world. If you enjoy eating out as much as I do, you should continue eating out in a variety of restaurants to keep you from becoming bored with your diet. To make your life easier, I offer examples of which foods to look for and which ones to avoid in the most popular ethnic restaurants. Since *The Restaurant Diet* is designed to get you to embrace losing weight while eating out, it is important to learn to be successful at any type of restaurant you choose from day one.

In a 2015 survey, Chinese was ranked the number-one most popular ethnic cuisine, closely followed by Mexican and Italian. Others in the top ten included French, Greek, Japanese/sushi, Indian, and Middle Eastern. Below are a number of examples of what to try and what to steer clear of in some of your favorite types of ethnic restaurants. By utilizing the strategies outlined in the preceding pages and plugging choices into a calorie counter, you'll be on your way to the tastiest and most fun weight-loss journey imaginable.

ITALIAN DINING

Italian food is my personal favorite, so I couldn't resist putting it first. Italian food can be an excellent, healthy choice, yet it can also be problematic—especially since many restaurants feature large portion sizes, fried foods, and lots of cheese (think parmigiana). Italian restaurants are usually home for great bread, often served with olive oil or a tasty dip. It's not hard to eat an entire loaf, especially if you are hungry. Resist the temptation. In later Phases, if calories allow, enjoy a piece of bread, and then ask your server to remove the tray. As far as food, look for: *Insalata Mista* (Mixed Salad), Arugula Salad with Shaved Parmesan (ask for the cheese on the side, so you can manage the amount), *Tricolore* Salad (arugula, radicchio, endive), Minestrone (vegetable soup), *Stracciatella* (chicken broth with spinach and egg), *Crudo* (raw seafood plates), grilled vegetables, grilled or pan-seared seafood (like Livornese with tomato, olives, capers), grilled Veal Chop, and Steak Pizzaiola. Pasta dishes are okay with a manageable portion size and as long as the sauce is tomato-based with no cream (such as Penne with Vodka Sauce); seafood and vegetables are fine add-ons. Avoid Parmigiana dishes (foods fried and topped with mozzarella cheese). Limit pizza to one thin crust slice and opt for vegetable toppings. Italian-style individual pizzas are also fine. Avoid large hero, hoagie, or grinder sandwiches (terminology depends on what part of the country you live in); you are better off with several meatballs and a salad than a meatball sub. For desserts, I recommend going with fresh fruit whenever possible in all types of restaurants, and saving other kinds of desserts for a taste once you are past Phase One.

CHINESE DINING

Chinese may be the most popular ethnic cuisine in America, but much of the Americanized Chinese food we regularly order for takeout or delivery is high in fat, calories, and sodium. Often it contains at least some MSG (monosodium glutamate), which is used to tenderize meat, but is high in sugar and known to give some people a headache. Hidden sugar and headaches are two things you don't need. Not that you shouldn't eat Chinese food. You just have to be selective, ask questions, and know what to choose.

Look for: Wonton, Egg Drop, and Hot & Sour Soups. Sometimes there are versions of all three with seafood and/or vegetables that are very satisfying. For starters, I like steamed dumplings (dim sum, which means "heart's delight").

Avoid things like egg rolls, spring rolls, fried shrimp balls, as all of these options are deep fried. Ask for brown rice, which has more nutritional value than white rice. Look for dishes like: Moo Goo Gai Pan (chicken with vegetables), Chicken or Beef with Broccoli or Snow Peas, Moo-Shu Pork (leave out the pancakes), and Chinese Broccoli. Dishes to avoid: General Tso's Chicken, Sweet and Sour anything (also deep fried), Lo Mein (large portions of mostly pasta), and Fried Rice.

FRENCH DINING

French offers a contrast of rich dishes and sauces versus some really light, healthy options. *Plateaus de Mer* (chilled seafood platters), *Huitres* (oysters on the half shell), and *Moules Marinieres* (mussels in a white wine broth) are all delicious choices. I know it's tempting, but skip eating an entire baguette to dunk in the broth of the *Moules Marinieres*.

Look for: steak or seafood tartare as a starter. If you love Onion Soup, try it without the bread and cheese. The broth with the onions alone is delicious. Look for Bouillabaisse (fish stew), Tuna Niçoise Salad, Dover sole, asparagus (Hollandaise on the side), steak (leave out the fries), Coq au Vin (chicken), and lamb. Avoid: the cheese cart, Duck (especially the skin), Pâté, Frog's Legs (often fried), *Pommes Frites* (fries), Pommes Dauphinoise (potatoes with melted cheese), and anything else saturated in butter, cream, or oil. If you are ordering a *Steak au Poivre* (peppercorn brandy sauce), ask for the sauce on the side and just dip each bite; you don't need all the sauce.

GREEK DINING

There are many wonderful options available at Greek restaurants. Start with the ubiquitous Greek Salad, which is typically loaded with feta cheese and creamy dressing. Ask for the cheese on the side (and add a sprinkle), as well as the dressing (or go with oil and vinegar). Avgolemono (Lemon-Chicken Soup) is also satisfying, though the calories add up fast if it contains pasta, rice, or orzo. Often the latter is served with rice, which you can ask to have left out. Skip the Spanakopita (spinach and feta baked in phyllo dough) and Saganaki (flaming cheese). Instead look for: Grape Leaves. Moussaka (Eggplant) is good to share. Go for grilled seafood and meats and limit things like Gyro's, Souvlaki, Lamb Shanks, and Pastitsio (Greek lasagna). Skip the Baklava for dessert. (Or, in later Phases, if you are with a group, you may have a bite and keep passing it around!)

In the New York area, there are "Greek diners" in practically every town. These are frequently open twenty-four hours a day and serve practically every kind of food imaginable. They are not typical "Greek restaurants" *per se*, as they don't focus on Greek food. The best advice for these—as with any restaurant—is planning in advance when possible and making good choices from the vast array of options.

INDIAN DINING

Indian food is full of great choices, as well as options that are loaded with sugar and fat. It is a fun cuisine full of great flavors and spices. It's easy, however, to get sidetracked with crispy bread known as papadum for starters; avoid this, unless it's prepared with dry heat and not fried. Skip the Poori (deep fried) in favor of a small slice of Naan (unbleached flour). A go-to starter is Mulligatawny or Lentil Soup. Avoid things like Paneer (cheese), Pakoras (fried), and Samosas (unless baked). Good entrée choices include Tandoori Chicken (without skin, marinated in yogurt and baked in a clay pot), as well as Chicken Tikka (also a tasty yogurt marinade), and curries with vegetables. Aloo Gobi is worth a try without the potatoes. If you are going to try Saag Paneer (spinach with cheese), skip the cheese and opt for the vegetable only.

JAPANESE DINING

Whether you prefer dining at a sushi restaurant or at a hibachi/teppanyaki grill, there are a plenty of healthy options. Look for: Miso Soup and Onion broth, Ginger or Avocado Salad, and sashimi (leave off the rice). For sushi rolls, avoid those with fried foods on top and any sauces that contain mayonnaise and cream cheese. These can add hundreds of unnecessary calories to a 6-piece roll. Also, a lot of sushi places offer brown rice instead of white for their rolls.

For hibachi-style, I suggest talking with your waiter and chef prior to starting preparation at the grill and requesting he use as little oil and butter as possible. See if he can replace regular soy sauce with low-sodium soy sauce. Choose a beef, chicken, fish, shrimp, lobster, or vegetarian dish (or a combo). These are also good to share, as hibachi restaurants typically serve a ton of food with extras, such as shrimp, vegetables, bean sprouts, and rice included. Always substitute the Fried Rice with brown rice (on the side) or ask for additional vegetables instead of rice. I am a big fan of green tea, which contains a lot of health benefits, and is a great accompaniment to a Japanese meal. Of course, I recommend skipping the fried ice cream.

JEWISH DELI AND BAGEL SHOP DINING

This didn't make the top 10 survey, but no doubt it would if only New York and South Florida were counted. Jewish deli food has always been a personal favorite of mine, having grown up in New York among Jewish relatives and having lived in South Florida. Jewish-style delis—many of which are famous in big cities, such as Katz's and the Second Avenue Deli in New York—offer a wonderful assortment of food that can work well in Phase One—but you must be especially careful of fatty meats and salty foods. Look for: Matzo Ball Soup, Split Pea, Stuffed Cabbage, Chicken in a Pot, and Gefilte Fish. Avoid fattier cuts of meat like pastrami, corned beef, tongue, and brisket in Phase One and limit them thereafter. Look for turkey (especially if roasted in-house) instead. If you are looking at deli meats, I recommend opting for just the meat without the bread or limiting the bread to one slice. As a condiment, use mustard instead of mayonnaise, ketchup, or Russian dressing. Avoid Reuben sandwiches, as the added fat and calories from the Russian dressing and Swiss cheese will likely blow any calorie budget (not to mention that both sides are sautéed in butter or oil). Smoked Fish, like Nova Salmon, Sable, and Sturgeon are fine as they are not high in calories, but watch carefully as they are high in salt content. Bagels should be avoided in Phase One and limited thereafter as they have between 250 and 400 calories and offer zero nutritional value. If you're doing cream cheese, go with light varieties and only spread on a thin *schmear*.

MEXICAN DINING

Recently ranked the #2 most popular ethnic cuisine in America, Mexican cuisine has never been more popular—and not just on Cinco de Mayo! Look for: freshly made guacamole (I love restaurants that prepare it at your table)—just limit the amount of chips to a handful. Many places offer veggies instead of chips, which is a much better option. Also look for items like Ceviche (raw fish in citrus juices), Chicken Tortilla Soup, and Grilled Fish Tacos. You'll need to hold off until Phases Three and Four for the occasional margarita. Avoid things like: Quesadillas, Nachos, Burritos, Fried Fish Tacos, Chile Rellenos, Refried Beans, and Enchiladas. Many places also offer lettuce wraps in place of taco shells. Many Mexican entrees include some sort of rice or potato. See if you can substitute this with a green vegetable. Chimichurri rubbed steak, grilled or roasted seafood, or chicken, are good choices.

MIDDLE EASTERN DINING

Middle Eastern cuisine offers an array of healthy, flavorful foods with exotic spices. Look for: salads, such as Fattoush (typically a lovely garden salad with pieces of torn pita) and Tabbouleh (parsley, tomato, mint, onions, and cracked bulgur wheat with lemon and olive oil), grilled meats, seafood, kebabs, couscous, and dips like hummus (chickpeas) and baba ganoush (eggplant). Limit the amount of pita bread to just a small slice or two or, better yet, ask if they have vegetables for dipping instead.

HOW TO HANDLE THREE POPULAR AMERICAN PASTIMES: BRUNCH, BUFFETS, AND HAPPY HOUR

BRUNCH

In addition to ethnic cuisines, brunch is a favorite American pastime worth addressing. Many brunches are served as lavish, all-you-can-eat buffets at fancy restaurants or hotels. Some restaurant brunches offer *Prix Fixe* menus or choices of everything from Eggs Benedict and omelets, to waffles, pancakes, smoked salmon platters, fresh fruit, oatmeal, avocado toast, ham, steak, and more. Some of these items can be healthy, but many are not conducive to weight loss. See below to determine which of these are good to eat (in moderation) and which to avoid entirely.

BUFFETS

If you're headed to a brunch buffet—or any buffet—you have to be especially careful to map out your strategy. There are so many choices, and it is very easy to go astray. I do not recommend buffets at all in Phase One. For later Phases, I would advise limiting "all-you-can-eat" food options to special occasions or once in awhile—even if you have reached a healthy weight.

For buffet dining, try practicing "The Two-Plate Rule." One plate should be your main course and some side dishes (such as an omelet or slice of beef, ham, or turkey), smoked fish, and healthy side dishes, like vegetables. Eggs can be a good bet; if you go for Eggs Benedict, skip the English Muffins and limit Hollandaise sauce. My favorite choices are vegetable omelets—either whole eggs, egg whites, or a combo. I ask for little or no cheese, since it is one-hundred calories an ounce. (Note: Feta is a bit less.) Smoked fish with slices of tomato and onion are okay—but avoid a bagel and cream cheese at the buffet. Salad with a fish, shrimp, chicken, or beef is a nice option. If they offer Avocado Toast or French Toast on sprouted bread, it is worth trying. Oatmeal and fresh fruit are safe and healthy options.

Breakfast foods like waffles, pancakes, blintzes, bacon, sausage, and hash browns may be tasty, but are high in fat and calories and do little to satisfy or provide nutrition, so they should be limited. The second plate should be a salad and/or some fresh fruit and berries. Many brunches have elaborate salad bars with lots of excellent items. Just be careful with the dressing; as always, simple oil and vinegar or oil and lemon are the best options.

Another buffet tip—don't overload your plates! Keep them simple so you can see everything on them if you are going to taste several different things. As overeaters, we are used to large portions—especially if we are able to choose from a seemingly endless bounty. If you are going to try a buffet situation, handle it with the utmost care. If you are doing lunch or dinner at a buffet, try some lean protein combined with some vegetables, fruit, and/or a salad. Try to leave some of the plate visible (don't pile the food on). If you can't resist the temptation of "all-you-can-eat," you can always leave. Anytime you find yourself in an uncomfortable situation, you can always excuse yourself. To quote Kenny Rogers' song "The Gambler": "know when to walk away, and know when to run!" Just because you encountered a problem doesn't mean you shouldn't try going out to eat again. Perhaps you should try a different restaurant or type of food if something proves to be problematic.

HAPPY HOUR

For those of us social creatures who like to dine out, Happy Hour can be an enticing, budget-friendly option. It can also, however, mean a lot of unnecessary temptation. If willpower is an issue, I would suggest you wait for Phase Two, so that you can first get comfortable with your new diet before heading to a Happy Hour. If you don't drink—and especially if you have issues with alcohol—Happy Hour is obviously not a good idea.

Many restaurants offer happy hours with not only drink specials, but also discounted bar bites as well. Some restaurants even offer a discount on meals from their regular menus during Happy Hour. As with all other restaurant outings, it is best to research online in advance or to call.

Some fair advice to keep in mind when at a Happy hour: do not eat high-fat, bar-centric food like wings (of any kind), jalapeño poppers, fried mozzarella sticks, and nachos. A preferable alternative would be shrimp cocktail. Ruth's Chris Steakhouse, a top nationwide chain, features a discounted USDA Prime Hamburger as part of Happy Hour and is one of the best burgers, and deals, around. At this upscale restaurant you can order a burger (skip the bun, fries, and ketchup), salad (light dressing only), and Happy Hour glass of wine and walk out feeling satisfied without having broken your calorie budget. The Seared Tuna with ginger-mustard sauce at Ruth's Chris Steakhouse is also excellent and available at a discount during Happy Hour.

It is especially important when you are in a bar setting to order some water, or a no-calorie beverage such as unsweetened iced tea, to sip on, in addition to any drink you may have. Take a sip from one, and your next sip from the other. This makes the beverage last longer, fills you up, and makes you less likely to order additional cocktails that you don't need. This is helpful in any social situation. If you are out with friends or coworkers who are drinking and you are trying to stick to one, or not drink all, ask the bartender to make you a water-based drink and serve it to you in a rocks glass, so you don't feel out of place. Any situation where people are overindulging should be handled with extreme care—it is always a good idea to excuse yourself and leave early if a get-together is beginning to go overboard.

A note of caution: it's easy to get carried away at happy hours and not even realize it, especially if you are drinking, which really adds up in calories (and cost). It's no coincidence that overeating and drinking too much go hand-in-hand, as they both have the same emotional and genetic roots. If you are in any danger of this trap, avoid happy hours altogether.

By this time, you should have a good idea how *The Restaurant Diet* works. I suggest reviewing this information, working on your Avoid List, and deciding where you want to go have dinner! Print out the menu, get out your app, and figure out what you're going to enjoy. Within no time, this should become second nature and you will be well on your way to enjoying losing weight by eating a variety of tasty foods in many wonderful restaurants.

OUT-PSYCHING RESTAURANT PSYCHOLOGY

We face the challenge that many restaurants, at least in the United States, serve portions that are simply too large. The ironic part is that the restaurants get blamed for doing this, but would likely face a backlash if they were to reduce their portion sizes. How many times have we complained that the portions are too small, or criticized *Nouvelle Cuisine*? People are obsessed with quantity and value for their dollar, which is understandable. People want to feel like they're getting a good deal instead of being ripped off. This is why the philosophy behind "supersizing" a meal works so well. For a fraction of the cost of a regular portion, you can add a significant amount to it, whether it's a drink or a dinner entrée. As savvy consumers, we need to understand that this kind of "gotcha marketing" appeals to our inner impulsivity and need to get a "deal" and find value. However, just because someone is giving away free samples of food at your local supermarket or warehouse store doesn't mean you have to try them.

Our eyes and minds also play tricks on us, encouraging us to go for the bigger portion because it looks better, appeals to the "reward center" in our brains, and offers better value. We can't change any of this. What we *can* change is how we deal with this reality. Let's face it. What looks more appealing—a 24-ounce Tomahawk Ribeye Steak or a 6-ounce Petit Filet Mignon? My advice, as someone who lost a ton of weight by learning to make better food choices, would naturally be to pick the Filet. It is a reasonable size for one person to enjoy in one sitting, it is a leaner cut of meat, and there is less room for temptation. True—the Tomahawk Steak is definitely more attractive, but could and should easily serve several diners. To be successful, you need to recognize this and make a choice: Are you going to pick the smaller steak, or consider sharing or taking home some of the larger steak? Another way to look at the size-value proposition of a potential dish, or to judge what is an appropriate meal, rather than a better-looking meal is to think back to anytime you over-ordered, gave into temptation, ate the wrong foods, or overate. Think how you felt—regretful, guilty, ashamed, angry, disappointed in yourself, and uncomfortably full. Do you ever want to feel that way again? I don't. I've found it is not worth the risk of temptation.

We need to realize that just because a restaurant offers an item for one person doesn't mean we need to order and eat it all ourselves. Restaurants have long been criticized for imposing "sharing charges" on their menus. While this might seem objectionable and profit-driven, it is actually advantageous in some instances for diners and dieters to pay the sharing charge. Keep in mind that many restaurants that include soup, salad, or a side dish with an entrée will serve these courses to each diner if they are charging extra for sharing. To be sure, just ask!

WINE AND ALCOHOL WITH WEIGHT LOSS

A key difference between my diet and the other plans I had tried before was that, in mine, I drank wine almost every day. You can too, but in Phase One and Phase Two, limit your intake to one glass of wine (red or white) with dinner per day, knowing that a typical 5-ounce glass of red or white wine is approximately 125 calories. In Phase Three, you may have a cocktail in place of wine if calories allow, and in Phase Four, you are allowed anything in moderation, subject to some guidelines we will address in Phase Four.

I recommend limiting alcohol to wine only and to one glass per day, since these are empty calories. Beer, spirits, mixed drinks, and liqueurs typically have more calories, and the type of calories from distilled grains and sugar go straight to the belly. On the other hand, studies have shown that wine in moderation offers health benefits. People have been enjoying wine for thousands of years, and there are many delicious wines that pair well with food. If you enjoy wine, you shouldn't stop just because you are trying to lose weight and get healthy. Learn to make wine part of your healthy lifestyle the right way.

If you are not into wine and prefer beer, but don't want to give it up, you might try a light or low-carb beer, like Michelob Ultra, which is considerably lower in calories and carbs than regular beer, and actually tastes good. Michelob Ultra has 95 calories and 2.6 carbs per 12-ounce serving, and is something I enjoyed in Phase Four. So, if beer is your thing instead of wine, I suggest having one light beer with dinner instead of the one glass of wine, during Phase One and Phase Two. When it comes to beer, go with the lighter option; regular Budweiser, for instance, has 145 calories and 10.6 carbs per 12-ounce serving, and most dark beers are even higher in calories and carbs, both of which work against weight loss. If you prefer to drink something other than wine with dinner during your weight loss, you might try to substitute with something calorically equivalent during the first two Phases (125 calories or under).

In this example, *The Restaurant Diet* can and should be flexible to accommodate individual tastes and preferences, enabling you to achieve a similar result while not feeling denied or deprived. For example, if you only drink vodka, where there are 64 calories per ounce, meaning that 2 ounces is roughly equivalent to an average glass of wine, that is something that could be adapted to work for you. Just remember that many bartenders serve martinis that are 4 ounces or even larger, which is a definite no-no in Phases One and Two. Find out the serving size before ordering anything to drink when you are out and get in the habit of measuring anything you may be pouring or mixing at home.

A word of caution: if you don't drink now, I don't recommend starting, and I would never encourage alcohol consumption for anyone who has a drinking problem or is committed to sobriety. We all should know our limits and what is best for us. If you are unsure, consult your doctor or nutritionist. Personally, my favorite alcoholic beverage is wine, so I designed a diet that allowed me, and others who feel the same, to enjoy wine with dinner in Phases One and Two, and the opportunity to enjoy something of similar caloric value in Phase Three.

When I began my weight loss, I reasoned that since I was drinking less, I should drink better at home and when dining out. I felt that I could upgrade my wine selection and spend a little more to enjoy a higher-end wine than I might have otherwise purchased. Learning to savor good wine with gourmet food allowed me to hone my passion and establish a healthier relationship with both. Rather than eating and drinking whatever I wanted, fine wine became something I learned to appreciate more and enjoy in moderation. During the year I lost the weight and years that followed, I sampled countless wines that I had never enjoyed before I learned to apply a refined way of thinking about wine: drink less, and drink better!

If you are a wine drinker, and want to learn more about wine and how to pair it with food, you might consider a wine appreciation class, subscribing to *Wine Spectator* and *Decanter* magazines, or checking out a wine dinner at a local restaurant, provided the paired food menu is within your calorie budget. If it isn't, ask if a reasonable accommodation can be made—most of the time restaurants are happy to substitute a fattening entrée for something healthier (like grilled

Surf and Turf and vegetables). While learning to enjoy wine in moderation, I enrolled in the level 1 sommelier class given by the Court of Master Sommeliers, based in Napa, California, which is typically taken by people in the service industry, and passed the examination. Wine appreciation is one of the many activities I have learned to enjoy and incorporate into my new and improved life. Instead of just drinking wine, I learned to better understand, appreciate, respect, and enjoy it—and you can, too.

KEEPING YOUR MOUTH BUSY WITH GUM OR ICE CUBES

Chewing sugar-free gum helps keep your mouth busy, and is a good distraction; a 5-calorie piece of gum is a better way to satisfy a munch craving than a bowl of chips or nuts.

Also, sucking on ice cubes helps keep you hydrated and lowers your core temperature, which speeds up your metabolism.

STAY HYDRATED: DRINK EIGHT GLASSES OF WATER A DAY

A glass of ice-water is not only free of calories, it actually helps you burn calories: cold water forces your body to speed up its metabolism, helps fill you up, and aids in digestion. I recommend 8 glasses (8 ounces each) of water per day, and even more if you are exercising and perspiring. Aside from water, another recommended beverage is unsweetened iced tea with lemon. Consider sparkling water, seltzer, or mineral water as well—especially if you are accustomed to having cans of soda or sugary beverages in the house. Look for naturally flavored sparkling water, such as Perrier and La Croix for a zero-calorie carbonated drink. To be environmentally friendly, consider a water filtration system or pitcher, so you can enjoy water right out of the tap, and a home carbonation system if you like bubbles. Mineral water is an integral part of life in places like Italy and France, where it is consumed passionately as a digestive aid that is good for the liver. I especially enjoy ice-water or bubbly water with lemon; lemon is a simple, healthy addition to water. They contain vitamin C, antioxidants, help neutralize your PH, resulting in a healthier inside, and speed up digestion by stimulating bile production. Try drinking water with lemon every morning, and enjoy sipping it between bites when eating, which helps you feel full sooner. Water helps keep you feeling full and helps flush out toxins that are known to accumulate in the body, especially in the excess fat on people who are overweight and inactive.

ENLISTING THOSE YOU LIVE WITH

If you live with other people, it is definitely more of a challenge to stick to a weight-loss routine, unless you are doing it together. You should kindly ask anyone you live with to be supportive, but you may need to realize that not everyone will be, and in fact, you may even come across people who want to stand in the way of your weight loss and attempt to regain control of your life and, in some cases, they might be the people closest to you. You may need separate places to store food, or even different dining hours if a cohabitant isn't willing to help you (by keeping things like chips and ice cream in the house, or is unwilling to cook something other than fried chicken). If you live with someone like this, you are better off eating out and making appropriate choices than trying to force change in this situation—people have the right to choose their own lifestyle. Of course, if you are living with your spouse or kids, it should be easier to make getting healthier a family affair, both at home and when you eat out. There is nothing better than positive reinforcement from those around us. But since we only spend a small percentage of each day actually sitting down for a meal, we need to find ways to stay motivated the rest of the time.

Hopefully your family or others you live with will be supportive, even if that means keeping things like chips and fattening desserts out of the house. However, if you happen to live with people who eat unhealthy foods and are unwilling to cooperate—in addition to eating out, you may be better off finding new roommates.

•

What About the Leading Commercial Diets?

Overweight consumers spend billions every year on shakes, bars, cookies, pills, supplements, and meal programs that may not taste good, and that ultimately, in many cases, don't work. When contemplating any weight-loss program, ask yourself if it is a program you can follow for the rest of your life. The problem with most commercial diets and products, aside from the fact that they are generally costly, is that they offer only a temporary means to an end. They appeal to our desire for instant gratification and quick, easy results with minimal effort.

While it is conceivable to lose weight, even a lot of weight, by trying any number of plans, ask yourself: do I really want to do it this way? Do I really want to be stuck at home microwaving frozen food? Do these "diet" foods taste as good as "the real thing"? Are the flavors right in ethnic cuisines that are designed for warming up at home? Do I really want to avoid eating out? Do I want to be so limited in my choices? Do I plan to stick with this kind of program even after I lose weight? My answer to all these questions was an emphatic NO! This is part of why so many people regain their lost weight. They focus on eating less, or eating foods they don't enjoy, and they fail to learn anything about eating better or making positive, permanent lifestyle changes. Many dieters become obsessed about reaching a certain number on the scale in a specific amount of time. They end up working against themselves and setting themselves up for failure or relapse. Most dieters don't learn how to cook better, shop better, or to make better choices when eating out. Instead, they follow a plan, hating every minute of it, hoping their next weigh-in will validate their suffering. Those who are fortunate enough to lose the weight end up scrapping the diet, and go back to eating the way they did before—they start making poor choices, exercise becomes less important, and the weight comes back. What diet has actually encouraged you to go out to eat, and taught you to do it better?

Often people start dieting without consulting a doctor, nutritionist, or working with a therapist to get to the core reasons they were overeating or overweight to begin with. The only successful way to permanently lose weight is to deal with every aspect of your life and change for the better.

Making positive, permanent changes is the key to lasting success. To succeed at weight loss and maintain the new you, your weight-loss and lifestyle plan must be something you are willing to follow forever. Before you spend any more money on typical "diets" or gimmicks, try my approach. If you make healthy, realistic, positive changes in your diet and lifestyle—while learning to enjoy food in restaurants and at home, and work through emotional issues that may be tiggering your overeating—the money you spend eating quality foods and improving your life will not be a waste. Consider it to be a sound investment in you.

•

SUGAR AND SUGAR SUBSTITUTES

The American diet today is full of sugar. We must recognize that sugar is everywhere—in sodas, sports drinks, snacks, desserts, salad dressings, and more. According to the U.S. Department of Agriculture, in 2015 the average American consumed 94 grams of sugar per day (3.32 ounces), which translates to 43 ounces of sugar per year. Sugar contains 110 calories per ounce, so Americans are consuming 365.2 empty calories per day from sugar, and a whopping 133,298 calories per year! Considering that 3,500 calories is equivalent to a pound of fat, this number could translate into an extra 38 pounds per year if not burned off by exercise. No wonder America's waistlines continue to grow.

If you are serious about losing weight and getting healthy, the number-one thing you need to cut from your meal plan is sugar. This doesn't mean you can't occasionally have a treat when you get to Phase Two or beyond. I'm not going to tell you to never have anything sweet again but, to be successful, you need to realize just how bad sugar is for all of us, and not only is it bad for our waistlines.

Sugar (glucose) as well as fructose (which is used as a sweetener) has been shown to have adverse consequences for health and diet. In fact, cancer patients are told not to eat sugar, as cancer cells thrive on it. Glucose and fructose products can stimulate cravings for more sugar, and have been shown to trick your body and wreak havoc on your metabolism and plans for weight loss by stimulating hunger. Sugars also convert to fat that is stored in the abdominal area.

What about the controversial sugar substitutes on the market, which claim to have zero calories? I suggest avoiding sugar substitutes such as Splenda and Aspartame (diet sodas, etc.). Your body does not know how to handle these chemicals and they may in fact lead to cravings for actual sugar. The best choice is to do without sugar or sugar substitutes completely during Phase One and, before long, you really won't miss them. Look for natural sweeteners other than sugar, such as stevia, agave nectar, and honey. In later Phases, you may reintroduce a limited amount of sugar, but you will likely find it not all that appealing after being "off it" for a while. I prefer to have a small amount of actual sugar on occasion and to look for ways to incorporate natural sugar substitutes, as opposed to using artificial sweeteners.

After a successful Phase One, the best advice I can give is to enjoy all things in moderation and with a healthy balance. If you are going to have dessert, make it a treat on a special occasion. Try sharing a dessert, or taking a taste and passing it along. Look for restaurants that feature desserts in shot glass-sized portions, like at Seasons 52, a popular, upscale, health-centric nationwide chain. I prefer occasionally having a bite or two of "the real thing" than deluding myself into thinking I am doing something "healthy" by eating something that contains artificial sweeteners. As you progress in your weight loss, you will want to reward yourself and learn to enjoy most foods in moderation so you won't feel deprived.

Phase One, the shortest and most restrictive of the four Phases, is designed to shock the body and send an unmistakable message: things are changing! Here, carbs are reduced while butter, sugar, cream, whole milk dairy products, and fried foods are eliminated. Unlike with most diets, a glass of wine with dinner is okay. Going out to eat is encouraged! Eating better doesn't mean a harsh diet of unpalatable foods. It means learning to love and respect food as a necessary, life-sustaining substance by establishing a realistic calorie budget, making better choices, learning to do research and plan in advance, and strategically navigate the restaurant experience.

FOOD SHOPPING AND COOKING AT HOME

Although this book is called *The Restaurant Diet*, and I ate out frequently while losing the weight, it is also helpful to employ many of the same strategies in your own cooking that *The Restaurant Diet* teaches you to do when dining out. Start by reducing your amount of fat and calories by measuring and calculating before you buy or prepare something, by plugging in the components of a recipe into a calorie analyzer. Initially, it may seem time-consuming and a little frustrating, but after doing it for a while became it will become second nature. You will actually have fun adjusting some of your favorite recipes by finding ways to "lighten" then up without sacrificing flavor! Save these recipes and calorie counts in an app or write them down in a journal for easy reference. When you revisit a recipe you already analyzed and prepared, it is like having the night off! Try to think of analyzing recipes to reduce fat and calories a game. It will be far better than any diet you've ever tried!

Whether you enjoy cooking or not, consider taking a cooking class where the emphasis is on healthy preparation. If you are working with a nutritionist, let him or her show you healthier ways of cooking. I enjoy reading cookbooks and magazines that focus on health, as I get many ideas for the dishes I make at home from these, and from online sites including Pinterest and Instagram. You may also want to search online for new healthy menu ideas and experiment with them. I went online and found websites which feature recipe analyzers that allow users to determine calorie counts in a recipe, making it easier to determine whether or not something is healthy, as well as how to potentially adjust the ingredients, preparation, or portion size to lower fat or calories.

Recipe analyzer/calorie estimators:
www.fitwatch.com/database/analyzer.php
http://recipes.sparkpeople.com/recipe-calculator.asp
www.caloriecount.about.com

As far as eating better at home, it all begins in the market. If it isn't healthy or happens to be on your Avoid List, don't buy it! Make your quest to lose weight a quest for the best. Only buy the freshest, best quality ingredients your budget will allow. Look for local, organic produce, free-range meat, and wild-caught fish when possible. Start on day one by cleaning out your refrigerator, freezer, and pantry. Donate or throw away any foods that could pose a problem for you, such as sweets, fattening foods, and processed foods.

Start visiting your local farmer's markets and specialty markets for a variety of fresh, seasonal, quality products—especially for fresh fruits, vegetables, and seafood. Many areas have local dairies and ranches. Once you start shopping this way, you will be amazed by the difference in flavor—everything will start tasting better without adding fattening cooking techniques, sauces, or dressings. Get to know your local merchants. When I started frequenting local shops and purveyors, I found most wanted to take care of me and see that I got the best, ensuring that I was a happy customer who would come back and refer others; it is mutually beneficial. Locally owned mom and pop stores and stands typically appreciate your business and want you to have the best.

Try growing your own herbs and vegetables. If you have a yard, gardening is a great form of exercise; working the earth and being out in the fresh air and sunshine is also therapeutic. If your space is limited, there are many herbs and vegetables that do well in containers on a balcony, patio, or even in a window. Produce grown without pesticides is far better than what you will find in most supermarkets, which often feature items that are picked before they are ripe and treated with chemicals so they arrive "ripe" at the store.

INCREASE QUALITY, DECREASE QUANTITY, AND SPEND LESS

When you reduce the quantity, you are consuming and focus on the quality, you can buy the best and actually spend less, because you are consuming less. People may think that a diet of "gourmet" foods and eating out frequently sounds expensive. Top restaurants and top-quality foods—those that are organic, local, and fresh—aren't inexpensive, but if you are mindful of what you are eating, especially with regard to quantity, the bills will be more reasonable than you might think.

Make your entire life a quest for the best. Tell yourself you deserve it, and have fun finding the very best. If the tomatoes don't look good at one store or market, go someplace else and find better ones. If you love food, you will enjoy this experience a lot more than any previous weight-loss attempts. Get informed about what you are eating and develop the mindset that you deserve the highest quality. Develop a positive, beneficial relationship with food as an enjoyable, life-sustaining substance. Your relationship with food will be better than ever because of it.

COMMIT TO A REALISTIC DAILY EXERCISE ROUTINE

If you are like I once was—someone who wanted to find an easy way to lose weight that didn't involve exercise, here's the bad news. There is no way around the fact that fitness is an essential component to weight loss and overall well-being. The key is consistency—doing something every day, and gradually increasing the duration and intensity of your exercise routine. For those of us who don't like to exercise, the first step towards making exercise an integral part of your daily life—just like eating food, drinking water, breathing, and sleeping—is to change your attitude; learn to enjoy exercise.

As we learn to love ourselves again and respect food and our bodies, we will *want* to exercise to keep it in better physical shape. Eventually we will feel better, be able to do more, and a greater variety of activities, and will feel more secure about ourselves. Building self-esteem is a great way to replace the self-loathing and feelings of emptiness that frequently plague overweight people—feelings that become more exposed when we stop overeating.

Start by being consistent—doing it at the same time every day for two weeks, then start to increase your amount and level of activity if you are able. Eventually, you will want and be able to include new activities. Mixing it up a bit as you go along by trying new things, or even doing the same things in different ways, such as walking in the park or on the beach instead of around your neighborhood, can help keep it interesting, and prevent you from becoming bored. Exercise, weight loss, and the inevitable results that will come from the effort you put in, is akin to climbing a mountain. It takes effort, but the view from the top is worth it.

In order to exercise, you need to take proper precautions so that you don't end up injured or worse. The very first thing you must do is to see your doctor for a complete physical. You need to know if you have any underlying health problems aside from being overweight that need to be dealt with, and that might preclude you from certain types of activity.

Once you have received medical clearance for exercise, talk to your doctor about what exercise is recommended given your situation, and start slowly with a realistic plan for daily activity. A personal trainer is a worthwhile consideration as well, especially if you are new to working out. A trainer can help design a program with you, show you how to use various equipment to achieve your results, minimize the risk of getting hurt, and motivate you to show up and work harder! Many trainers even come to your home, and can help design a program to fit your needs if you are working at home; or meet you at a gym and show you routines that you can easily take with you when you travel, whether or not a gym is available. At a minimum, you should try several sessions, especially if you are new to working out. As an overweight person, you stand at a greater risk of getting injured by exercising improperly. Let a professional help design an appropriate program with you, show you how to do various exercises, and how to use various equipment, so you don't get hurt. If you are someone who especially hates exercise and needs motivation, or someone to drag you out of bed, a personal trainer is a team member to definitely consider. He or she should hold you accountable for keeping your appointments and sticking to your exercise regimen.

Joining a gym is a must for anyone serious about losing weight, keeping it off, and getting in better shape. A gym is like an added insurance policy. Certainly, we can all exercise without a gym, but in the event of inclement weather, having a gym nearby is a big help to anyone wanting to live a healthier lifestyle. Most gyms offer a variety of different equipment that works different muscles and helps us achieve different results. Consider working with someone at your gym to help design a program that will best help you achieve your goals and is best suited to your current physical condition.

Consider a gym that is conveniently located near your home or office, clean, has good hours, and offers the kind of clientele, staff, and equipment you desire. There are local YMCA's nationwide that are typically convenient and inexpensive. Especially if you live in a cold, hot, or wet climate, a gym is an excellent idea so that you can exercise indoors, rain or shine. Also, many facilities offer fun classes, including aerobics, Pilates, and yoga. The healthier you get, the more likely it is you will want to try different classes and activities. Most full-service gyms have knowledgeable staff that can answer questions, show you how to use the equipment, and design a program that works for you—don't hesitate to ask!

Consider using the "Buddy System"; you may wish to find an exercise buddy to plan workouts with and help motivate each other. This could be your spouse, friend, neighbor, family member, or someone you meet at the gym. I enjoyed several running events in which I had a buddy to train and participate in the event with. Just be careful not to rely too much on another person for your success. It is great to have a walking or workout buddy, but you need to lace up your shoes and show up, whether your buddy does or not! Many companies now have gyms onsite and offer incentives for their employees to get healthy—something that benefits everyone. If your workplace has a gym or offers access to a nearby facility, see if any coworkers use the facility and join them.

Two exercises that are typically recommended early on when you are the most out of shape are walking (which is much easier than running) and swimming, which is non-weight bearing, and often best suited to people who are very overweight. My doctor recommended walking and swimming, and to simply start by doing 20–30 minutes a day of either or both, gradually increasing the duration and the intensity as the weight came off and the activity became easier.

In my case, since I was very overweight, I started by simply taking a walk in the morning and a walk after dinner. There was no reason I couldn't have started off with swimming too, except I was self-conscious in a bathing suit. I would eventually start swimming by the time I reached Phase Three, when I was also ready to get to the gym and start doing weights. I will caution that every individual's situation is different, depending how overweight and out of shape a person is, so don't beat yourself up if you are not able to do what another person is doing at any point in your weight loss.

I began Phase One by walking to the end of my street and back twice a day: first thing in the morning, and again after dinner. This took approximately 20 minutes each time. In order to make something a habit, you must do it daily for fourteen days. If walking is your exercise of choice, be sure to wear comfortable sneakers or walking shoes, as well as comfortable clothing. As time goes on and walking becomes easier, you will begin walking faster, further, and for longer durations.

It is especially important for procrastinators, or those of us who are not especially fond of exercise, to get the majority of our workout out of the way, first thing in the morning, if possible. In the past, I typically hemmed and hawed when it came to lacing up my shoes to go for a walk or head to the gym and—as one thing often led to another–I ended up not going. If this sounds at all like you...

Try exercising when you get up in the morning, before breakfast, to start your day off right. Consider finishing your day with some light exercise, like a leisurely walk, or swim after eating dinner. Working out before breakfast helps rev your metabolism in the morning, and keeps it going, to facilitate digestion while you sleep. Try doing the most intense activity you can handle early in the day, and take a more leisurely walk or swim an hour or two after finishing dinner. Before long, this new lifestyle will become second nature, as you continue adding good habits to your daily routine and repeating the process day after day. Also, you will be proud of yourself for making the commitment to a healthier, better-looking you—and motivated to keep going!

KEEP TRACK OF YOUR PROGRESS

Start by getting on the scale the first day you decide to change your life. Write down your weight either in a journal or log it into an app. During Phases One, Two, and Three, you should weigh yourself once a day, preferably first thing in the morning when you get up, before you eat or drink anything, and before you exercise, for consistency, and to ensure you are headed in the right direction. In Phase Four, you should weigh yourself every three days to monitor your progress.

During the first several weeks in Phase One, you may not lose a lot of weight. There are bound to be times during your weight loss where you may lose several pounds in one week, and then not lose anything for two weeks. There may even be times you get on the scale and your weight goes up—don't get discouraged. Remind yourself: *"Good things take time."* If your weight remains stuck in a plateau or begins to creep back up, you need to examine whether you are in fact following the routine, or whether you may have overeaten or not exercised enough. Getting stuck in a plateau could be an indication you are ready for just a little more exercise; try to walk an extra five or ten minutes a day, or swim an extra few laps every day for a week, and see what happens. If you are experiencing any concerns about going in the wrong direction, definitely talk to your doctor.

Contrary to other diets you may have tried, this is not about setting a record. Telling yourself you need to lose twenty pounds before Memorial Day is a nice goal, but you only end up competing with yourself. Your goal should be getting healthier, both inside and out, however long it takes, so long as you keep moving forward.

Eventually, you will get the hang of this and exercise will become something you look forward to doing, and something you will feel good about, especially as you start to lose weight and feel better physically. Even though your weight loss may be slow at first, and you will likely encounter plateaus, if you continue to put one foot in front of the other, you will be successful.

During Phase One, after a successful first month of exercise, and having lost a few pounds, I increased my walking from twenty minutes twice a day to thirty minutes twice a day. As my level of fitness improved, I was already walking further than I had when I began. For exercise to work with your weight-loss goals, you should plan to gradually increase the duration and intensity of your activity. Measure how far you are walking or how many laps you are completing in a given timeframe, and you will likely see an improvement as you go along.

This has become much easier with devices like the Fitbit and various exercise apps and monitors. Log your daily activity into an app or journal to help you keep track. The key is to do some activity every day! I don't buy into plans that say you can take a day off—you can if you want, but there is no reason you can't find twenty minutes to take a walk every day. This is especially important if you have a history, like I did, of procrastinating and avoiding exercise. One day off could lead to two, and then three.... Of course, if you are under the weather or injured (which we will talk about later), that's a different story. The good feeling of accomplishment you will get from actually committing to a plan, doing it consistently, and seeing positive results will be your incentive to keep going.

DEALING WITH EMOTIONAL OVEREATING, SELF-CONTROL, AND WILLPOWER ISSUES

I learned the hard way by losing weight before (and gaining it all back) that for any diet to be successful, not only do the food choices have to be palatable, we also must deal with our emotions and work to develop better coping skills for how to handle the inevitable stresses of life—without turning to excess food. Many overweight people overeat as a way of coping with anger, anxiety, frustration, pain, and sadness. Many of us realize this on a subconscious level, but prefer to avoid dealing with any of it; hence, we overeat. Typical diets leave us feeling like out of control failures that are being punished. We starve, eat foods we hate, and struggle with exercise we find painful and unpleasant. We are left feeling empty and powerless, as we struggle to overcome our compulsion to use food to stuff down feelings of discomfort. Even after successful dieting, some outside stressor comes up—as they always do in life, many of us go off the wagon and binge. I've done it many times in my life.

First, overeaters and anyone looking to lose weight need help dealing with our emotions. The best advice I can give is to find a qualified therapist who specializes in dealing with food-related issues. Some insurance plans even cover such therapy. If not, keep an open mind and try to make it a priority in your life and budget. You should be spending less on food than you were. Consider investing some of that in helping yourself deal with your emotions and why you overate to begin with, so you will hopefully not feel compelled to ever again.

Anyone losing weight and dramatically changing his or her lifestyle after years of gluttony is bound to feel a sense of loss and deprivation. This inevitable grief process should be worked through with a professional. A lot of emotions are likely buried beneath the fat, and you should have someone to help you through them, as you are vulnerable during this time. If you decide on giving therapy a try, go in with an open mind and to be honest with your therapist. You are not doing yourself any favors by holding things back.

The best ways to deal with your emotions and maintain self-control and willpower are:

1. **Attend a support group—there are many worldwide.**

   It can be helpful to share your story with other people who are in a similar situation and are bound to strict principles of anonymity and confidentiality. It was not easy to go to my first meeting. It took me several weeks to finally muster up the courage, and a lot of second-guessing before I got out of the car and walked in. Speaking for the first time was not easy but, once I did it, there was no looking back. I now realize we aren't meant to do this alone— sure it can be done, but the more support we get, the more we can talk about ourselves and our issues, especially any setbacks and struggles (everyone trying to lose weight experiences them). We gain strength by knowing we are not alone, that there are millions of people struggling with the very same issues. Listening to others share their personal struggles helped me to open up and share. Perhaps something you share will resonate with and help someone else. We're all in this together.

2. **Get a sponsor and call him or her when you need to talk (preferably before you consider bingeing).**

   In the beginning, it felt as though the phone weighed more than I did. I looked for every excuse to avoid getting a sponsor, and for every reason not to call them. Once I did, it was an enormous relief. Finding someone who is compassionate, available, willing to devote time to you, and is dealing with the same issues will not let you get away with making excuses most important.

3. **Consider a qualified therapist who specializes in dealing with food-related issues.**

   You should discuss this with your primary care physician; perhaps he or she can recommend someone. A therapist can help you understand things about yourself and your behavior in ways that friends, family, coworkers, and even similarly situated folks in your support group just can't. I have learned a lot about myself in therapy, and I'll be the first to tell you that my progress would not likely have been as fast or as successful had it not been for my determination to commit to seeing a therapist.

4. **Find trusted people.**

It is important to get things off your chest outside of your weight issues. A word of caution: Only do this with people you totally trust. If someone judges you—whether a friend or therapist—that person is likely neither a good friend nor a good therapist. If there are things you feel you can't share with trusted friends, or do not wish to tell people you know, then share them only with a therapist who has an ethical duty of confidentiality. Other possibilities include a priest, rabbi, or minister. Odds are, whatever you're going to tell a therapist or leader of your church or synagogue, he or she probably already heard something similar, and thus may be better able to offer you guidance and support than a family member or friend.

5. **Write in a journal to express your thoughts.**

Letting your thoughts and emotions all out on paper is a great way to let off steam. But not only is a great way to de-stress, it is also a good way to acknowledge that these feelings are there. Burying negative emotions and issues will only make them worse, and by keeping a journal you will be avoiding any potential setbacks in your progress. Also, it a great way to remember your weight-loss journey so that, when you look back, you can reflect on how far you have come!

6. **Try prayer or meditation.**

Whatever your religious beliefs, or even if you have none, you may find it helpful to take time every day to quiet down and simply pray and/or meditate. Spending a few minutes each day in total solitude can do wonders. In fact, a lot of inspiration can come to you when you take time out to meditate. The beach is a favorite place for me. Learning to enjoy and appreciate nature and take time out to "smell the roses" is crucial in our hectic world. You may also find that you can meditate when you are walking, running, and even swimming, so long as you are in a peaceful, calm, quiet state of mind. It is very helpful to turn off the chatter in our minds and to just "chill out." Part of my personality is constantly thinking, analyzing, or obsessing about things. Learning to shut this down and just *be* was a very important first step towards achieving a sense of balance. When my analytical mind would stop, I often found inspiring thoughts and messages from my subconscious—things I would have never perceived had I not taken the time to find peace within. I suggest making time each day just for you. Even take an entire day and dedicate it to enjoying spending time with yourself.

7. **Enjoy new activities.**

During the weight-loss process, I strongly recommend getting out and exploring new activities. Consider things like a group sport or league. Bocce and pickleball are very popular and don't require a lot of intense activity. Perhaps join a book, art, or garden club, play cards, take dance lessons, or volunteer. The best thing is to start getting out there, trying new things, and meeting new people. It is very hard to step out of our shell or comfort zone, especially after many years of being overweight. Our perspective becomes completely distorted. Once we start trying new things and meeting new people, we begin to open up and enjoy a whole new world of possibility that doesn't center around food. Many of us will discover things about ourselves we never knew before our weight-loss journey.

8. **If you ever binge or fall off the wagon (everybody does), accept it.**

Don't beat yourself up. This is not to give you permission to cheat or go back to bad habits. You need to realize, however, that you are human and should explore why you went off the wagon, rather than punish yourself over it. This way, you are more likely to avoid a problem in the future.

9. **Anytime you feel compelled to eat take a moment to explore may have triggered your emotional hunger.**

When you stop overeating and start listening to your body, the connection between your emotions and overeating should become pretty clear.

I suggest making therapy sessions an integral part of your weight-loss journey, as well as attending several support group meetings each week, to listen to others share their experience and to realize you are not alone. This, plus getting involved in other activities, is a great way to take your mind off food. Soon, you should begin to realize you don't need excess food, or unhealthy foods in your life.

10. **Reward your progress.**

A great way to keep motivated is to reward yourself for reaching certain milestones, such as: exercising daily for two weeks, not slipping for two weeks, losing 10 pounds, 25 pounds, 50 pounds, etc. Treat yourself to something like a new outfit (you will likely need new clothes if you're planning to lose a lot of weight).

11. **Love yourself!**

I know this may sound corny, but it's true. This process is about much more than simply dieting, exercising, and dealing with emotions. At the very foundation of losing weight and getting healthier is learning to love ourselves. Call it an journey in self-love. Having been overweight for years, I didn't think very highly of myself. In fact, I didn't even like myself, and couldn't imagine anyone else liking me, let alone loving me. These were major reasons why I overate, and kept myself from things like dating for many years. I didn't like myself and couldn't imagine anyone else liking me, so being overweight ensured nobody else could prove me right by rejecting me.

We will discuss these and other codependent behaviors in a later chapter, but my self-perception and self-defeating attitude was part of a vicious, self-destructive cycle that led to my compulsive overeating and feelings of worthlessness. Learning to accept ourselves at our heaviest is the first step. Diets don't typically foster self-love or acceptance. They remind us of all the reasons we don't like ourselves in the first place. This time, you are going to diet and work on yourself at the same time.

●

Rating Hunger and Fullness

As you lose weight, you will learn to distinguish between actual hunger and emotional hunger. You will eventually eat only when you are hungry, and stop before you are stuffed. Try eating healthier snacks and smaller meals, so you are never ravenous or stuffed. To maximize your body's use of the calories it consumes, think of eating as "fueling a furnace." The furnace burns best when there is a steady supply of fuel, not too much at once, and it should never run out.

A simple way is to rate your hunger or fullness on a scale from 0–10. Think of your hunger gauge like a gauge for an automobile's gas tank. A rating of 0 means you are starving or your tank is completely empty. A rating of 10 means that you are stuffed, or your tank is completely full. And a rating of 5 indicates you are neither full nor hungry. As you learn to listen to your body you should strive to keep your hunger levels between 3 and 7. If your hunger gets to the point that you notice it, you should have something to eat, to bring your level back up, but you should never eat to the point of being stuffed. In fact, I recommend eating slowly and even ordering only one dish or course at a time in restaurants. Your body gets "full" roughly 20 minutes before your head suggests you are full, so slow down. If you eat and order more slowly, you will likely spare yourself as much as 20 minutes of eating more than you need in order to be satisfied. Putting the fork down between bites and taking a sip of water takes some practice, but it can help prevent you from overeating.

Whenever your focus turns to food, or you find yourself wanting to eat when it is not mealtime, ask yourself how you are you feeling: Anxious? Tired? Angry? Lonely? Depressed? Craving food is a warning light on your dashboard, indicating something isn't right inside.

●

EXAMINE TOXIC RELATIONSHIPS AND YOUR ROLE IN THEM

As someone who used food to cope with painful emotions, the therapeutic process helped me begin to recognize there were situations and relationships in my life that were harmful repetitions of my childhood, where I had desperately sought acceptance and approval, denied my own needs and feelings, and felt empty, hurt, and betrayed. I learned in therapy that these were some of the hallmark traits of codependency, a psychological condition, which left me hungry for acceptance I never seemed to get, and would try to compensate with too much food; I needed the help of a professional to work through this.

AVOID DIFFICULT PEOPLE AND SITUATIONS

Part of losing weight is learning to handle difficult people and situations that can threaten to sabotage our success. If there are people in your life who also overeat, you obviously shouldn't eat with them when you are losing weight or trying to keep it off. You should avoid anyone who tries to push food on you at any time. If you find a certain restaurant, food, person, or situation uncomfortable, avoid it. All-you-can-eat buffets, dessert places, bakeries, sports bars, fast food establishments, and restaurants that specialize in fattening foods are not good choices, especially if you have issues with self-control. Remember, you are emotionally vulnerable, especially if you have been overeating for a long time. Old habits, patterns, and tendencies aren't easy to break, and it is easy to fall back into these familiar habits. If a situation is not avoidable—such as a special event, party, or work-related dining situation—and you are feeling uncomfortable, it is always okay to excuse yourself and take a time-out from the situation, or leave early if necessary.

THE HOLIDAYS AND WEIGHT LOSS

Not long into my Phase One came the holidays, which are typically a difficult time for keeping weight off, and an especially challenging time to be on a weight-loss program. Many people gain 5 to 10 pounds between Thanksgiving and New Year's Eve, even those who aren't considered overweight or obese. It is common for people overindulge during the holidays, between holiday parties and family celebrations, with too much eating and drinking, vowing to take it off in January. How many people gain 5–10 pounds during those 6–7 weeks, and then struggle for months to take them off? How many people's New Year's resolutions to get healthy go bust? The best strategy, regardless of whether it is Thanksgiving, Christmas, Hanukkah, New Year's, Easter, Passover, etc., is sticking to your program, whatever phase you may be in. It's perfectly fine to partake in normal activities and eat traditional foods, but in moderation, if you are able. Continue to count calories, and even try a *latke* for Hanukkah!

Use a holiday, celebration, or event as a test to see if you are able to handle the situation sanely. If you aren't, don't beat yourself up. Just realize you need to take more time to get used to Phase One, and you may need to discuss the issue with a therapist or in your support group for some guidance. It is not valid to use a holiday as an excuse to overdo it.

In my case, Thanksgiving was the first test. I stuck to my plan on Thanksgiving Day and managed to consume only 1,500 calories when it would have been easy for me, or anyone for that matter, to consume thousands of calories. After that, Christmas and New Year's Eve were also tests, though I managed to eat a small piece of lasagna on Christmas and remain within my calorie budget for the day, not craving more. I was pleased that I was able to pass this test, only having to make an exception to Phase One's pasta restriction. My ability to handle this, combined with my progress thus far, signaled I was ready to move on to a new phase, where I could try to reintroduce things like pasta, pizza, and bread, in exchange for additional activity.

MOVING ON TO PHASE TWO

After two successful months in Phase One without a slip, getting through the holidays, passing my test of being able to eat a small portion of lasagna like a sane person, and losing 30 pounds (10 percent of my body weight and 20 percent of the total weight I was looking to lose), I was ready for the opportunity to eat additional foods. I was walking an hour every day, not missing a day of exercise for two months, and felt ready for the opportunity to increase my level of activity. After speaking to my doctor, we agreed that I should be able to add 100 additional calories each day, in exchange for increasing the intensity of my activity. I also decided it was time to reintroduce pasta, pizza, bread, and an occasional dessert, so long as they were within my calorie budget.

Although every person is different, consider using this as a guideline for whether or not you are ready for Phase Two. My recommendation is you should not progress to a new phase until, or unless, you have gone at least two months without a slip in either your food plan or exercise routine.

Chapter Three
Phase Two—Opportunity

In Phase Two, you will reward yourself for successfully completing Phase One and enjoy the *opportunity* to add an additional 100 calories to your daily budget. In my case, I was allowed 1,600 calories per day. You could, however, continue to enjoy a glass of wine with dinner if you so desire, and should continue with one cleanse day per week. In Phase Two, you have the opportunity to enjoy one serving of pasta, pizza, and bread each week, as well as one dessert, other than fruit or yogurt, of your choosing; so long as you don't have a particular problem with it, the quantity is within your calorie budget, and your carb and dessert are not on the same day. Keep in mind that any item you've had a specific problem overdoing, that is on your Avoid List, should remain on your Avoid List. Another change is that you may eat foods which contain a small amount of butter in their preparation, though I recommend asking for the amount to be reduced at a restaurant and to limiting its use at home.

One major caveat with Phase Two: since you are allowing foods back into your life that, when eaten in large quantities, can be very high in calories, such as dessert, in the event you have a problem and go over your calorie budget on any particular item (such as a large a piece of apple pie), you should consider adding that item to your Avoid List and forego the dessert treat the following week. This should not be viewed as a punishment, but rather as a means of slowing down, and guarding against any relapse of bad habits.

You should stick with Phase Two for a minimum of two months; in my case, I spent three months in Phase Two. My recommendation is to go a minimum of two months without any slips in either your food plan or exercise routine, in order to progress. Also, to move on to Phase Three, you should be ready and able to do considerably more exercise, such as jogging, bike riding, swimming, and moderate weight lifting. When I began Phase Two, I had made considerable progress but, at just under 300 pounds, I still had a ways to go before I was able to exercise vigorously enough to enter Phase Three.

FOOD IN PHASE TWO

Phase Two allows you the opportunity to reintroduce bread, pizza, and pasta, but you need to limit the quantity of each, as they are relatively high in calories for the nutrition they provide. Whether you are eating out or at home, limit pasta to 4 ounces, which equates to about 400 calories plus sauce; in a restaurant, you should always remember to ask what the portion size is so you know how much to order. For pizza, limit your portion to 2 New York-style slices (approximately 300 calories per slice for thin crust with plain cheese); for bread, stick to one bagel or an equivalently sized sandwich, if calories allow. With all of the above foods, how you dress them is critical.

When you are ordering pasta in a restaurant or preparing it at home, go for the simplest preparations—either a tomato sauce or tomato-based sauce like Puttanesca (tomato, garlic, olives, capers, anchovies), meat sauce (like Bolognese), or seafood (like Linguini with Clams). Avoid sauces that contain cream, and limit the amount of cheese you use. Stay away from sauces like Carbonara (bacon and eggs) and Alfredo (which in American restaurants is often butter, cream, and Parmesan cheese—not how they make it in Italy—don't get me started)! If you want something like lasagna, whatever the typical restaurant portion, a suggestion is eating half of it and taking the rest home for another meal—lasagna can easily be frozen and reheated.

Typical restaurant portions for pasta entrees are often at least twice as large as you really need, so first find out how large the serving is and, if it is larger than 4 ounces, either ask for a half portion (some restaurants accommodate), and take the other half home, or consider sharing it with a dining companion. If you have a problem with leftovers being in the fridge, then you are better off requesting a half-priced half portion, than taking a chance you will go home and overeat.

For pizza, I suggest sticking with thin crust, either New York-style or individual pizzas from wood burning or coal oven places. Go for vegetable toppings that are grilled, roasted, or plain, like peppers, onions, eggplant, mushrooms, spinach, and broccoli. You are better off at a family-owned pizza place than at most chains, in so far as product quality and fat content. If a slice appears greasy, blot it with a napkin before eating to remove excess fat and calories.

Individual pizzas made by wood burning or coal oven spots are a good option, though size may vary, making it tougher to calculate calories. Try to envision a typical New York-style slice when estimating calorie count for an individual pizza. Most large New York pizzas are 18 inches in diameter, and are cut into 8 slices. Therefore, each slice should be approximately 9 inches long by 4.5 inches wide at the crust. If you are in a pizza parlor, order one slice, and a maximum of two. As always, stop eating before you are full. You can always share a whole pizza with others but limit yourself to two slices. Avoid toppings like pepperoni, sausage, bacon, and extra cheese, which only add fat and calories. If you are going to make your own pizza at home, consider buying "00" flour that is imported from Italy, which has not been genetically modified. Opt for part-skim mozzarella or fresh mozzarella cheese (refrigerate first). If you are using fresh mozzarella, you don't need to load it on—in Italy, an individually sized Pizza Margherita (fresh mozzarella, tomato sauce, and basil) typically has plenty of exposed sauce, since they put a handful of thin slices of cheese on it, so it is balanced, not soggy.

For bagels, limit yourself to one bagel or, better yet, half a bagel, (average plain bagel is 250 calories), preferably not a variety with added sugar, like cinnamon raisin. Bagels are great with eggs, light cream cheese spread yourself (don't let the bagel shop spread it on, they usually put way too much), or with smoked salmon, tomato, and onion.

For bread, allow yourself an occasional sandwich that is no bigger than a typical bagel. For sandwiches, what you put on it is often the biggest problem, aside from portion size. Many delis and sandwich shops often put a pound of meat, loads of cheese, dressing, and things like globs of mayonnaise, which can be anywhere from 6 inches to one foot long! For an appropriate lunch portion in Phase Two, a 6-inch sandwich is probably more than you need. You can order one, but you need to be specific and ask for no mayonnaise or butter, go for light dressings, and light on things like cheese. For cold cuts, opt for sliced freshly roasted turkey if available, as opposed to processed meats, like baloney or fatty meats like salami and pastrami. Ask them to be generous with the vegetable toppings (lettuce, tomato, onions, peppers, etc.), which are all very low in calories. Continue, however, to avoid the breadbasket when you are eating out.

Lastly, when it comes to dessert, which is typically at the end of a meal and at the end of the day, be sure your calorie budget allows it. As in Phase One, I recommend continuing to pre-plan your meals and log in prospective items you wish to enjoy into your calorie counting app to see if they are appropriate, and then go sit down at your restaurant of choice and stick to your plan. On the day you are planning a dessert for your weekly treat, try planning out the entire day so your budget will allow it. For example, if you wish to have a slice of plain cheesecake for your weekly dessert treat, look up cheesecake in your app. If for example you want to try a regular slice of cheesecake from The Cheesecake Factory, Livestrong says a slice contains 707 calories. You may want to rethink your choice, share it, or perhaps eat only half of it. If you are dining alone, and are afraid you can't resist the temptation to eat the whole thing, maybe cheesecake should be on your Avoid List. You should ask your server to allow you to cut the slice in half and either let them keep the other half, or take the rest to freeze at home. It's your call. This is why it's so important to pre-plan—know in advance what you are going to order and consume, as it's very easy to get sidetracked and go overboard. Just think, if you wanted an entire slice of cheesecake and your calorie budget was 1,600 per day, you would only be able to eat less than 800 additional calories that day—which should include something for breakfast, lunch, and dinner! I suggest keeping your dessert treats small and be very careful about reintroducing them.

EXERCISE IN PHASE TWO

In Phase Two, continue with one hour of physical activity per day, or the maximum duration you have reached, in the morning and some after dinner. Further, you should increase the speed at which you are walking or swimming. In my case, I began to incorporate brief jogging intervals into my walks. During my two thirty-minute walks per day, I would briefly jog a few times (approximately twenty to thirty seconds each time, at first) to get my heart rate up and further rev my metabolism. A great way to power through this is by picking a target, such as a lamppost or a mailbox, and jogging to that spot.

Continue to gradually increase the intensity of your activity as you work through Phase Two. By the second month of Phase Two, your walks, which should already be considerably faster than when you started Phase One, will be more like "power walks." By power walking, you can try working up to a point where you are able to do a mile in twenty minutes, or three miles in an hour, while you are moving your arms and walking with a purpose, rather than just getting out and moving. Your goal in Phase Two is to increase the intensity of your activity, step outside of your routine, and gradually begin to try new things (running intervals if you are able, going for a bike ride, add in a short walk during the day, etc.). Of course, every person is different; power walking at a greater speed or jogging intervals may not be suitable for you, so check with your doctor first. The key is that you improve, and try to gradually increase your level of activity.

DEAL WITH EMOTIONAL ISSUES AND SETBACKS

Just as an occasional slip is inevitable, so is an occasional cold or illness that could prevent you from exercising. My best advice is to be honest about it. If you truly feel too sick to get out of bed (aches, pains, running a fever), then stay in bed, rest, drink fluids, call your doctor, and get better. The gym and your exercise routine won't miss you for a day or two. Just remember that if you are not able to engage in physical activity for any reason (illness, injury, etc.), you should dial your eating plan back to Phase One for both calorie and food allowance, until you are better. If you really don't feel that bad, you may want to try taking your walk and seeing how it goes. In my case, during Phase Two, I came down with a cold for several days. The first day I was up to doing my walk (no jogging), and the second day I took off and rested. For both days, I dialed my food and calorie allowance back to Phase One, which really wasn't a problem, as I made a pot of chicken-vegetable soup and had only that on those two days. My advice is to always be totally honest and don't beat yourself up or get discouraged, even if you are sick or injured and have to miss a few days or more of activity. If you are too sick or hurt in any way to exercise, then don't! You are working on creating a new life by gradually losing weight and getting healthier. Don't blame yourself for missing a few days for a legitimate reason that is beyond your control. Remember, this is a marathon, not a sprint. You are getting healthier for the rest of your life, not trying to lose so much weight by a certain date.

During Phase Two, I suggest continuing to seek professional counseling to deal with emotional issues that come up; in my case, this included dealing with the frustration of working through several plateaus that lasted at least a week each. The best advice is—slow and steady wins the race. Also, continue attending your support group meetings for added reinforcement.

WEIGHT LOSS AND TRAVEL

After over four months of successful weight loss at home, I was ready for a big test: my first trip out of the country to an unfamiliar destination. As someone who has always enjoyed travel, I needed to prove that I could take my program anywhere and be successful. As travel is loaded with potential problems, it required additional planning. If you enjoy travel or need to travel for business, don't let the fact that you are trying to lose weight cause you any needless anxiety. With a little planning, you will be just fine.

When packing, bring your exercise clothes, sneakers, headphones, and whatever else you may need to exercise at your destination in your carry-on bag so that, in the event the airline loses your luggage, there would be no excuse to not exercise. Second, research any restaurants you plan to visit, just like you would at home. Third, investigate any opportunities for fitness, both indoors and out. If you like to swim, find out if the hotel or area you are visiting has a convenient pool (indoor or outdoor), or gym, that you may use, and what the hours are. Look into local parks and trails for walking, biking, or running. Another great way to get exercise while exploring your new surroundings, is joining a walking or biking tour. If you have an early meeting, plan to get up a little earlier to exercise, or schedule time later in the day to get your activity in. With a little planning, you will be able to take your success with you.

MOVING ON TO PHASE THREE

Bottom line with Phase Two: seize the opportunity to increase your physical activity, while enjoying additional food options, as a reward for the progress you made in Phase One. Advance to Phase Three only if, having cleared it with your doctor, you are comfortable doing a variety of physical activities, started lightweight training if appropriate in your situation, and have managed to go on without any slips for at least two months in your eating or exercise routines. Only then will you be ready to tackle the next challenge.

Chapter Four
Phase Three—Challenge

By the time you reach Phase Three, you should feel excited and determined, proud of your progress, and ready to *challenge* yourself to take your exercise routine to the next level—as if your body wants to jump out of its skin and do more activity. In exchange, you will get to enjoy 100 additional calories per day, as well as more food and beverage options. Of course, you should talk to your doctor before making any major increases in your activity level, such as lifting weights, or jogging more than a handful of brief intervals during an hour-long walk.

FOOD AND PHASE THREE

In Phase Three, you will continue to enjoy eating out and at home as you have all along. The only difference is you may enjoy a few additional calories in exchange for an increase in your ability to exercise. In my case, my doctor and I determined that 1,800 calories per day was a realistic goal given my level of activity. In addition to allowing an extra 100 calories, there are two major differences from Phase Two. First, in Phase Three you may substitute a cocktail for the glass of wine with dinner, provided it was approximately the same number of calories; it is also okay to enjoy a beer or a Manhattan on occasion instead of the glass of wine. Secondly, in Phase Three, you can also reintroduce *lightly* fried foods and whole milk cheese on occasion, provided they are within your calorie budget. I do not recommend deep fried foods, or items like fried chicken with the skin on. You may also allow, but limit, butter (use sparingly in cooking) and a small amount of bacon, as part of a sauce or dressing.

EXERCISE AND PHASE THREE

By this point, you will have lost a good deal of weight and are able to do a wider range of activities, such as walking, bike riding, jogging, swimming, as well as lifting weights at the gym. Of course, every individual should evaluate their own situation and consult with their doctor before increasing their activity level, or the kinds of activities they are going to enjoy. Phase Three is essentially a preview of what the rest of your life is going to look like as far as exercise. Phase Three will last until you reach your goal weight.

In addition to the hour of walking, biking, jogging, or swimming each day, you should start going to the gym several days a week to lift weights in order to help build muscle and tone your body.

Everyone's pace will be different but, in my case, I would remain in Phase Three for seven months and lose a whopping one-hundred pounds! No matter what number you are at though, you will also be amazed at the things you can accomplish. I was astonished that I was doing things I never dreamed I would be able, or even want, to do, like running three miles without stopping, or taking an hour-long bike ride. Once this "diet" was "over," I felt prepared for what would come next, or so I thought.

Chapter Five
Phase Four—Achievement

Congratulations! You've made it to Phase Four—the permanent "Achievement" Phase! You've reached what you and your doctor determined is a realistic, healthy weight. In Phase Four you need to do the following twelve things:

1. Congratulate yourself on a job well done!

2. Enjoy a glass of champagne or sparkling wine if you wish. You deserve it.

3. Establish a realistic weight range to stay in.

4. Establish a realistic daily calorie budget, given your level of activity.

5. Continue to calculate and log calories into your app for six months, and thereafter you should at least estimate and write them down in a journal.

6. Continue to exercise daily.

7. Continue to deal with emotional issues, stress, and triggers that come up. Also, continue to see a therapist and participate in a support group if you have been doing so.

8. Weigh yourself every three days at a minimum, first thing in the morning.

9. If you reach the top end of your weight range, go back to an earlier phase for as long as you need to get back into the middle or bottom of your healthy range.

10. If you are under the weather or are injured, go back to an earlier phase commensurate with your ability or inability to exercise.

11. If you slip or "fall off the wagon" by bingeing, exceeding your weight range, stopping exercise, or counting calories, deal with why it happened and what you need to do better—don't beat yourself up, we are all human. Immediately go back to an earlier Phase and follow that phase for as long as it takes to get back where you belong.

12. Help others by sharing your success and wisdom, but only if they want to be helped. Don't push, though—people may resent it.

As I said earlier, my doctor and I determined my realistic weight range should be 180–190 pounds and, as a protective buffer, should not exceed 200 pounds. We also decided that my daily calorie budget should range between 2,000 and a maximum of 2,500, depending on my level of activity. If, after 6 months of success in Phase Four without a slip, you decide to discontinue plugging everything you eat into your app, make sure you still adhere to your calorie budget each day and keep track by estimating and noting it down. Anytime you need to dial back to an earlier phase for any reason, go back to plugging each item into the app for the time you are in the phase.

In Phase Four you should take everything you have learned and continue to use it forever, maintaining your exercise routine and healthy, balanced approach to eating. You should also continue to learn constructive ways to deal with emotions and stress that threaten to sabotage our success and send us back to where we came from. Now that you are no longer looking to lose weight, you need to focus on maintaining it. This starts by establishing a reasonable calorie budget for each day, based upon the amount of exercise you are doing, and continuing to make healthy, informed food choices.

One important thing I recommend is having a metabolic study done. Talk to your doctor about the timing. When I did mine, I was surprised to learn that my metabolism was actually slower after losing the weight than it was when I was obese, and considerably slower than a typical person my weight who had never been obese. If you have a study done, you need to take this kind of information into account when determining how best to live your life and maintain your weight loss.

After reaching your weight-loss goal, you should establish and strive to stay in a realistic weight *range*, rather than focusing on a specific target number, which can make people crazy. The most important part of Phase Four is remembering to immediately go back to an earlier phase for a "tune-up" in the event you ever reach or exceed the top of the range for any reason. My advice is to deal with weight gain openly, honestly, and immediately. You've come way too far to throw it all away!

After so much effort, Phase Four is all about appreciation for your remarkable achievement, but it is definitely not a time to rest on your laurels. Phase Four is about continuing to build on what we learn about ourselves through the weight-loss process. Perhaps surprisingly, some of the biggest challenges come after the weight is gone, as you learn to adjust to the new life you've created.

Physically, though you may feel better than ever, don't be surprised if emotionally you still have a lot of healing to do. In my case, I loved how good I looked, but I had a hard time adjusting to my new life. Only one year before, I was morbidly obese and miserable. I was anxious about my future and terrified of going back to where I had been.

FOOD AND PHASE FOUR

The Golden Rule for Phase Four—you can now enjoy almost anything in moderation, so long as:

1. It is within your calorie budget.

2. You can eat/drink it like a civilized person.

3. You do not obsess over it.

4. You do not crave seconds.

5. You do not wolf it down.

Any foods that prevent you from being able to control yourself should not be part of your life, and need to remain on your Avoid List in Phase Four. Remember, you have gradually reintroduced certain foods during Phases Two and Three into your diet, like a small portion of pasta, bread, an occasional dessert, as well as the occasional lightly fried food, whole milk cheese, and cocktail. But the foods on the Avoid List remain in play for the rest of your life. You have come a long way and worked too hard to let a few potentially problematic foods send you spiraling backward.

For example, you should continue to avoid the following in Phase Four: candy, chips, soda (regular and diet), sugary sports drinks and beverages, artificial sweeteners and anything else artificial.

As for alcohol, Phase Four does not restrict the type of alcohol you have, provided it is within your calorie budget and subject to the following guidelines: first, 6 days per week, you enjoy the maximum of only 250 calories per day (about 2 wine glasses) from any type of alcoholic beverage or cocktail. Second, 1 day per week, you only consume a maximum of 20 percent of your daily calorie budget from alcohol (about 400 calories out of 2,000 total).

Federal guidelines suggest alcohol should account for somewhere between 5–15 percent of a healthy daily allowance (100–300 calories out of 2,000). Unfortunately, however, adhering to only 5 percent alcohol would not even allow a 5-ounce glass of wine, which is not realistic for many people. As a typical 5–6-ounce glass of wine is still within a healthy range—my rule is, a glass of wine a day (or the equivalent) is fine in any phase of your diet.

WHY THE FORMERLY OBESE MUST BE EXTRA VIGILANT

As we discussed earlier, it is *very* easy for someone with a history of serious weight problems to slip, and for their weight to rapidly get out of control again. In fact, people who have been morbidly obese have a much greater susceptibility to becoming overweight or morbidly obese again than those who haven't been. While in many cases, people resort to bad habits, regaining weight is much more than an issue of self-control or willpower. Studies show that a person's adipocyte, or fat, cells divide in two once you reach the point of morbid obesity (BMI above 40). These are the cells that store fat and expand. Therefore, even though you are no longer overweight or obese, you will always have double the number of cells that attract and store fat than you would have at your current weight, had you not been obese before. Therefore, it is imperative that you keep your weight and diet in check.

Just as a recovering alcoholic may not ever be able to drink like someone without a previous problem with alcohol, you can never eat like a person without a history of being overweight or obese. You can still eat the foods you used to in moderation, and can even enjoy a moderate amount of fattening things, like dessert, on occasion. You cannot, however, eat loads of fast food, or hang out at the sports bar, drinking pitchers of beer and eating things like chicken wings and loaded nachos, or have a fattening dessert every night, regardless of how much you exercise. Your additional fat cells will always be craving any fattening foods you consume and will want to try to make you fat again. This is why it is so much easier to gain weight after eating just one fattening meal than it is to lose weight—and a major reason why many people regain the weight after they finish dieting.

Unfortunately, as a formerly overweight or obese person, your body will always be working against you. But in addition to exercising self-control, this self-knowledge should help you understand why you have to eat differently than other people. In my case, a balance of healthy gourmet food with a reasonable amount of daily exercise is required for continued success. I would also come to learn that, while training to run a marathon, even extreme amounts of exercise and calorie burn cannot be treated as a license to eat. Overdoing exercise does not afford us the ability to eat more—once it reaches a certain point, it actually has the opposite effect, which we will discuss later.

The other reason is that, even after losing a ton of weight, folks like me who were once extremely overweight or morbidly obese are prone to having their metabolic rates diminished substantially from what they once were. Although losing 150 pounds certainly isn't an easy task, what would prove the biggest challenge was keeping the weight from creeping back! I did a metabolic study both before and after I lost the 150 pounds. It turns out that, like most people who lose a lot of weight, I have a suppressed metabolism, and actually burn fewer calories than I did at over 300 pounds, and fewer than most people my age, weight, and sex should.

Given my body's fat cell makeup and its slow metabolic rate, I know I will need to eat less and exercise more in order to maintain my results than another person at my weight would have to do, had they never been severely overweight. I saw this in action after I ran my last marathon. Within a week, I had gained five pounds. Within a year of regular outdoor exercise, going to the gym several times a week, and sticking to a reasonable calorie budget given my level of activity once I was no longer training for a marathon, I was up 15 pounds! It became painfully obvious that the simple "calories in, calories out" formula does not work if you were once obese, even if you managed to lose the weight!

Due to the number of fat cells we have and physiological reasons we don't completely understand about our metabolism, many people who lose a lot of weight have their metabolic rate reduced, meaning that they need to exercise a lot more than an average person—even if they just want to eat an average amount of calories. The flip side is, if we exercise too much, our bodies go into survival mode and are predisposed to storing any calories we consume as fat. It is a tightrope walk and something we all need to be aware of, as recovering overeaters and formerly obese people.

Throughout the years of working to stay in my healthy weight range, I have struggled to fight my biology, physiology, and my overweight past—and will for as long as I live. Armed with this knowledge makes it a little easier to deal with, though it is one more painful dose of reality, and a reminder to anyone who has struggled with eating issues and weight problems that they can never totally leave their past behind. They will forever need to be especially mindful of their food intake and committed to a reasonable amount of exercise. Let this also be an added incentive for people who are overweight, or even obese, to keep from ever reaching the point of morbid obesity!

What is a person to do? Losing weight is a lot easier than keeping it off, for these very reasons, in addition to the more obvious issues of willpower, and one's history of emotional overeating. I have personally learned by seven years of trial, error, and trying to understand how my body works on all levels, that I need to exercise more, eat less, make adjustments as needed, and continually monitor my weight more than the average person my weight, if I want to maintain my weight. You may or may not have to keep the same things in mind.

Unfortunately, we are all set up to gain back some of the weight we have lost, even if we are living an active lifestyle and not overeating. Imagine if we go overboard or exercise less for a few days or weeks. You may even have to contend with exercising less several times out of necessity for medical reasons, which is an added challenge. These possibilities are something we all must continue to contend with for the rest of our lives, so I am giving you a word of caution that this is something you too will need to stay on top of.

EXERCISE AND PHASE FOUR

In Phase Four, you will continue to exercise as you have been doing all along in Phase Three, which means a minimum of one hour per day of cardio (power walking, running, biking, or swimming), plus lifting weights several times a week.

You may also want to challenge yourself further to participate in new activities. In my case, I signed up for a Thanksgiving Turkey Trot (5K) just three weeks after completing my weight loss, which was my first organized running event. You may even want to sign up for something like this before you've lost all your weight—it amazed me to see how many out-of-shape people were brave enough to participate, when I would have been too self-conscious.

Two months later, I ran a half marathon in under two and a half hours without stopping, and went on to run four full-length marathons in the following several years. My advice is to make sure your fitness goals are proactive and not rooted in fear, as mine partially were. For several years after losing the weight, I woke up at 5:00 in the morning to go run and reached the point within a year that I was eventually running more than ten miles per day. Sure, I was training to run a marathon and to stay in marathon condition, but the level of activity took its toll—I ended up injuring my Achilles tendon and had to stop running for months, which was depressing, and led me to exceed my weight range as I struggled to deal with this setback. Fortunately, I was able to heal and find a reasonable balance, and the weight dropped back into its healthy range and I no longer felt I needed to overdo exercise out of fear of regaining the weight.

To give you an idea of a varied exercise routine, this is what my typical week workout schedule looks like, now that I am no longer training for a marathon.

- Daily: sixty minutes of any of the following: walking, jogging, biking, swimming, though preferably a combination of two (walk and run, bike and swim, run every other day, etc.). It is best to do this in the morning before breakfast, whenever possible. I like to do a minimum of thirty minutes when I get up in the morning and, if I don't get to do the hour in the morning, I make time later in the day to complete the hour of activity. Try to do at least ten to twenty minutes of walking after dinner as part of this daily total.
- Several times a week: sit-ups and push-ups.
- Several times a week: weight lifting—a full-body machine weight circuit at the gym (average twelve reps per machine) and occasional concentrated areas with free weights such as upper body, lower body, or core (multiple sets with multiple reps).
- Occasionally: Yoga, Pilates, aerobics, and so on, in place of one of the above workouts. The key is to keep it regular, yet to also keep it interesting. Some days, I walk to the beach or elsewhere for a change of scenery. I have discovered that I enjoy hiking, especially in the mountains, and like to plan vacations to places that offer a variety of opportunities for recreation and physical fitness, as well as a great dining scene! Two of my favorite destinations I discovered after losing the weight were Aspen, Colorado, and northern Michigan (Traverse City, Petoskey, and Mackinac Island), which I have written about extensively on my blog.

DEALING WITH EMOTIONS IN PHASE FOUR

No weight-loss journey would be complete without addressing any and all emotional triggers for why we overate. Failure to do so leaves us vulnerable the next time a "familiar" situation presents itself, in which we previously used excess food for cover. Although I mention "codependency" throughout the book, I felt it best to save a brief background discussion of how my codependency led me to become an emotional overeater for this part of the book, for ironically it is here, after losing all the weight, that I was best able to see how my codependent behavior had helped me become an overeater, and threatened to derail my progress. I needed to deal with this once and for all.

I learned during this process that I had been codependent since childhood, though this is not a term I had any real understanding of until I began to lose weight and entered therapy. Codependency is a psychological condition often caused by traumatic events or unhealthy relationships during one's formative years, that is often at the root of most addictions and compulsive behaviors: a person seeks fulfillment from external substances to compensate for feeling incomplete, unloved, or unappreciated by those around him or her.

I would learn to keep the good aspects of my personality, namely the inherent kindness and compassion, and learn to love myself enough to make better choices in selecting whom I chose to associate with and bestow my kindness upon. What I learned by working through it is that codependency, especially in romantic relationships, is more challenging for me to deal with and overcome than to lose 150 pounds and keep it off for six years and counting. Even after losing the weight and looking great, I still struggled with feeling inadequate.

"Codependency," as defined by *Merriam-Webster,* is "a psychological condition or a relationship in which a person is controlled or manipulated by another who is affected with a pathological condition (as an addiction to alcohol or heroin); broadly: dependence on the needs of or control by another." In other words, codependency is characterized by unhealthy relationships with other people.

Codependency is often at the root of many addictions and compulsive behaviors, including overeating, alcoholism, drug addiction, and abusive relationships whereby the needy codependent person uses excessive quantities of food or other substances, and even emotionally or physically abusive partners, to attempt to "fill" what they perceive to be lacking in themselves.

The hallmarks of codependent behavior are as follows:

- Low self-esteem.
- Denial.
- Intense fear of abandonment.

- Dependence upon others for emotional gratification.
- Excessive caretaking of others to feel important or to boost ego.
- Low priority on the codependent's own needs.
- Decreasing interest in one's own life, activities, interests, and feelings. Often a severe codependent gets to the point where they have no idea how to have fun or enjoy life, and feel that life is a never-ending series of unpleasant tasks they often begrudgingly do for others, feeling that only they can handle them. A severe codependent can be furious about something and respond, "Everything is fine" and actually believe it.
- Unclear boundaries. There's no idea where one's own personal space and business begins/ends (often intrudes into others' business and allows others to intrude into theirs).
- Excessive preoccupation with the needs and feelings of others.
- Playing the victim or martyr in an attempt to control others or to try to get their needs met.
- Inability to speak up or state one's own needs.
- Often pick and stay in abusive relationships.
- Often angry and resentful they do not get the recognition or acceptance they feel they deserve.
- Negate praise when received.
- Difficulty accepting generosity from others since it doesn't feel deserved.
- Feel they have to "do more" or bring something extra to the table to be on an equal footing with another person (codependents do not feel adequate).
- Engaging in behaviors that negatively impact one's quality of life.

Codependency is often a coping mechanism used to survive in a family dynamic which is experiencing an extreme amount of emotional pain, such as with an addiction, abuse, a divorce, or otherwise unhealthy structure. Codependents are typically kind, emotionally needy, overly caring people who are willing to do almost anything for the acknowledgement and acceptance of another person with whom they are preoccupied. Codependents by habit tend to choose to associate with people who are abusive, addicted, or unavailable, setting up an impossible situation in which they cannot win.

Codependents are obsessively afraid of being alone and are constantly looking for acceptance. They feel they need to go out of their way to make others like them and seem to always be running to put out the next fire whether or not they are asked. They often play the victim in an argument and when they stand up for themselves, they feel guilty, or when they try to leave the relationship, they feel lost.

Codependents are frequently more concerned about how the other person perceives them, and may go out of their way to try to manipulate, control, or change another person with whom they are preoccupied to try to get that person to acknowledge, love, or appreciate them, which usually backfires, resulting in the codependent feeling angry, hurt, used, or rejected.

Looking back, I see how so many relationships in my life have been codependent, going back to childhood, and that, even as an adult and even after losing all the weight and spending years in therapy examining and dealing with my behavior, my tendency has been to choose one-sided interactions that ultimately did me more harm than good. The end result was I often felt used and unappreciated. In some cases, if I "stopped" a harmful behavior, such as excessive giving, interfering, or caretaking, the other person ended up resenting it, possibly lashing out at me, blaming me, and ultimately walking away from me, only to leave me feeling "abandoned," which was exactly what I was trying to avoid in the first place.

I needed to look at my role in every relationship I had. Also, I needed to realize I didn't have to go overboard to buy affection or acceptance and that I shouldn't be doing things for others that they could do for themselves.

I had to learn to modify my kind and generous behavior, just as I had to learn to modify my eating habits. Like with food, relationships with other people cannot be avoided in this world, so it is imperative for a codependent overeater to make peace with both food and him or herself so they can live a more peaceful, productive life. When I began to realize that I was good enough, deserved better, and stopped being the victim, the need for excessive food, caretaking, exercise, or anything in excess became less. I was accustomed to always being "on call" for people who were never there for me, and typically never expressed one shred of gratitude for anything I did for them. Just like I needed to change my relationship with food, I needed to change how I dealt with people and how I treated myself. If you have a similar experience, you should do the same.

It is not bad to occasionally put others first, of course, but people who are codependent *habitually* put others first to their own detriment. Remember, you can't control the other person's selfish behavior, but you can control your own behavior. Advice to anyone in a codependent relationship, where they come last, if at all: stand up for yourself, know you deserve better and, if necessary, walk away! Once you believe you deserve better, you will find it, and you won't need excess food or other substances to compensate for what may be lacking in your relationships.

APPLY A 15-MINUTE H.A.L.T.

Apply a fifteen-minute H.A.L.T. to everything related to food. If you are in a hurry, angry, lonely, or tired, wait fifteen minutes before eating anything! Go for a walk, make some tea, have a glass of water, call a friend, or go on your way without grabbing something to eat. Most cravings pass within fifteen minutes. If you feel you must have something to eat, have a piece of fruit or a low-fat yogurt (something under 100 calories).

BE MINDFUL OF EXTERNAL CUES

Be especially mindful of food advertisements on television. Listen to your body, not to the advertisements. Also watch for subtle reminders or food cues, like the delicious aroma emanating from a restaurant you pass on your way home. Things like this can trigger cravings even if we are not hungry. Overeaters' brains are wired to respond to food. The mere smell, sight, or even thought of food can send us over the edge, something we always have to be mindful of, even years after we've stopped overeating. Studies have shown that for some of us, food, especially certain kinds of food, affects the pleasure center in our brains in the same way that drugs do.

LEARNING TO ENJOY THE HERE AND NOW

Despite learning to lose weight without expecting instant gratification, somehow I felt I was entitled to a dream life now that I had done the unthinkable. For years, I had wished and hoped for a magical way to lose weight without a lot of effort. I wanted a roadmap to a great life that was effortless and painless. I expected the girl of my dreams to knock on my door and for life to suddenly be perfect. I learned the hard way that this is not how it works—we have to put in the effort and the results will be well worth it. We all learn as we struggle through our lives that good things take effort, dedication, and persistence.

When I started to write this book, and had my initial manuscript ready to publish, it was early 2011. I expected a book deal within a few months and to for my story to be out on the shelves by the end of the year! Despite many things going for me, there were times when it looked like my journey with trying to publish this book had reached a dead end. Still, I was determined. I started blogging online, writing for *Venu Magazine*, and I continued to speak, travel, introduce myself to countless chefs and restaurant owners, and help others get on the right track with their own weight-loss journeys. Just when I was ready to finally surrender—to accept that the outcome of whether or not this book ever gets published was in God's hands, that I had done everything I reasonably thought I could, and perhaps it wasn't meant to be, I got a call from my agent, saying *"The Restaurant Diet* has found a home!"

DEALING WITH SABOTAGE AND IGNORANCE

After losing a lot of weight, you may be shocked to hear that people around you (some may be good friends or even family) become somewhat hostile or ignorantly concerned. Be prepared. The same people who used to call you fat may actually tell you that you are "too skinny!" Some people might even suggest that you need to put some weight back on! People might even ask if you have become anorexic or bulimic—let's hope not, as this is an extremely destructive form of behavior that happens too often to people who were once overweight. You might be asked if you have cancer and people might even gossip about you, spreading rumors that you may have had gastric bypass surgery and didn't tell anyone.

Sadly, people think it is "open season" to pick on, harass, ridicule, or make fun of overweight people. Once we are no longer overweight, many of these same people feel they still have a right to invade our space and make insensitive comments. My best advice to anyone condemning an overweight person or picking on someone who is losing weight: if you don't have anything nice to say, don't say anything—mind your own business! My advice to people trying to lose weight: be prepared to be extra vigilant, ignore the shameful and ignorant behavior you will likely be subjected to, and don't be discouraged. The ignorant comments and behavior are *their* issues, not yours, and many people will be jealous of your success and find it easier to continue to criticize you or question your success than applaud you. You may have to completely detach from certain people, which is not easy. Some of the same people who may have criticized you for being overweight may now criticize you and question your success. People close to you may actually try to push food on you. They may bake you cakes, try to tell the waiter or waitress you need to eat more, change your order, or serve you an inordinate amount of food at their home. The best advice is to be aware in advance and, if you find yourself in such an uncomfortable situation, you need to be firm, and excuse yourself if necessary. What you eat and your weight are not anybody else's business!

The sad reality is people have their own issues, and many people just won't be used to seeing you as anything other than fat. It will take you time to adjust to the new you—it will take other people time as well. Just don't be upset or disappointed if not everybody gets the new you right away. Many people don't seem to care that their comments and behavior, especially related to food, threaten to sabotage dieters' success. I use the analogy of how a recovering alcoholic must feel when his old friends at the bar don't understand him and want nothing to do with him. The old friends might tell him to just have one drink for old-time's sake. They have no frame of reference for sobriety and don't realize that all it could take is walking into a bar, or one small sip, for someone in recovery to completely fall off the wagon. It is the same thing with food. One bite of the wrong thing at the wrong time, one poor choice, or even one comment could cause weight loss or a healthy lifestyle to go bust. Just like learning how to eat differently and exercise, we have to learn to stay positive, ignore any negative comments, and stay in control of our success, especially in the face of negativity.

So, there you have it—my Four-Phase Gourmet Weight-Loss Program. As you've learned, at the heart of it all is learning to enjoy and appreciate food, make better choices, and deal with emotional issues and past regrets. I hope that through the general guidelines provided for each phase, as well as the personal accounts of my experiences through the four Phases, you now have a good idea of how to move ahead—and that you are motivated to do so.

Chapter Six
Summary of Key Weight-Loss Tips

TAKEAWAY

Organized into three basic groups and four Phases, The Restaurant Diet works like a multicourse menu that nourishes body and mind.

THE RESTAURANT DIET—TAKE OUT MENU

Food Fitness	*Body Fitness*	*Mind Fitness*
	Phase One— BEGINNING—Do it for 2 months OR after losing 10 percent of total body weight OR 20 percent of total weight you want to lose.	
Meet with a nutritionist.	Get a complete physical (cardiac, blood work, hormones, etc.) and medical clearance before starting exercise.	Meet with a therapist.
Shock your body with a 1,500-calorie limit, or limit determined by your doctor.	Shock your body with reasonable daily exercise in the morning and after dinner, once medically cleared.	Shock your mind by opening up and being totally honest.

Lower your carbs and fat intake—eliminate butter, sugar, bread, white flour (pasta/pizza), white rice, white potatoes, bacon, fried foods, chocolate, alcohol (except a glass of wine with dinner), and desserts, excepting fruit & yogurt. Add salads to fill you up and enjoy lean protein (beef, chicken, turkey, seafood, lamb, pork, etc.). AVOID: all chips, candy, soda (regular and diet), sugary sports drinks, and other sugary or artificially sweetened beverages. Limit fruit juices, even those that contain only natural sugar. Get your carbs from beans, barleys, and whole grains (quinoa, barley, tabbouleh, etc.). Enjoy light salad dressings.	Start simple—walk it off! Swimming is another consideration. Start with 20 minutes of physical activity in the morning and 20 minutes in the evening and gradually work your way up to one hour per day.	Start simple—begin to love yourself. Work with affirmations, slogans, meditation, or whatever feels right.
Stick with it—your body will try to hold onto its fat reserve in the shock phase.	Stick with it—it may take a few weeks before the pounds start dropping.	Stick with it—it will take a while to recognize codependency.
Make it enjoyable. Don't beat yourself up with awful, tasteless meals. Learn to eat out in your favorite restaurants and lose weight. Preview restaurant menus online. Plan and strategize your meals with a calorie counter such as Livestrong.com. This will soon become second nature. Learn strategies to make dining out and losing weight second nature. Talk to your server and the chef and explain to them what you're doing—get them on your side!	Make it enjoyable—walk in scenic areas to keep exercise from getting boring.	Keep a positive outlook.
Learn to shop for fresh, healthy ingredients in supermarkets.	Don't place a time limit on your weight loss—let it occur naturally. Don't rush it.	The combination of eating better, exercise, massage, and emotional therapy will change your perception of life.

Take one day a week as a "Cleanse" day: only fruits, vegetables, water, green tea.	Regular massages with a licensed therapist helps loosen up a body not used to moving, improving circulation, flexibility, and reducing inflammation.	Join a support group.
Eat healthy snacks: fruit, low-fat yogurt, and berries. Choose healthy salad ingredients and light dressings.		
This is the shortest phase— so have no fear. I only spent two months on Phase One.		

Food Fitness	*Body Fitness*	*Mind Fitness*
	Phase Two— OPPORTUNITY Continue for as long as you need until you are comfortable with your regimen, you haven't had a slip for at least two months, and you are ready for additional exercise, as well as weight training.	
Increase calories slightly to 1,600 per day.	Offset the increase in calories with longer exercise period.	Learn to deal with the naysayers once the weight starts coming off.
Allow, but limit, the following: butter (use sparingly in cooking), sugar (as part of an occasional dessert), bread & white flour (on occasion) pasta/pizza max (as a treat and in moderation), 4-ounces pasta, 2 slices pizza. Occasional bacon as part of a sauce or dressing, fried foods (sparingly), chocolate as part of an occasional dessert treat (small amounts) Still no white rice and white potatoes. Alcohol still limited to one glass of wine with dinner. Allow a couple of treats each week, like a small dish of pasta, a slice of pizza, or a dessert, so long as it is within your calorie budget.	Walk longer distances. Power walk. Incorporate jogging intervals if you are able. Swimming is also a good choice.	People will tell you that you looked better with the weight on! Don't listen.

Continue logging and tracking calories.	Begin to combine walking and jogging.	There are people out there who will try to sabotage you with "just one scoop of ice cream." Be strong....
Continue to enjoy a glass of wine with dinner. Try eating better quality foods and drinking better wine.	Measure your steps using a pedometer, an app on your smartphone, or a device like a Fitbit.	Realize that people working in restaurants will want to help you.
Ask for smaller portions in restaurants. Ask for portions to be cut in half before the food is served, with half immediately going into a doggie bag. Continue one cleanse day per week in Phase Two.	When you've lost at least 10–30 pounds, take a dumbbell of that weight with you on a short walk. Notice the heaviness of the extra weight you'd been carrying.	Begin to overcome self-consciousness. It's okay to go out in public, to walk/jog outdoors during daylight hours, or to swim at a public pool.

Food Fitness	*Body Fitness*	*Mind Fitness*
	Phase Three— CHALLENGE Do this for as long as it takes to get into your healthy, desired weight range.	
Calories can increase to 1,800 a day, or the amount determined by your doctor. It will feel like a license to feast. Same food restrictions/allowances as Phase Two, except that alcohol is no longer limited to just wine. You may substitute one cocktail or other alcoholic beverage for the glass of wine if it is in your calorie budget.	Change up the cardio: add bike riding and swimming to the mix.	Forgive the people who hurt you.
Get to know restaurant chefs and work with them. Take a cooking class to learn how to cook healthier!	Now it's time to join a gym and begin to tone it up with weights.	Forgive yourself.
Continue logging and tracking calories.	Begin to combine walking and jogging.	Continue keeping a journal to record your progress, thoughts, and emotions.
Take your time eating—enjoy every bite. Slow down, put your fork down between bites, and have a sip of water.	Stick with Phase Three until ideal weight range reached.	Learn to ride out the plateaus.

Make peace with food. You'll find it empowering. Occasionally enjoy whole milk cheese, something that is lightly fried, or use a small amount of bacon in a sauce or dressing, if you so desire.	Cleanse Day discontinued in Phase Three.	Shop for new clothes—but keep one item from your heaviest weight so you'll have a visual reminder of how much you're losing.

Food Fitness	*Body Fitness*	*Mind Fitness*
	Phase Four—ACHIEVEMENT In the event you reach or exceed the high end of your healthy weight range, or are unable to exercise due to illness or injury, dial it back to an earlier phase until you are back in the middle of your healthy weight range or you have recovered from your illness or injury and are able to resume activity.	

Calorie limit settles in at 2,000 per day (or a high 2,500 per day, depending on activity level, height, and age). Higher allowance for days when you work out (lift weights) or are running extensively (such as training for a marathon).

All foods and beverages are now permitted, with emphasis on the foods that were allowed during the weight loss. My golden rule is anything in moderation—so long as you can eat it like a civilized person! If you crave seconds or wolf it down, stop eating it!

As for alcohol, you do not have to restrict a type of alcohol, provided it is within the calorie budget. For example, 6 days per week, allow yourself only 2 glasses of wine per day (or the equivalent 250 calories from any other type of alcohol), and 1 day per week in Phase Four alcohol may be to be 20 percent of your daily calorie budget (400 calories out of 2,000 total).

A piece of bread is okay, so long as you enjoy it, and it is within your calorie budget! Choose olive oil over butter.

CONTINUE TO AVOID: candy, chips, soda (regular and diet), sugary sports drinks and other sugary or artificially sweetened beverages.

Any foods that you have had or have trouble with should be on your Avoid List or Limit List.

All the strategies you've learned during your weight loss should be second nature and you should continue to practice your healthier lifestyle.

Be careful not to replace excess food with excess anything else, such as alcohol, tobacco, spending, gambling, or other potential addictive behaviors.

Continue to count and track calories, logging them on an app for the first six months. Thereafter, continue to write down and keep track of calories, looking up items if needed.

Continue to visit and enjoy the restaurants that have been a part of your success! By now you will know how to eat anywhere you go!

In the event of a slip or problem, be accountable! Deal with it both on the food end (avoid, limit, go back to an earlier Phase).

Continue to cook at home and buy the best quality!

Maintain exercise routine.

Enjoy a wide range of activities, and even try new ones! Best to be consistent as far as time of day you exercise.

Always best to include aerobic activity (cardio) with weight training.

Best to enjoy a variety of activities so you won't get bored. This will also help keep your body in better condition.

In the event of a slip (getting lazy, missing a day or days of exercise), don't let it become a habit! Consider getting a trainer anytime you need fitness motivation. Alternately, consider a fun fitness-centered event you can enjoy with a friend or your family (such as a fun run or charity walk).

Enjoy activities that are pleasurable that were difficult or impossible before: hiking, golf, tennis, etc.

Consider getting involved with a local group or league that participates in a sport so you have consistency.

You are strong, and will be accepted for who you are. You depend on yourself, not anyone else.

Ironically, Phase Four is the biggest challenge of all! Pat yourself on the back, get some stylish new clothes, show off your new appearance, but DO NOT REST ON YOUR LAURELS and think you don't need therapy or to exercise, or to be mindful of what you eat! For many reasons, you have to be more mindful than ever, forever.

Continue to see a therapist regularly and deal with any issues, feelings, emotions, or difficulties that may arise.

Continue to go to support group meetings for added encouragement and to encourage others!

In the event of a slip or any beginning to regress, you MUST talk to your therapist, doctor, sponsor, and support group. No making excuses!

Target weight range should be achieved. Talk with your doctor to help determine an appropriate range for you to stay in.	Mix in an aerobics class, yoga, or Pilates once in awhile. Consider taking up dancing—it's a great form of exercise!	It's time to try dating again.
If your weight moves up to reach the top of your range, go back to an earlier Phase for a tune-up. If you go back to an earlier Phase, go back to tracking and logging calories with your app.	Your exercise routine can take you to unexpected places. Mine took me to running in the New York City Marathon.	Recognize that it will take time for your emotional age to catch up to your chronological age, especially if your weight problems were during childhood, adolescence, or young adulthood.
Achievement is about finding a healthy and permanent balance, not about going back to eating whatever you want like you used to. Continue to employ all that you have learned during the previous three Phases. Remain vigilant and recognize that, although you should be able to enjoy food, you will never be able to eat like a person who did not have a weight problem due to physiological reasons.	Caution not to "overdo" exercise out of fear of regressing. If you are obsessed about exercise and losing more weight, or are exercising for more than 2 hours a day for any reason, you may need to examine why. Continue to monitor your weight, weighing yourself several times a week at the same time. Do not become obsessed or focused on a specific number.	Learn how to deal with sabotage and ignorantly concerned people. Deal with codependent behaviors linked to overeating. Learn to remove yourself from troubling situations whether it be food or people-related.

RECAP OF THE FOUR PHASES

Although I didn't set out initially with this specific timeline, my goal was to shock my system in the beginning and get used to my new way of eating and exercising until the food plan became second nature, exercise became easier, and I lost 10 percent of my body weight and 20 percent of the total I would end up losing. Phase One ended up lasting me 2 months, but these Phases should be used as a guide and should be considered flexible and geared to your specific situation. In the event you have any slips along the way, definitely don't progress to a later phase until you have gone at least 2 months without another slip.

PHASE ONE: BEGINNING

In Phase One you will decrease your calorie consumption and avoid certain foods and beverages. Do this strictest phase for two months or until you have lost either 10 percent of your body weight or 20 percent of your total goal, and you are able to tolerate more exercise and increase your activity level. In Phase One, you will focus on lean protein, vegetables, limited carbs (no pasta, pizza, white bread, white potatoes, white rice), no butter, cream, or whole milk dairy products, no fried foods, and no sugar or sugar substitutes. You may also enjoy a glass of wine with dinner. Observe one cleanse day per week. Begin seeing a therapist you like who specializes in weight loss and is willing to help you explore the reasons for your overeating and develop better coping strategies for dealing with emotional issues, such as codependency.

Begin an exercise program. Remember to get medical clearance from your doctor first. You may be able to start with twenty minutes in the morning and twenty minutes at night and gradually increase to thirty minutes in the morning and thirty minutes at night. Starting the day with exercise and end by taking a walk after dinner, it revs your metabolism in the morning and aids in digestion after dinner.

PHASE TWO: OPPORTUNITY

Phase Two is an intermediate phase where you will reward yourself by allowing some additional food choices and a few more calories after you have successfully completed Phase One by demonstrating proficiency with your new eating and exercise plan and gone two months without a slip. I did this for three months, until I was ready to introduce additional forms of physical activity in exchange for slightly more calories and food choices.

In Phase Two, you may reintroduce foods such as a limited amount of pasta, pizza, and an occasional dessert in exchange for additional exercise. You may also enjoy foods that contain a limited amount of butter in their preparation. Do this for at least two months.

PHASE THREE: CHALLENGE

This is the final weight-loss phase you will enjoy once you are able to do additional physical activity and you will be rewarded with a slightly higher calorie allowance, as well as the ability to enjoy a cocktail instead of the glass of wine with dinner. Do this for as long as it takes to reach your healthy, desired weight.

You may occasionally eat foods that contain limited amounts of butter, whole milk dairy, as well as occasional fried foods. Continue to follow all of the other recommendations for Phase One.

You may discontinue the weekly cleanse day in Phase Three.

If you hit a plateau, or start seeing the numbers go up instead of down, dial back your dietary routine to an earlier phase for as long as you need to get back to losing, or consider increasing your activity.

PHASE FOUR: ACHIEVEMENT

This is your Forever Phase. This is all about maintaining. You will continue to remain within your calorie budget and continue to exercise regularly. Follow all of the "quality over quantity" guidelines throughout this book. At this point, it is not about limitations; it is about choices.

Phase Four allows for an increased daily calorie allowance over the preceding three Phases based on height, age, current weight, and activity level. Consult with your doctor. Continue to make healthy choices, based upon your continued adherence to your Avoid List, limiting certain foods that are not the healthiest, and to allow yourself to eat pretty much anything not on the Avoid List, in moderation.

The key to maintenance is to stay within your weight range and to use the upper end of your range as a protective buffer. If you approach the upper limit of your weight range, go lighter for a few days or weeks by following one of the earlier Phases to drop a few pounds, with the goal of getting back to the middle of your healthy range.

In the event of an injury or illness, which would preclude or limit exercise, temporarily drop back to the appropriate phase, based on your level of activity. In dropping back to earlier Phases in the event of illness or injury, you should track your foods for the duration of that phase, using your calorie counter. For example, if you are unable to exercise much or at all, definitely drop back to Phase One until you are able to resume a greater level of activity. Don't allow an injury or illness to become an excuse for weight gain.

HEALTHY LIFESTYLE PRINCIPLES I LEARNED ON MY TRAVELS IN ITALY

Much about my new and improved lifestyle has been inspired by my travels in Italy, where the emphasis is on quality over quantity, both when cooking at home and when dining out, and exercise is a built-in part of daily life. The following principles helped form the foundation of my diet and lifestyle plan.

PRINCIPLE #1—USE THE FRESHEST, HIGHEST-QUALITY, LOCAL INGREDIENTS WHENEVER POSSIBLE.

The fruit and vegetables in Italy are exceptional—everything is exquisitely fresh, ripe, and flavorful. Most of the produce is grown close to where it would be consumed. Thus, the Italian diet truly is "regional and seasonal," as it draws on the local bounty with the focus on fresh and local whenever possible. The same holds true for their seafood, meats, and other items: fresh, top-quality, and local when possible. Italians feel it is their birthright to find and enjoy the very best, whether it be from their own garden, in a restaurant, or a market.

At home in America, you can explore local farmers' markets and buy the best organic produce, wild-caught seafood from reliable sources, and high-quality meats and poultry from trusted suppliers. Read labels and try to avoid processed foods and items that contained ingredients you can't pronounce. While the *quantity* you consume will decrease considerably, the *quality* will improve. As they say, "You are what you eat!" Make your life a quest for the best!

PRINCIPLE #2—MONITOR AND CONTROL PORTION SIZE

Italian-American families are known for generous portions. "Family-style" meals at many Italian restaurants in the States means there's a tendency to eat a lot more than we need in order to be healthy. In Italy, the portions are generally smaller than in America. Also, Italian meals are much more balanced, featuring small servings of pasta, when combined with a meat or fish course and a side of vegetables, a small but delicious salad, and fresh fruit, or a serving of pasta simply with some salad or vegetables and fruit.

In Italy, most lunches and dinners feature a light and healthy Mediterranean *tricolore*, or *mista* (mixed) salad. The salad helps fill you up so you're not as ravenous for the more fattening offerings like meats, cheeses, bread, pasta, and dessert. Pasta portions in Italy are generally around 3 to 4 ounces (80–100 grams) and is not over-sauced or mushy. In the States, however, it is not uncommon to be served half-a-pound or even a pound (16 ounces) of pasta covered in high-calorie cheese and sauce, as a single serving. Pasta is relatively inexpensive, so many restaurants serve large portions, thinking their customers will appreciate it!

Italians enjoy dessert, such as gelato, or a pastry, but they typically walk to get it! Fresh fruit is frequently a part of each meal. If you eat a healthier combination of foods in reasonable portions, as they do in Italy, and simply start walking, you will be off to a very good start.

PRINCIPLE #3—REDUCE FAT AND CALORIES

In Italy, I noticed that day-to-day, people tend to eat more simply than they do for holidays, and in smaller quantities than their American counterparts. For instance, fish is often served whole, baked or broiled with a lemon, sea salt, fresh herbs, and olive oil; dishes are typically not overly sauced. Salads are light and fresh, and portions are considerably smaller than Americans are used to. However, the Italian portions are actually more appropriate portions. We have to change our perspective!

In addition to smaller portions, there are numerous other ways to cut calories, as well. First, choose baked, broiled, grilled, roasted, or poached, instead of fried. We can do this in restaurants and when we cook at home. We can learn to "lighten up" our favorite dishes. For example, try making *eggplant parmigiana* by roasting the eggplant slices instead of frying them, and topping them with sauce, a sprinkle of Parmesan cheese, and a little thinly sliced fresh mozzarella, rather than a lot of shredded mozzarella. I tried making my meatball recipe by poaching the meatballs in the simmering tomato sauce, rather than baking or frying them first in oil—they came out moist and delicious! I prepared my "healthy" meatballs before a live television studio audience in 2015—people in the audience proclaimed them to be "the best meatballs ever!" The recipe is featured in the Recipes section so you can make them too! Making lighter versions of typical dishes makes a big difference, as eliminating just 100 calories per day from our diet translates into 10 pounds lost in a year, and eliminating 500 calories per day from our diet translates to a pound lost per week.

PRINCIPLE #4—*FARE UNA PASSEGGIATA!* (TAKE A WALK!)

Even if you can't stand exercise, or it is painful or unpleasant, the only way to ensure successful weight loss is by getting up and moving! Exercise doesn't need to be unpleasant. Just by simply taking a walk as opposed to sitting on the couch after dinner, you are doing yourself a huge favor. Italians typically do a lot more walking than Americans since, in Italy, walking is considered a fast, convenient way to get around in a city or small village. This is not as easy in America, especially in suburban or rural areas where things are so spread out and mass transit is not as reliable. In addition to walking to get from place to place, taking a leisurely stroll, or *passeggiata*, after dinner is a time honored Italian tradition. Rather than sitting at home and watching television, Italians like to walk around their city or village after dinner to socialize and help digest a meal. Wherever you live, simply taking a walk in your neighborhood is an easy way to help jump-start a healthier lifestyle, and something that can easily become part of a permanent, healthy lifestyle! If you have dogs, walk with them! It will be good for you and your four-legged family member. Instead of looking at exercise as torture, learn to appreciate and enjoy the walk, whether you are alone, with your dog, a spouse, or a friend. Take in your surroundings and feel good about yourself, knowing you are doing something good for you!

A recent study by A.C. Nielsen, a marketing research center at the Wisconsin School of Business, revealed the average American watches 4 hours of television each day (including adults and children), which adds up to 28 hours per week, and 2 months per year! In 65 years of living, the average person would have spent 9 years watching television! If every American spent just thirty minutes each day doing some form of cardiovascular activity, like taking a walk after dinner, our nation's weight problems would be greatly reduced. If you don't want to miss your favorite program, consider getting a treadmill and placing it in front of the television, or doing some light weights or squats during commercials. Also, most gyms offer cable television directly on the cardio equipment, so you can burn calories while watching TV! You can bring a book, an e-reader, or an iPod and listen to music as well. This is especially convenient for bad weather.

Find ways to add additional activity to your day. Walk from your office to lunch. Take the stairs. Park further away. If you have several errands in close proximity to one another, leave the car in one spot and do a little more walking as opposed to moving the car each time.

PRINCIPLE #5: ADOPT A POSITIVE ATTITUDE

Italians, for the most part, have a positive attitude and a passion for life. They live life with *gusto*, or enthusiasm. They don't just take a walk. They take *una bella passeggiata* or "a beautiful walk." They don't just prepare a meal. They make it into art. They enjoy life, but the key is *enjoyment*, not *excess*. They enjoy a glass or two of wine with dinner, but typically not to the point they can no longer appreciate it. This attitude is exactly the kind of mindset we need to adopt in order to be successful, not only at losing weight, but successful at mastering life. We need to relearn the art of loving and savoring life, not just obsessing about food.

Chapter Seven
Conclusion

In November 2013 I ran the New York Marathon, which was one of the most exhilarating experiences of my life, and something I will never forget. Going back to where I grew up was especially triumphant. Crossing that finish line in the cold, blustery, late autumn twilight with leaves swirling around in Central Park, I realized that anything is possible if we dare to dream it, and dare to take the first step and to keep going!

Today, it is 2017—over seven years since I began my quest to lose weight and transform my life. I am finally living the life I was meant to—my healthy, gourmet version of *"La Dolce Vita."* Today I enjoy food—dining in great restaurants, traveling and experiencing new destinations, preparing meals and entertaining friends and family at home, and doing things I never before dreamed were possible. I believe the best way to keep what I've worked so hard to earn is to share it, so I may help others. I've found that I could have an exciting, amazing life beyond anything I could have imagined.

Since I began my new life, I have had the courage to go after and achieve some of my dreams. To begin, I recently attended the prestigious Toscana Saporita Cooking School in Tuscany. Learning to cook authentic Italian cuisine while staying at a working *agriturismo* (farm) and attending cooking school in Italy was another dream of mine. I have included several signature recipes from Chef/Owner Sandra Lotti in the Recipes section, and highly recommend this school to anyone who especially enjoys Italian food, cooking, and wants to learn more and have a blast! Next, I had the pleasure of starting my own company, Fred Bollaci Enterprises in 2014, and have been working with hundreds of top chefs and restaurant owners to promote living my trademark Golden Palate® lifestyle exemplified in *The Restaurant Diet*. To date, I have had the privilege of naming hundreds of Golden Palate Partners in the United States, Italy, and elsewhere, and over 100 Platinum Palate™ establishments, whose owners, chefs, and staff go the extra mile to anticipate their clients' needs, and make a healthy, gourmet lifestyle possible. I have been fortunate to coach and help many people lose weight by making positive changes to their lives. Seeing others benefit from my experience has been very rewarding.

My advice to everyone: weight loss and transforming your life is not an easy task, but it can and should be one of the greatest experiences you'll ever have—a process through which you will get to know the real you and improve every aspect of your life! Losing weight and getting healthy should be an exercise in self-love and empowerment, where you face food and your demons, rather than avoiding them and feeling deprived. Weight loss should be a positive experience and, if you like to eat out, you shouldn't have to stop. For dieting to work, it should never be a temporary, unpleasant, goal-oriented means to an end. Without learning to eat better in your favorite restaurants and at home, learning to embrace and enjoy exercise, and learning to deal with anxiety, stress, and emotional triggers along the way, the likelihood of you being able to maintain your weight loss will be very slim.

It is with a positive attitude and much gratitude that I keep moving forward. I have taken a lot of lemons and made *limoncello*, a favorite expression of mine.

Whatever your situation, you alone hold the keys to changing your life for the better. Life should be enjoyed and appreciated, just like food. No matter how tough it may seem to lose weight and get healthy, if I did it, so can you! A better life is waiting for you to claim it. Why not start by making today the first day of your exciting journey to a new and better life?

PART TWO

RECIPES

Chapter Eight
Recipes from Some of My Favorite Restaurants

I am proud to feature an extensive collection of recipes from many of my favorite restaurants nationwide, from exciting destinations like northern and southern California, Aspen, Colorado, Florida's east and west coasts, Atlanta, Michigan, New York City, Long Island, Connecticut, Massachusetts, Vermont, and Maine, as well as a bonus section featuring two favorite destinations in Italy, Toscana Saporita Cooking School, and Hotel Santa Caterina in Amalfi (my favorite hotel in the world)! Now, you will not only know many of my favorite places to eat, you have a great collection of recipes at your fingertips so you can cook like a gourmet chef at home! For your convenience, I have grouped the restaurants alphabetically by state, followed by recipes from two great establishments with multiple locations in many states (Ocean Prime and Truluck's) and three "Hall of Fame" chefs/restaurateurs (Silvano Marchetto of Da Silvano in New York City, Renzo Sciortino of Renzo's of Boca, and Tony May of The Rainbow Room, San Domenico and SD26 in New York City) who have retired from the restaurant business, but who generously contributed recipes before closing their doors. Their cuisine has had a profound influence on my culinary perspective, and I am honored to include them in this book. To make the recipes more user-friendly, I have listed the appropriate phase(s) for each recipe, and included nutritional information, as well as tips on how a recipe can be adjusted at home—both in terms of reducing fat and adjusting portion size, as well as helpful suggestions and alternatives—some offered by the chefs/ restaurateurs themselves. *Buon Appetito!*

INDEX OF RESTAURANT RECIPES

California

Four Seasons Resort The Biltmore, Santa Barbara
Coconut Chia Pudding (Breakfast or Dessert) (All Phases)

Geoffrey's Malibu, Malibu
Spicy Shrimp Salad (Salad/Entrée) (All Phases)
Lobster and Scallop Ceviche (Starter or Entrée) (All Phases)

The Girl and The Fig, Sonoma
Heirloom Tomato & Watermelon Salad (Salad) (All Phases)

Left Bank Brasserie (locations in Larkspur, Menlo Park, and San Jose)
Pernod Prawns (Entrée) (Phases Two–Four)

Perbacco, San Francisco
Agnolotti Dal Plin (Pasta Filled with Roasted Meats and Savoy Cabbage) (Entrée) (Phases Two–Four)

The Ritz-Carlton Bacara, Santa Barbara
Tomato Soup with Goat Cheese Crème (Soup) (Phases Two–Four)

Valette Restaurant, Healdsburg
Burrata & Peach Salad with Pickled Green Peaches, Char Grilled Peaches, & Peach Leaf Vinaigrette (Salad) (Phases Two–Four)

Colorado

Campo de Fiori, Aspen and Vail
Linguine Diavola with Lobster (Entrée) (Phases Two–Four)

The Little Nell, Aspen
Ajax Tavern and Element 47
Ajax Tavern's Brussel Sprouts with Pomegranate Molasses (Side/Vegetable) (Phases Two–Four)
Mountain Mojito Recipe (Cocktail) (Phases Three–Four)

Connecticut

Finalmente Trattoria, Westport
Squaletto Isolano (Halibut with Sun-dried Tomatoes, Artichokes, Capers, Olives, & Prosecco) (Entrée) (All Phases)

Homestead Inn/Thomas Henkelmann, a Relais & Châteaux Luxury Resort and Restaurant, Greenwich
Roasted Stuffed Rabbit Loin (Entrée) (All Phases)
Salmon in Brick with Russian Ossetra (Entrée) (Phases Two–Four)

Florida

Abe and Louie's, Boca Raton and Boston, MA
See recipe for Roasted Beet, Poached Pear, and Goat Cheese Salad, and recipe for Beef and Mushroom Barley Soup in Boston, MA.

Addison Reserve Country Club, Delray Beach
Chilled Curry Cauliflower Soup (Soup) (All Phases)

The Beach Bistro, Holmes Beach (Anna Maria Island)
Bouillabaisse (Entrée) (All Phases)

Ben's Kosher Deli, Boca Raton and New York locations
See recipe for Ben's Israeli Salad in New York.

Bern's Steakhouse, Tampa
Grilled Wild King Salmon with Asparagus & Lobster Vinaigrette (All Phases)

Bice Ristorante, Palm Beach, Naples, and Orlando (with locations worldwide)
Branzino alla Griglia con Vegetali Misti e Salmoriglio (Grilled Mediterranean Sea Bass with Mixed Vegetables and Lemon-Olive Oil Dressing) (Entrée) (All Phases)
Minestrone di Verdure alla Cas*arecchia* (Minestrone Soup) (Soup) (All Phases)

Bijou Café, Sarasota
Chilled Tomato-Tarragon Soup (Soup) (Phases Two–Four)
Mixed Greens and Goat Cheese Salad with Confit Tomatoes (Salad) (Phases Two–Four)

Bistro Chez Jean-Pierre, Palm Beach

Snapper with Herb Sauce and Ratatouille (Entrée) (All Phases)

Sautéed Pink Key West Shrimp with Citrus Sauce and Endive Salad (Entrée) (All Phases)

Bleu Provence, Naples

Chilled Vegetable Salad with Honey Key Lime Dressing and Eggplant Caviar (Salad) (All Phases)

Boca Raton Resort & Club, Boca Raton

Preserved Lemon and Spinach Risotto with Basil Blaze (Entrée) (Phases Three–Four)

Summer Sun Watermelon Salad (Salad) (All Phases)

The Breakers, Palm Beach

Grilled Vegetable Salad with Lemon-Tomato Vinaigrette from The Flagler Steakhouse (Salad/Entrée) (All Phases)

Three-Minute Sicilian Calamari from The Italian Restaurant (Starter/Entrée) (All Phases)

Buccan, Palm Beach

Grilled Shrimp Scampi (Entrée) with Mango Salsa (Snack/Accompaniment) (All Phases)

The Café at Books & Books (Coral Gables, Miami Beach, and Miami)

Café Shrimp Mango Mojo (Entrée) (All Phases)

Café Chardonnay, Palm Beach Gardens

Crab Cakes with Hearts of Palm (Entrée) (Phases Two–Four)

Macadamia Nut-Crusted Snapper with Tropical Fruit Salsa (Entrée) (Phases Three–Four)

Café L'Europe, Palm Beach

Peruvian Shrimp Ceviche with Guacamole (Starter/Entrée) (All Phases)

Café Martorano, Fort Lauderdale, FL (also in Las Vegas, Nevada and Atlantic City, NJ)

Bucatini Amatriciana with Guanciale and Onions (Entrée) (Phases Two–Four)

Café Sapori, West Palm Beach
Potato-Crusted Baked Orata (Mediterranean Sea Bream) with Taggiasche Olives (Entrée) (Phases Two–Four)

Caffé Luna Rosa, Delray Beach
Florida Yellowtail Ceviche (Starter) (All Phases)
Dijon Mustard-Horseradish Aioli (Suggested with Florida Stone Crab Claws) (Dip) (All Phases)

Casa D'Angelo, Boca Raton, Ft. Lauderdale, FL, and Atlantis, Paradise Island, Bahamas
Pan-Seared Sea Scallops with Endive, Orange, and Mint Salad (Starter/ Entrée) (All Phases)

Charley's Crab, Palm Beach, FL, and Grand Rapids, MI
Chilled Gazpacho with Charley's Crab's Fat-Free Italian Vinaigrette Dressing (Soup/Entrée) (All Phases)

Chop's Lobster Bar, Boca Raton, FL and Atlanta, GA
Chop's Lobster Bar's Spinach Salad with Creamy Basil Dressing (Salad/ Entrée) (Phases Three–Four)

City Fish Market, Boca Raton and Atlanta, GA
Hong Kong-Style Fish (Phases Two–Four)

Columbia Restaurant, Tampa, Sarasota, Clearwater Beach, St. Augustine, and Celebration (Orlando)
Columbia's Original "1905" Salad™ (Entrée) (All Phases)

Cucina dell'Arte, Palm Beach
Snapper Livornese (Entrée) (Phases Two–Four)

CUT 432, Delray Beach
USDA Prime Steak Tartare (Starter/Entrée) (All Phases)

Donatello, Tampa
Ossobuco alla Milanese (Braised Veal Shank) (Entrée) (Phases Two–Four)
Vitello Dolce Vita (Veal with Ham, Sage, and Mushrooms) (Entrée) (Phases Two–Four)

Euphemia Haye, Longboat Key
Zucchini Fettuccine with Tomato Sauce (Entrée or Side/Vegetable) (All Phases)

Cauliflower Mash (substitute for Mashed Potatoes) (Side) (Phases Two–Four)

The French Brasserie Rustique, Naples

Salade Niçoise (Entrée) (All Phases; Phases One–Three)

Henry's, Delray Beach

Turkey Burger with Cranberry Relish with a cup of Magical Low-Fat Split Pea Soup (Soup/Meal/Entrée) (All Phases)

Jack Dusty at The Ritz-Carlton, Sarasota

Jack Dusty's Signature Cornmeal Blinis and Lemon Crème Fraiche, Served with Mote Marine Sustainable Sturgeon Caviar Raised in Sarasota (Appetizer) (Phases Two–Four)

Joe's Stone Crab, Miami Beach

Joe's Crab Cakes (Entrée) (All Phases) and Joe's Vinaigrette (All Phases)

Kathy's Gazebo Café, Boca Raton

Dover Sole Meunière (Entrée) (Phases Two–Four)
Salmon Tartare (Starter or Entrée) (All Phases)

Limoncello Ristorante, Palm Beach Gardens

Stuffed Artichokes (Starter/Entrée) (All Phases)
Chicken Pappagallo (Boneless Chicken Breast with Agrodolce- Sweet and Sour Sauce with Grapes and Olives) (Entrée) (Phases Two–Four)

Louis Pappas Fresh Greek, Clearwater, Lakeland, and Tampa

Louis Pappas Famous Greek Salad™ (without Potato Salad) (Salad/Entrée) (All Phases)

Marcello's La Sirena, West Palm Beach

Scaloppine di Vitello Sciue (Veal Escalopes with Grape Tomatoes, Gaeta Olives, & Fresh Mozzarella) (Entrée) (Phases Two–Four)

Mario's Osteria, Boca Raton

Flounder Vesuvio (Entrée) (Phases Two–Four)

Matteo's, Boca Raton and Hallandale (also in Huntington and Roslyn, NY)

Shrimp alla Wendy with Burned String Beans (Entrée) (All Phases)

Mediterraneo, Sarasota
Veal Milanese with Arugula & Tomato Salad (Entrée) (Phases Two–Four)

Michael's on East, Sarasota
Grilled Skirt Steak with Chimichurri, Grilled Red Onions & Roasted Roma Tomatoes (Entrée) (All Phases)

Mystic Fish, Palm Harbor
Chilean Seabass with Hijiki Sauce (Entrée) (Phases Two–Four)
Bermuda Fish Chowder (Soup) (Phases Two–Four)
Kona-Seared Salmon with Pistachio-Dill Pesto (Entrée) (All Phases)

Nino's of Delray, Delray Beach
Flounder Francese (Entrée) (Phases Two–Four)

Ophelia's on the Bay, Sarasota
Seared Sea Scallops with Sesame Buckwheat Noodle Stir-Fry and Baby Bok Choy (Entrée) (Phases Two–Four)

Osteria Tulia/Bar Tulia, Naples
Florida Black Grouper *all' Acquapazza* "Crazywater-style" (Entrée) (All Phases)

Paradiso Ristorante, Lake Worth
Fig & Chestnut Risotto (Entrée) (Phases Two–Four)

Renato's, Palm Beach
Grilled Marinated Veal Chop (Entrée) (All Phases)

Simon's Coffee House, Sarasota
Raw Beet Ravioli & Jicama Slaw (Entrée) (All Phases)

Ta-boo, Palm Beach
Ta-boo Wellness Salad (Entrée) (All Phases)

32 East, Delray Beach
American Lamb Loin with Wild Mushrooms, Asparagus, and White Wine (Entrée) (All Phases)

Tramonti Ristorante (see also Angelo's of Mulberry Street in New York, NY)
Zucchini Flowers (Starter/Entrée) (Phases Three–Four)

Trattoria Romana, Boca Raton

Eggplant Pie (Starter/Entrée) (Phases Two–Four)

Trevini, Palm Beach

Orecchiette con Polpa di Granchio e Asparagi (Ear-Shaped Pasta with Crabmeat and Asparagus) (Entrée) (Phases Two–Four)

Georgia

Atlanta Fish Market, Atlanta

See recipe for Hong Kong-Style Fish at City Fish Market in Boca Raton, Florida.

Buckhead Diner, Atlanta

Butternut Squash Soup (Soup) (All Phases)

Chop's Lobster Bar, Atlanta

See recipe for Chop's Lobster Bar's Spinach Salad with Creamy Basil Dressing in Boca Raton, FL

Kyma, Atlanta

Kyma's Slow-Cooked Eggplant Stew with Sweet Onions and Tomatoes (Soup) (All Phases)

La Grotta Ristorante, Atlanta

Granchio con Avocado e Pompelmo (Lump Crabmeat with Grainy Mustard over Avocado, Orange, and Grapefruit Segments) (Salad/Entrée) (All Phases)

Pricci, Atlanta

Grilled Lamb Chops with Mushroom Funghetto (Entrée) (Phases Two–Four)

Maine

Balance Rock Inn, Bar Harbor

Shrimp and Lobster Cakes, with Preserved Lemon Aioli & Lobster Oil (Entrée) (All Phases)

Natalie's at Camden Harbour Inn, Camden

Black Bass with Gnocchi and Vegetables (Entrée) (Phases Two–Four)

Massachusetts

Abe & Louie's, Boston, MA, and Boca Raton, FL
Roasted Beet, Poached Pear, and Goat Cheese Salad (Salad/Entrée) (All Phases)
Beef and Mushroom Barley Soup (Soup or Entrée) (Phases Two–Four)

Wheatleigh, Lenox
Butternut Squash Soup (Soup) (All Phases)
Seared Tuna with Broccolini, Couscous, and Squash (Entrée) (Phases Two–Four)

Michigan

Charley's Crab, Grand Rapids and Palm Beach, FL (See Florida)
See recipe for Chilled Gazpacho with Charley's Crab's Fat-Free Italian Vinaigrette Dressing at Charley's Crab in Palm Beach, Florida.

Chateau Chantal, Traverse City
Baby Portabella Mushroom Caps with Caramelized Shallot & Fontina (Starter) (All Phases)
Fruit, Avocado, and Goat Cheese Roll (Starter) (All Phases)

Grand Traverse Resort and Spa, Acme (Traverse City)
Aerie Restaurant
Vegetable Terrine (Vegetable/Side) (All Phases)

Nevada

Café Martorano, Las Vegas
See recipe for Bucatini Amatriciana with Guanciale and Onions in Fort Lauderdale, FL.

New Jersey

Café Martorano, Atlantic City
See Bucatini Amatriciana with Guanciale and Onions in Fort Lauderdale, FL.

New York

Almond, Bridgehampton and New York, NY
Monkfish Cioppino (Entrée) (All Phases)

The American Hotel, Sag Harbor
Seared Tuna a la Nage (Entrée) (All Phases)
Bison Carpaccio (Starter/Entrée) (All Phases)

Barbetta, New York, NY
Roasted Peppers alla Bagna Cauda (Appetizer/Side/Snack) (All Phases)

Ben's Kosher Deli, Manhattan, Bayside, Carle Place, Greenvale, Scarsdale, and Woodbury, NY, and Boca Raton, FL
Ben's Israeli Salad (Salad or Entrée) (All Phases)

Dario's, Rockville Centre
Mussels Fra Diavola (Entrée) (All Phases)

Estia's Little Kitchen, Sag Harbor
Whole-Wheat Pancakes (Breakfast) (Phases Two–Four)

The Frisky Oyster, Greenport
Montauk Tuna with Cilantro Walnut Pesto, Mushrooms, and Bok Choy (Entrée) (All Phases)

Gabriel Kreuther, New York, NY
Baked Black Sea Bass, Fennel seeds-Coriander Broth, Green Tomato Marmalade (Entrée) (Phases Two–Four)

The Golden Pear Café, Southampton, Bridgehampton, East Hampton, and Sag Harbor
Grilled Fresh Wild Salmon Salad (Entrée) (All Phases)
Citrus Veggie Tuna Salad (Entrée) (All Phases)
Garden Vegetable Egg White Omelet (Breakfast) (All Phases)

La Bussola, Glen Cove
La Bussola's Combination Salad (Salad) (All Phases)
Pork Chop Scarpariello (in the style of the Shoemaker) (Entrée) (All Phases)

La Ginestra, Glen Cove

Mixed Grilled Vegetables and Marinated Grilled Jumbo Shrimp (Starter/ Snack/Entrée) (All Phases)

La Grenouille, New York, NY

Grilled Chicken Paillard with Summer Vegetables and Aged Balsamic Vinegar (Entrée) (All Phases)

Matteo's, Huntington and Roslyn (also in Boca Raton and Hallandale, FL)

See recipe for Matteo's in Boca Raton and Hallandale, Florida.

Mirabelle Restaurant at The Three Village Inn, Stony Brook

Escabeche of Red Snapper (Entrée) (Phases Two–Four)

Noah's, Greenport

Noah's Local Fluke Crudo (Starter/Entrée) (All Phases)
Noah's Local Seafood Bouillabaisse with Saffron Fennel Broth (Entrée) (All Phases)

The Plaza Café, Southampton

Pan-Roasted King Salmon with Frisee, Roasted Shallots, Haricots Verts, Red Bliss, and Mustard Seed Vinaigrette (Entrée) (All Phases; Phase One)

Red Bar/Brasserie, Southampton

Grilled Prawns with Romesco Sauce (Entrée) (All Phases)

1770 House, East Hampton

1770 House Meatloaf (Entrée) (Phases Two–Four)

75 Main, Southampton

The "Spa Burger" (Entrée) (All Phases)
The "Chop-Chop" Salad (Salad/Entrée) (All Phases)

Starr Boggs, Westhampton Beach

Grilled Harissa-Marinated Calamari (Appetizer) (All Phases)

Stone Creek Inn, East Quogue

Chilled Zucchini Soup with Lobster Tail and Avocado (Soup/Starter) (All Phases)

Vermont

The Perfect Wife, Manchester Center
The Perfect Wife's Famous Howling Wolf Vegan Special (Entrée) (All Phases)

Nationwide

Ocean Prime (locations in Phoenix, AZ, Beverly Hills, CA, Denver, CO, Naples, Orlando, and Tampa, FL, Indianapolis, IN, Boston, MA, Detroit, MI, New York, NY, Columbus, OH, Philadelphia, PA, Dallas, TX, and Washington, DC)
Tangerine Tuna (Entrée) (All Phases)

Truluck's (locations in La Jolla, CA, Boca Raton, Fort Lauderdale, Miami, and Naples, FL, Austin, Dallas, and Houston, TX, and coming soon to Chicago, IL)
Chimichurri Sauce (All Phases) and Cioppino (San Francisco-style Seafood Broth) (Entrée) (All Phases)

Hall of Fame

The following outstanding restaurateurs have since retired and closed their doors but have contributed so much to my culinary appreciation and were generous enough to provide recipes. It is an honor to include them!

Da Silvano (Silvano Marchetto), New York, NY
*Spiedino di Pesce Ri*minese (Seafood Skewers with Squid, Swordfish, and Shrimp—Inspired by Rimini) (Entrée) (All Phases)

Renzo's of Boca (Renzo Sciortino), Boca Raton, FL
Renzo's Yellowtail Snapper Oreganato (Entrée) (Phases Two–Four)

San Domenico/SD26 (Tony May), New York, NY
Vignarola (Spring Vegetable Soup) (Soup/Entrée) (All Phases)

Italy

Hotel Santa Caterina, Amalfi

San Pietro (John Dory) and Artichoke Roll with Asparagus Bundles and Potatoes (Entrée) (All Phases)

Toscana Saporita Cooking School, Chef Sandra Lotti, Massaciuccoli (Lucca)

Pasta Fatta in Casa – Basic Pasta (Entrée) (Phases Two–Four)
Insalata di Farro – Farro Salad (Starter/Entrée) (All Phases)
Branzino in Cartoccio – Sea Bass Marinated in Orange Juice & Cooked in Parchment with Vegetables (Entrée) (All Phases)

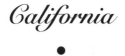

California

•

Four Seasons Resort The Biltmore, Santa Barbara

1260 Channel Drive, Santa Barbara, CA 93108

(805) 969-2261 • www.fourseasons.com/SantaBarbara

The luxurious Four Seasons Biltmore faces one of the most beautiful beaches in California, with private bungalows and terraces overlooking the Pacific Ocean and Channel Islands. Set amongst twenty-two acres of lush jungle and tranquil gardens, the resort is the epitome of world-class service and amenities. Enjoy gourmet fine dining at Tydes, which offers intimate indoor and outdoor oceanfront dining, exclusively to Resort guests and members of the Club, with panoramic views atop the Pacific Ocean through floor to ceiling windows. Experience local seafood with Mediterranean flavors and fresh, seasonal preparations created by Executive Chef Marco Fossati and his culinary team. The highlight is the new Coral Reef Bar, an outdoor twenty-eight-foot oval seawater aquarium bar with a living coral reef. Bella Vista Restaurant is Santa Barbara's most beautiful premier *al fresco* oceanfront dining experience. Bella Vista, the resort's Italian restaurant also features panoramic ocean views, showcasing fresh California ingredients inspired by Chef Fossati. The expansive terrace features Italian marble, indoor fireplaces, an outdoor fire pit and a retractable glass roof. Bella Vista is one of only twelve restaurants in California (the only one in Santa Barbara) licensed to cure its own meats. The shared charcuterie plate is the most popular appetizer on the menu.

Recipe courtesy of Emilie Plouchart, Director of Public Relations.

. . . .
Coconut Chia Pudding

Breakfast or Dessert • All Phases • Serves 2

INGREDIENTS

½ cup Chia Seeds
½ cup coconut flakes or ground
2 cups Coconut milk
3½ Tbsp. honey or Agave nectar
  (Vegan)

Optional: any diced seasonal fruit any
  favorite nuts or seeds (pumpkin
  seeds, sunflower, pistachios,
  macadamia, etc.)

INSTRUCTIONS

Mix all items and let it sit overnight in the fridge. Add your favorite selection of seasonal fruit and nuts/seeds. Garnish with fresh mint.

NOTE

The above nutritional analysis was calculated using honey. With agave nectar, the number of calories would be 556, so from a caloric standpoint they may be used interchangeably based upon preference. Analysis is done without any added fruit or nuts. I suggest a smaller serving for dietary purposes.

Nutrition Facts (per serving)
Calories: **552** • Calories from fat: **46%** • Fat: **28g**
Saturated fat: **14g** • Cholesterol: **0mg** • Carbohydrates: **62g**
Protein: **14g** • Sodium: **36mg** • Fiber: **22g**

•

Geoffrey's Malibu, Malibu

27400 Pacific Coast Highway, Malibu, CA 90265
(310) 457-1519 • www.geoffreysmalibu.com

Geoffrey's, the legendary southern California landmark restaurant, is situated in one of the most spectacular locations anywhere in America, high on a bluff overlooking the Pacific Ocean, where guests can dine al fresco, watch the whales, catch a few rays of California sunshine, and enjoy excellent cuisine. Geoffrey's pedigree is as impressive as its location, first opening as the Holiday House resort and watering hole to the stars in 1948. It immediately became THE destination, hosting the likes of Frank Sinatra, Shirley MacLaine, Lana Turner, John F. Kennedy, and Marilyn Monroe. In 1983, Harvey Baskin, a financier/ gourmand/nature lover purchased the Holiday House and created Geoffrey's, first by redesigning the restaurant so every seat had a view of the ocean. In 1999, Geoffrey's was purchased by Jeff Peterson, who started as a busboy at the restaurant eleven years before, and expanded the restaurant's presence in the community, by hosting numerous charitable benefits. Geoffrey's still attracts Hollywood celebrities, politicians, ambassadors, world travelers, and locals, and was featured on the HBO hit series, *Entourage*.

Recipes courtesy of Emily Richardson, Director of Public Relations, Geoffrey's, Malibu.

. . . .

Spicy Shrimp Salad

Salad/Entrée • All Phases • Serves 4

INGREDIENTS

Shrimp Salad:

16 U-12 shrimp

¼ package tamarind paste

2 Tbsp. canola oil

4 ears yellow corn

½ pound baby arugula

1 medium-sized jicama

1 cup pear tomatoes

4 ounces Spicy Asian Vinaigrette
  (see below)

1 package fried wonton skins (omit for
  weight-loss purposes)

Spicy Asian Vinaigrette:

2 Tbsp. Sambal Chili Sauce

1 tsp. fish sauce

½ bunch finely chopped cilantro

2 Tbsp. rice wine vinegar

1 egg yolk

¼ tsp. sesame oil

¼ cup canola oil (reduced from ½ cup
  for home/weight-loss preparation)

INSTRUCTIONS

Shrimp salad:

- Mix ¼ package tamarind paste with oil and toss shrimp to marinate.
- Shuck and clean corn, lightly oil, and grill; let cool and cut kernels off ear.
- Peel and julienne jicama.
- Grill marinated shrimp.

Vinaigrette:

- In a medium bowl mix Sambal, fish sauce, cilantro, vinegar, and egg yolk.
- Whisk in sesame and canola oils until emulsified.

Assembly:

In a large bowl mix baby arugula, grilled corn, Jicama, and pear tomatoes with vinaigrette. Evenly divide among 4 bowls. Arrange shrimp around salad and top with fried wonton skins.

NOTE

Calorie count excludes fried wontons and uses ¼ cup oil in the dressing.

Nutrition Facts (per serving)
Calories: **393** • Calories from fat: **53%** • Fat: **24g**
Saturated fat: **3g** • Cholesterol: **90mg** • Carbohydrates: **25g**
Protein: **23g** • Sodium: **319mg**

. . . .

Lobster and Scallop Ceviche

Starter or Entrée • All Phases • Serves 4

INGREDIENTS

Lobster and Scallop Ceviche:

6 ounces fresh Maine lobster
6 ounces day boat scallops
pinch salt, to taste
1 ounce diced shallots
1 ounce diced mango

3 ounces Mango Habanero Chili Water
  (see below)
16 mini taco shells
½ ounce micro cilantro

Mango Habanero Chili Water:

1 whole mango, cleaned and diced   ½ cup distilled water

1 habanero pepper

INSTRUCTIONS

Lobster and Scallop Ceviche:

- Start with a whole/live fresh Maine lobster.
- Fill large stockpot with water adding a pinch of salt.
- Bring to a boil.
- Place live lobster in boiling water and cook for 3 minutes.
- Remove lobster from water and place into ice bath.
- Once lobster is cool, remove from ice bath and clean (remove head from tail; crack shell on tail and remove meat).
- Clean lobster and cut into ¼-inch dices.
- Clean scallops and cut into ¼-inch dices.

Mango Habanero Chili Water:

- Place all ingredients in a blender, purée, and then strain. Set aside.

Assembly:

- Mix diced lobster, scallops, shallots, mango and Mango Chili Water in a bowl, add pinch of salt.
- Let mixture (ceviche) marinate for 30 minutes.
- Fill mini taco shells with ceviche mixture and top with micro cilantro.

Nutrition Facts (per serving)
Calories: **204** • Calories from fat: **23%** • Fat: **5g**
Saturated fat: **1g** • Cholesterol: **28mg** • Carbohydrates: **23g**
Protein: **16g** • Sodium: **213mg**

The Girl & The Fig

110 W. Spain St., Sonoma, CA 95476 • (707) 938-3634 • www.thegirlandthefig.com

The Girl and The Fig, by Chef/Owner Sondra Bernstein has been a favorite in the heart of downtown Sonoma since 1997, featuring exceptional Provence-inspired seasonal farm-to-table cuisine, a wonderful antique bar with French *aperitifs*, unique cocktails, an award-winning wine list, notable house-cured charcuterie platters, and outdoor garden patio seating. She named her restaurant for the fruit that symbolizes passion, the fig—representing her passion for locally-grown ingredients and French cuisine. Twenty years later, it is still one of the hottest spots in wine country. Also, check out The Fig Café in Glen Ellen, CA.

Recipe courtesy of Chef/Owner Sondra Bernstein.

. . . .

Heirloom Tomato & Watermelon Salad

Salad • All Phases • Serves 6

This is one of the most popular menu items at The Girl & The Fig. You don't normally think of pairing tomatoes with watermelon, but peak tomato season is usually the same for watermelon. The two fruits are somewhat similar in texture and color, as well. The watermelon's sugar content, though higher than a tomato's, ties the two fruits together. The addition of the salty sheep's milk feta and a sprinkling of sea salt create a nice contrast to the sweetness of the salad. We use fresh oregano as the main herbal flavor, but it would be just as good with fresh basil or thyme.

INGREDIENTS

Vinaigrette:

1 medium yellow tomato, blanched, peeled and seeded

1 Tbsp. Dijon mustard

1 Tbsp. champagne vinegar

½ cup extra-virgin olive oil

Salt and white pepper to taste

Salad:

½ cup feta cheese

3 Tbsp. extra-virgin olive oil

1 pound seedless watermelon,
rind removed, sliced into ½ x
2-inch rounds
2 pounds assorted heirloom tomatoes,
sliced into ½-inch pieces

2 Tbsp. fresh oregano leaves,
for garnish
Sea salt, for garnish

INSTRUCTIONS

Vinaigrette:

- Place the yellow tomato in a blender.

- On medium speed add the mustard and then the vinegar.

- Slowly add ½ cup of olive oil. Taste and season with salt and white pepper as needed and set aside.

Salad:

- In a separate bowl, crumble the feta and mix it with 3 tablespoons olive oil.

- Divide the heirloom tomato slices and the watermelon slices equally among 6 plates.

- When plating, alternate the slices and garnish with a bit of feta. Drizzle the vinaigrette over each portion and garnish with the oregano leaves.

- Add a touch of sea salt to the salad if desired.

> **Nutrition Facts (per serving)**
> Calories: **319** • Calories from fat: **85%** • Fat: **0g**
> Saturated fat: **7g** • Cholesterol: **17mg** • Carbohydrates: **12g**
> Protein: **4g** • Sodium: **672mg**

Left Bank Brasserie

507 Magnolia Ave., Larkspur, CA 94939 • (415) 927-3331
635 Santa Cruz Ave., Menlo Park, CA 94025 • (650) 473-6543
377 Santana Row Suite 1100, San Jose, CA 95128 • (408) 984-3500
www.leftbank.com

One of the top French restaurants in northern California, this popular trio known as Left Bank Brasserie is named after *La Rive Gauche* (The Left Bank), the southern bank of the River Seine in Paris. *"Rive Gauche"* or Left Bank generally refers to the Paris of an earlier era: the Paris of artists, writers and philosophers. The phrase implies a sense of bohemianism, counterculture, and creativity. While it remains a haven for artists and bohemians, it is also the site of many wonderful and famous brasseries, including Les Deux Magots, Café Flore, and Brasserie Lipp. Chef proprietor, Roland Passot epitomizes this fun French Culture with three locations in the San Francisco Bay area.

Internationally acclaimed for his exceptional French cooking, Chef Passot has designed a simple, French brasserie-style menu that changes with the seasons. A native of Lyon, known as France's gastronomic capital, Roland began his restaurant career by simultaneously going to school and working as apprentice to many fine chefs, including Jean-Paul LaComb at Leon de Lyon. At the age of nineteen he became the chef de cuisine at Pierre Orsi.

After two years at Orsi, Jean Banchet, chef/owner of Le Français in Wheeling, Illinois, persuaded Roland to come to the United States and join his award-winning restaurant team. During this period, Le Français was regarded as the finest French restaurant in north America. Roland remained in Chicago for four years. In 1980, Roland relocated to San Francisco as the opening chef of Le Castel. In 1981 Jean Banchet appointed Roland as chef at The French Room at the Adolphus Hotel in Dallas, Texas. In 1988, Roland returned to San Francisco and opened La Folie with his brother George and his wife Jamie. Since that time, La Folie has achieved tremendous critical acclaim.

In 1990, Roland himself was awarded the coveted James Beard Rising Star Chef award. As a result of Roland's culinary prowess and his contributions to French cuisine, he was inducted as a Maître Cuisiner of France in 1991. Roland is one of the most popular instructors at nationally acclaimed state-of-the-art

Draeger's Culinary Center in both Menlo Park and San Mateo. In July 1994, in partnership with long-time food service executive Edward Levine, Left Bank in Larkspur opened to much anticipation. Four years later in 1998, the second Left Bank opened in Menlo Park. San Jose opened in 2003 and remains a favorite for a Parisian-style snack (oysters and a glass of champagne or wine) or something heartier.

Recipe courtesy of Chef Roland Passot.

. . . .

Pernod Prawns

Entrée • Phases Two–Four • Serves 1

INGREDIENTS

6 prawns, shelled & deveined
½ Tbsp. olive oil
1 shot of Pernod (1½ ounces)
½ Tbsp. sweet butter
8 toy box tomatoes or sweet 100 cherry tomatoes

zest of 1 lemon
4 leaves of basil, chiffonade (thin strips or shreds)
¼ tsp. finely chopped Italian parsley
½ clove garlic, peeled and minced

INSTRUCTIONS

Prawns:

- Season prawns with salt and pepper.
- Sautée in hot pan in olive oil for about 15 seconds.
- Flip and de-glaze with Pernod.
- Add butter, tomatoes, lemon zest, garlic, basil, and parsley.
- When the butter melts, the prawns are ready. Do not over-cook.

Crouton Garnish:

- Slice 4 pieces from a baguette. Toast until crisp. (Optional, may omit for weight-loss purposes.)

Assembly:

- Plate the shrimp with cooking juices in a shallow, wide soup bowl.
- Tuck the croutons in at an angle, just touching the sauce.

NOTE

If you choose to omit the bread, the recipe will be approximately 150 calories less (75 calories per ounce, assuming 2 ounces).

Nutrition Facts (per serving)
Calories: **573** • Calories from fat: **22%** • Fat: **13.5g**
Saturated fat: **4.5g** • Cholesterol: **15.5mg** • Carbohydrates: **38g**
Protein: **5g** • Sodium: **2,115mg** • Fiber: **1g**

●

Perbacco

230 California St., San Francisco, CA 94111 • (415) 955.0663 • www.perbaccosf.com

"*Perbacco*" is an Italian word to accentuate positive comments. It can also be an expression of pleasure and surprise, and is a reference to Bacchus, God of Wine and "good times." Perbacco the restaurant is thoroughly steeped in the traditions of Italy, yet has a refreshingly modern feel and attitude. Perbacco introduces urban San Francisco to the full range of flavors found in the northern Italian regions of Piemonte and Liguria, with a touch of France via Provence. Chef/Owner Staffan Terje and Owner Umberto Gibin have been sharing their passion for the food and wine of Italy with Americans for nearly three decades.

With the opening of Perbacco, Terje and Gibin, culinary stars who rose to prominence at some of California' s finest Italian restaurants, including Scala's Bistro, Chianti and Poggio, as well as the esteemed San Francisco dining destinations Fifth Floor and Masa's, ensure that each guest gets a taste of an authentic Italian dining experience. Swedish-born chef/co-owner Staffan Terje, chose to open an Italian restaurant because "Italian food is the food that talks to me. You don't choose who you fall in love with. It just happens." Following high school, Staffan enrolled at the Hotel and Restaurant School in Stockholm, completing his apprenticeship at the Michelin-starred restaurant, Gourmet. In 1982, after working in Stockholm for a few years, Staffan was offered a job in Sarasota, Florida. "My friend and I planned to work there for a year and come home with bragging rights that we had worked in 'The U.S.,'" Staffan says. "We're both still here." After a couple of years, Staffan headed west and worked in several restaurants in Orange County, CA, before ending up in Napa Valley in 1986. There he worked at Sherry Oven, a restaurant housed in a historic winery in downtown Napa. Other career highlights include a seven-year stint at San Francisco's famed Scala's Bistro and cooking at the James Beard House in New York City.

"These days, chefs are taking back the skills required to master the craft of cooking," Staffan explains. In January 2010 Staffan, along with partner, Umberto Gibin, opened barbacco eno trattoria, next door to Perbacco. At barbacco, he maintains the same quality-driven tenants to form the seasonally changing menu. Born in Venice, Italy, and raised in Torino, in the Piemonte region, Umberto Gibin was naturally introduced to the pleasures and traditions of the Italian table at a very early age. Gibin began to learn the hospitality trade at several prestigious European restaurants and hotels, such as Villa d'Este in Lake Como, The Palace in St. Moritz, and The Caprice in London. He arrived in the United States in 1979 where he began his U.S. career at the venerable Ernie's and Ciao in San Francisco. After a stint as General Manager at Spectrum Foods' Chianti Restaurant on Melrose Avenue in Los Angeles, he returned to San Francisco as one of the founding team members of Il Fornaio. With Il Fornaio Gibin was instrumental in the successful opening of six restaurants. In 1999 he joined Kimpton Hotels, at The Grand Café, and later as a Director of Restaurant Operations, where he oversaw several restaurants including The Fifth Floor, Masa's, and Splendido. In 2004 he re-joined his old friend and mentor Larry Mindel to open Poggio in Sausalito as Managing Partner, where he remained through spring of 2006. To Perbacco, Gibin brings his Italian hospitality, enhancing the already authentic Italian experience. "I am personally devoted to every guest's enjoyment. Every single person entering our restaurant is greeted as if they are our friends and family. The overall experience is enriched with personal touches, from a little complimentary *aperitivo* to 'let me go to get your car for you.' We want our guests to leave with the thought of 'How soon can we return to Perbacco?'"

At Perbacco, Umberto is able to really embrace his love of wine. Hours of research and countless tastings have resulted in a classical yet diversified wine list with an emphasis on the wines of the Piemonte region in northern Italy, such as Barolo, Barbaresco, Dolcetto, and several fruity, aromatic whites. The extensive list is rounded out by a selection of bottles from elsewhere in Italy and an appealing collection of New World options. Gibin explains, "The wine list at Perbacco is designed to enhance the overall experience. I have chosen wines that will complement the dishes that Staffan has created, particularly those from small producers and with a good balance of fruit, acid and tannin. At Perbacco, the wine service is simple yet sophisticated. It will give our guests the opportunity to enjoy wine in many different ways."

Recipe courtesy of Umberto Gibin.

. . . .

Agnolotti Dal Plin (Pasta Filled with Roasted Meats and Savoy Cabbage)

Entrée • Phases Two–Four • Serves 8

INGREDIENTS

Dough:

3 cups Italian "00" flour or all-purpose flour

5 whole large eggs, plus 5 egg yolks

Filling:

2 Tbsp. butter

1 garlic clove, thinly sliced

1 sprig fresh rosemary; leaves only

2 pounds roasted veal shoulder or breast, chopped in food processor

2 cups Savoy cabbage, cut into 1" pieces

½ cup reduced veal or beef broth

1½ cup freshly grated Parmigiano-Reggiano

Freshly grated nutmeg, to taste

Salt and freshly ground black pepper

INSTRUCTIONS

Pasta:

- Sift and mound the flour in the center of a large wooden cutting board.

- Make a well in the middle of the flour and add the eggs.

- With a fork, beat together the eggs and begin to incorporate the flour, starting with the inner rim of the well.

- As the well expands, continue pushing the flour up from the base of the mound to retain the well shape. The dough will come together when half of the flour is incorporated.

- Start kneading the dough with both hands, using the palms of your hands.

- Knead for about 15 minutes, adding any of the remaining flour if necessary to create a cohesive mass.
- Once you have a cohesive mass, remove the dough from the board and scrape up and discard any leftover bits.
- Lightly re-flour the board and continue kneading for 6 more minutes. The dough should be elastic and a little sticky.
- Wrap the dough in plastic and allow to rest for 30 minutes at room temperature.
- In a 12-inch saucepan, add 1 tablespoon of butter over high heat until hot but not smoking.
- Add the garlic and rosemary and let cook until the garlic is light golden brown; about 5 minutes.
- Add the veal, and cook for 8–10 minutes.
- Season with salt and pepper, to taste.
- Do not be afraid to let the meat begin to caramelize a bit.

Filling:

- In a fitted pot, melt butter and add Savoy cabbage and ¼ cup of water.
- Cover with a lid and cook until cabbage is very tender.
- Chop in food processor until almost smooth.
- Let the veal cool to room temperature and place in a large mixing bowl.
- Stir in the Parmigiano, cabbage, veal broth, a pinch of nutmeg and salt and pepper, to taste.
- Use a wooden spoon to mix until well combined. Set aside.
- Cut the pasta dough into 3 equally sized pieces.
- Re-wrap 2 of the pieces in plastic wrap and set aside.
- Begin working with the 1 unwrapped piece of dough.
- On a lightly floured work surface, use a floured rolling pin to roll out the pasta dough until it is ⅛-inch thick (you can also use a pasta machine and roll out the dough on its thinnest setting).
- Lay the resulting pasta sheet on a lightly floured surface with a long side facing you.
- Trim the edges so they are straight.

- Using a tablespoon, scoop equally-sized spoonfuls of the filling and place along the bottom half of the pasta sheet, leaving a 1½-inch border of dough at the bottom and sides: each dollop of filling should be approximately 1½ inches away from the next.

- Pull the top edge of the pasta up and over the filling. The dough should form 1 large pocket over the dollops of filling.

- Seal the agnolotti by gently and carefully molding the pasta over the filling and pressing lightly with your index finger to seal the edge of the dough to the pasta sheet; don't drag your finger along the dough to seal, or you risk ripping the dough.

- When sealed, there should be about ½-inch of excess dough visible along the bottom of the mounds of filling (where you sealed it). Be certain that you are sealing tightly while pressing out any pockets of air. Seal the left and right ends of the dough.

Agnolotti:

- Starting at one end of the dough, place the thumb and forefinger of each hand together as if you were going to pinch something and, leaving about 1-inch of space between your hands and holding your fingers vertically, pinch the filling in 1-inch increments, making about ¾-inch of "pinched" are between each pocket of filling.

- Run a sharp knife or crimped pastry wheel along the bottom edge of the folded-over dough, separating the strip of filled pockets from the remainder of the pasta sheet. (Don't cut too close to the filling, or you risk breaking the seal.)

- Separate the individual agnolotti by cutting the center of each pinched area, rolling the pastry wheel away from you.

- Working quickly, place the agnolotti on a baking sheet dusted with a thin layer of cornmeal, which will help prevent sticking. (Don't let the agnolotti touch.)

- Repeat with the 2 remaining dough balls until the entire bowl of filling has been used.

- Let the shaped agnolotti rest for 24 minutes.

Assembly:

- Bring 6 quarts water to a rolling boil, and add 2 tablespoons salt.

- Add the agnolotti to the water and cook until tender, about 4 minutes total.

- Drain well and toss with a sauce or ragu of your choice or a combination of beef broth and butter.
- Sprinkle with freshly grated Parmigiano-Reggiano and serve immediately.

Nutrition Facts (per serving)
Calories: **430** • Calories from fat: **47%** • Fat: **23g**
Saturated fat: **10g** • Cholesterol: **270mg** • Carbohydrates: **28g**
Protein: **28g** • Sodium: **320mg** • Fiber: **1g**

●

The Ritz-Carlton Bacara,
Santa Barbara

8301 Hollister Avenue, Santa Barbara, CA
(805) 968-0100 • www.ritzcarlton.com/en/hotels/california/santa-barbara

Situated on a beautiful seventy-eight acres overlooking the Pacific Ocean just north of Santa Barbara, Bacara offers a luxurious, peaceful retreat, featuring a world-class spa, excellent dining in their signature restaurant Miro, or more casual fare at the Bistro. Bacara features sumptuous guest rooms in beautiful mission-style buildings, and sprawling, beautifully landscaped, impeccably manicured grounds. Bacara is the ideal getaway with several pools, fitness center, horseback riding, and golf, as well as the opportunity to explore beautiful Santa Barbara and the nearby wine country of Santa Barbara County.

Recipe Courtesy of Executive Chef David Reardon.

Tomato Soup with Goat Cheese Crème

Soup • Phases Two–Four (see Note) • Serves 12

INGREDIENTS

5 Tbsp. olive oil

2 Tbsp. minced garlic

2 large onions

8 pounds of Bacara Ranch Heirloom Tomatoes or 10 pounds canned peeled plum tomatoes

1 Tbsp. finely chopped fresh oregano,
   or 1 ¼ tsp. dried
1 Tbsp. finely chopped fresh thyme, or
   1 ¼ tsp. dried
¼ tsp. minced chives
3 Tbsp. chopped fresh basil

8 cups water
1 cup heavy whipping cream
salt and pepper, to taste
3 ounces goat cheese
12 ¼-inch-thick basil brioche slices
   (see Note)

INSTRUCTIONS

- Heat 3 Tbsp. oil in large pot over medium-high heat.
- Add garlic and onion and sauté until fragrant, about 2 minutes.
- Stir in tomatoes, oregano, thyme, chives, and basil.
- Add water and bring to boil. Reduce heat and simmer uncovered until soup thickens slightly, about 25 minutes.
- Stir ½ cup of cream and remove from heat.
- Place soup in blender and blend until you reach a smooth consistency.
- Season to taste with salt and pepper.
- Meanwhile, pre-heat broiler. Brush both sides of brioche slices with remaining 2 Tbsp. oil.
- Transfer to large baking sheet. Broil croutons until golden, about 2 minutes per side.
- Serve with soup.
- For the goat cheese cream, place ½ cup heavy cream in a chilled bowl and whip until the cream is just thick. Crumble the goat cheese into the cream and continue whipping until it becomes thick. Place a small quenelle of the cream on each crouton.
- Place 6 ounces of soup in each bowl, center with the crouton and goat cheese crème, and serve immediately.

NOTE

For calorie analysis, we are assuming each crouton is a slice of a baguette, which is approximately 80 calories. If you want to enjoy this soup in Phase One, simply omit the goat cheese, cream, and baguette—it is still delicious!

Nutrition Facts (per serving)
Calories: **276** • Calories from fat: **64%** • Fat: **14g**
Saturated fat: **6g** • Cholesterol: **30mg** • Carbohydrates: **17g**
Protein: **5g** • Sodium: **546mg**

•

Valette Restaurant

344 Center St., Healdsburg, CA 95448 • (707) 473-0946 • www.valettehealdsburg.com

The dream of Valette began nearly two decades ago between two brothers. While enjoying a glass of wine on their father's porch overlooking the beautiful Alexander Valley vineyards of Sonoma County, Dustin Valette and Aaron Garzini envisioned opening a restaurant together which would provide a place for Sonoma County farmers, winemakers, and artisans to showcase their craft. The restaurant would be located in Healdsburg, the heart of Sonoma County— and the location where their great-grandfather operated bakeries. They would serve high-quality, yet honest food, offer warm and impeccable service, and house a collection of boutique, small-production wines. At the time, Aaron was establishing himself as a dynamic server and sommelier in Sonoma County and Dustin was in New York learning the culinary craft. They never lost sight of their dream.

In 2015, Valette Restaurant opened its doors, showcasing the brothers' combined forty-seven years of restaurant experience and a deep dedication to Sonoma Country and its food and wine community. Chef Dustin Valette honed his craft in some of the most celebrated restaurants on the west coast, including the Michelin-starred Aqua in San Francisco and Napa Valley's Bouchon. Additional credits include Hokus at the Mandarin Oriental Hotel Honolulu, a five-star, five-diamond property; the exclusive North Ranch Country Club in Westlake Village, California, and VOX Restaurant & Wine Lounge in Henderson, Nevada. Most recently, Valette spent six years as Executive Chef of Dry Creek Kitchen, a Charlie Palmer restaurant in downtown Healdsburg. At Dry Creek Kitchen, he gathered great acclaim for the strong relationships he cultivated with local farmers and purveyors in order to provide the restaurant with the area's freshest and most unique ingredients.

Valette was known for his exceptional ability to pair some of the country's best wines with his intense, flavorful, and dynamic cuisine. Valette is a graduate of the Culinary Institute of America in Hyde Park, New York. Aaron refined his skills in the art of providing first class service at John Ash & Co., spending a decade with this pioneer in world-renowned wine country cuisine. A desire to expand his leadership and service talents led Aaron to the San Francisco restaurant scene, gaining several years of invaluable experience at Betelnut Restaurant on Union Street. Aaron then returned to his Sonoma County roots as the restaurant manager at Rustic Restaurant, Francis Coppola's restaurant at his famed Geyserville, CA-based winery.

Recipe courtesy of Chef/Owner Dustin Valette.

. . . .

Burrata & Peach Salad with Pickled Green Peaches, Char Grilled Peaches & Peach Leaf Vinaigrette

Salad • Phases Two–Four • Serves 4

This dish is a fun spin off a classic and utilizing the 'whole peach'. The aromatic Sauvignon Musque clone adds an amazing floral note to the wine and blend harmoniously with the aromatic kaffir lime vinaigrette.

INGREDIENTS

½ cup peach leaves, medium-sized and young
2 ounces Champagne vinegar
6 ounces canola Oil
6 kaffir lime leaves
1½ tsp. Dijon mustard
2 cups green peaches, the size of an almond and young
½ cup cane sugar
1 cup Champagne vinegar
4 ripe peaches, washed
4 4-ounce balls burrata Cheese
½ loaf sourdough baguette
1 cup red endive leaves, washed

4 cups baby wild arugula, washed
extra-virgin olive oil, drizzle to lightly coat baguette

INSTRUCTIONS

Pickled Peaches[1]:

- Start by cleaning the baby peaches in warm water.
- Blanch them in boiling, salted water for 2 minutes.
- In a medium saucepot combine the sugar, vinegar and a pinch of salt; bring to a boil and pour over the blanched peaches and cool.
- Refrigerate for 3 days and up to 1 month. Once pickled slice very thin.

Peach Leaf Vinaigrette:

- Pick medium-sized young peach leaves and wash them vigorously. Place the leaves and the vinegar in a small pot and gently warm, allow to infused strain and discard leaves.
- In a small pot combine the kaffir leaves and canola oil; warm over low heat until around 115 degrees; steep for 45 minutes.
- Once infused, strain and discard leaves.
- In a blender place the mustard, peach leaf vinegar and flesh of one peach.
- Purée until smooth then slowly add the kaffir lime oil.
- Adjust seasoning with fresh pepper and salt.

Grilled Peaches:

- Start by taking ripe peaches and cutting into wedges.
- Toss in extra-virgin olive oil, salt and fresh pepper.
- Grill them over a wood burning grill or BBQ approximately 2 minutes.
- Slice the baguette into 8 long croutons, toss with extra-virgin olive oil, salt and pepper; lightly grill until golden brown.

Assembly:

- In a small bowl combine the endive and arugula, toss with the peach leaf vinaigrette and season with salt and pepper.
- In the center of the plate make a line with the salad, place the warm grilled peaches on top, sprinkle with the sliced green peaches and the grilled bread to one side.

---

1   If baby peaches are not available you can substitute pearl onions.

- Finish with the burrata, drizzled extra-virgin olive oil and a little sea salt. Repeat with the remaining dishes.

NOTE

May reduce sugar (or substitute with agave nectar for dietary purposes), and omit bread for dietary purposes, and may serve ½ portion of burrata (90 calories per ounce).

Nutrition Facts (per serving)
Calories: **686** • Calories from fat: **60%** • Fat: **46g**
Saturated fat: **18g** • Cholesterol: **80mg** • Carbohydrates: **36g**
Protein: **23g** • Sodium: **479mg** • Fiber: **4g**

Colorado

•

Campo de Fiori, Aspen and Vail

205 S. Mill St., #24, Aspen, CO 81611 • (970) 920-7717
100 East Meadow Dr., Vail, CO 81657 • (970) 476-8994
www.campodefiori.net

Campo de Fiori uses the freshest local ingredients and imported cured meats and dried goods from Italy to create exceptional authentic Italian cuisine, paired with an excellent wine list. The team's personalized care and service create a festive and vibrant atmosphere that feels like a party! Chef Luigi Giordani (also of Acquolina) grew up in Italy watching his uncle, a Chef, create magnificent dishes for guests. Luigi obtained a degree from an esteemed culinary school in Rome. When he arrived in the U.S., Luigi had already worked at several fine eateries throughout Europe and established his stellar reputation while working as the Executive Chef of Prego Ristorante in Irvine, California. In 1992, Luigi along with his wife Elizabeth Plotke, who loved food and cooking since childhood, planned to move to Italy, via a six-month detour through Aspen, Colorado. It was then that a love affair with the Colorado mountains and Aspen began. Using their entire life savings and tapping into the creativity of their friends and family, they started Campo de Fiori (Field of Flowers) in Aspen. In 1995, the first year of operation Campo won an award for one of the top new restaurants in the country. In 1997, applying the successful techniques and exemplary standards, Luigi and Elizabeth focused on opening Campo de Fiori Ristorante in Vail, and later Acquolina in Aspen.

Recipe courtesy of Elizabeth Plotke.

· ·

Linguine Diavola with Lobster

Entrée • Phases Two–Four • Serves 4

INGREDIENTS

2 28-ounce canned peeled tomatoes (do not drain)

4 medium-sized fresh lobsters (for nutritional analysis we used 1¼ pound lobsters, which typically yield about 20 percent of their shell weight, or about 3–3½ ounces of meat)

8 garlic cloves, very finely chopped

1 16-ounce box of dried linguine from Italy—or fresh if you have access (see Note)

2 tsp. fresh mint, finely chopped

1 tsp. of crushed red pepper

4 Tbsp. olive oil

4 Tbsp. cold pressed extra-virgin olive oil to drizzle at the end (see note)

½ tsp. salt (for sauce)

Kosher salt (one handful for pasta cooking water)

INSTRUCTIONS

· Chop the tomatoes and set them aside in their juice.

· In a large sautéed pan, heat the olive oil over medium-low heat.

· Add garlic and about a ½ teaspoon of salt and cook until the garlic is translucent.

· Add chili flakes and cook for another minute, all the while gently mixing the garlic and chili with a wooden spoon.

· Add the tomatoes and tomato juice. Raise the heat to medium and let the tomato juice begin to simmer. Once it's bubbling a little, turn the heat back down to low and simmer for about 2 hours. The tomatoes will dissolve into the sauce in this time. Once the sauce is complete, check if salt is needed. Set everything aside.

· Steam the lobsters for about 15–20 minutes and then remove from heat and allow them to cool down a little.

· Bring a large pot of water to boil. Add a medium handful of kosher salt to the water for flavor. Add the linguine, stirring occasionally and cook until it is still firm or *al dente*.

· Drain the pasta, saving about 1 cup of the salted pasta water on the side.

· Break down the lobsters, removing all the meat from the tail, claws, etc. Discard the roe and green goop. All the other meat is great and usable.

Set all the large pieces of meat aside in a deep bowl, so the meat remains warm but is no longer cooking. Take all the small pieces and chop them up and set them in a small bowl.

- Begin to reheat your tomato sauce in its same pan over medium heat adding a few large spoonfuls of the pasta water.
- Toss in the cooked linguine and stir.
- After about 1–2 minutes, add in all the small pieces of chopped lobster meat. Stir everything together, adding pasta water and olive oil for proper moisture and consistency.
- After another 1–2 minutes, distribute portions of pasta with sauce into 4 pasta bowls. Take all the large lobster meat pieces and place the meat on top of the linguine.
- Drizzle everything with the cold pressed olive oil (optional) and sprinkle the fresh mint.

NOTE

For weight-loss purposes, I suggest the following: make 3 ounces of pasta per serving (pasta is 100 calories per ounce, so you save 100 calories). Also, omit the additional olive oil at the end (120 calories per Tbsp.). By reducing the amount of pasta to 3 ounces and eliminating the additional Tbsp. of olive oil, the calorie count is down to 632 per serving.

Nutrition Facts (per serving)
Calories: **752** • Calories from fat: **36%** • Fat: **30g**
Saturated fat: **4g** • Cholesterol: **0mg** • Carbohydrates: **96g**
Protein: **18g** • Sodium: **2,154mg**

The Little Nell

675 East Durant Ave., Aspen, CO 81611 • (970) 920-4600 (Main Number)
Ajax Tavern : 685 East Durant Ave., Aspen, CO 81611 • (970) 920-6334
element 47: (970) 920-6330
www.thelittlenell.com

The Little Nell has the honor of being Aspen's only five-star, Five-Diamond hotel (also a Relais & Châteaux resort). Prominently situated at the base of the famed Aspen Mountain gondola, the setting is unparalleled. Enjoy Aspen's best après-ski at the casual-chic Ajax Tavern on the sun-drenched patio facing the slopes. Savor a gourmet meal in element 47, featuring a 20,000-bottle *Wine Spectator* Grand Award-winning wine cellar and program led by Master Sommelier Carlton McCoy. Before arriving at The Little Nell in 2011, McCoy worked at Thomas Keller's Per Se, Marcus Samuelsson's Aquavit, Tom Colicchio's Craft Steak in New York, and Eric Zeibold's CityZen at The Mandarin Oriental in Washington, D.C.

Carlton was drawn to The Little Nell by the notable wine program and the property's exciting reputation. In May of 2013, Carlton became the 10th Master Sommelier to come through The Little Nell's famed wine program. Considered the top dining destination in all of Colorado, element 47's Executive Chef, Matt Zubrod, began his career with Ritz-Carlton, initially working in Aspen, Naples, and Boston before moving on to the historic Hotel del Coronado in San Diego as Executive Sous-Chef. In 1999, he took over The Vail Cascade Resort as Executive Chef and opened The Ritz-Carlton, Aspen Highlands as Executive Chef in 2001. He next moved to Hawaii where he opened Monette's at Mauna Kea Resort and then California at Rancho Valencia Resort & Spa before returning to Aspen in 2013 to serve as Executive Chef at BB's Kitchen until joining The Little Nell.

"Matt's style of cooking encompasses a variety of flavors informed by Alpine and coastal influences from his time working in the Rocky Mountains and by the Pacific Ocean," said The Little Nell's Managing Director, Simon Chen. As Executive Chef, Matt's main objective is "to continue establishing The Little Nell as the culinary hub of Colorado." Named after a mining claim originally located not far uphill from where the hotel sits today, The Little Nell attracts a diverse international clientele, including celebrities, dignitaries, Fortune 500 magnates and political leaders. Enjoying *"La Dolce Vita"* at The Little Nell calls to mind the kind of stylish, international scenes depicted by the late LeRoy Neiman. For the ultimate in world-class luxury, service, and amenities, look to The Little Nell.

Recipes courtesy of May Selby, Director of Public Relations, The Little Nell.

. . . .

Ajax Tavern's Brussel Sprouts with Pomegranate Molasses

Side/Vegetable • Phases Two–Four • Serves 2

INGREDIENTS

20 Brussels sprouts

1 pomegranate

2 ounces pomegranate molasses
  (see Note)

1 ounce fresh lemon juice

2 ounces chestnuts

1 Tbsp. olive oil

2 Tbsp. butter (see Note)

INSTRUCTIONS

• Take Brussel sprouts and cut them in half lengthwise.

• Blanch them in boiling, salted water for 5 minutes or until tender. Then shock in ice-water to cool.

• In a large sauté pan, heat up olive oil until the smoke point. Remove from heat and add Brussels. Add butter to even out browning color to Brussels.

• Once golden-brown, remove from pan and add pomegranate molasses, pomegranate seeds, lemon juice, and crushed chestnuts to finish on top.

NOTE

If you can't find pomegranate molasses, you can buy pomegranate juice from the store and reduce it in a pan on a low flame until it reaches a syrupy consistency. You may choose to reduce quantity of butter in half for dietary purposes.

Nutrition Facts (per serving)
Calories:**360** • Calories from fat: **47.5%** • Fat: **19g**
Saturated fat: **8g** • Cholesterol: **31mg** • Carbohydrates: **30g**
Protein:**4.5g** • Sodium: **27mg** • Fiber: **3.5g**

Created by By Ricardo Leyvas, Bar Manager at The Little Nell.

. . . .

Mountain Mojito Recipe

Cocktail • Phases Three–Four • Serves 1

INGREDIENTS

1½ ounces Montanya platinum rum

½ ounce fresh lime juice

½ ounce agave nectar

½ ounce blood orange purée

4 fresh mint leaves (at The Little Nell, these are clipped from the gardens)

splash of soda water

INSTRUCTIONS

- Muddle the mint along with the lime juice and agave in a Collins glass
- Add ice and the rest of the ingredients
- Top with soda water (club soda, seltzer, or mineral water)
- Garnish with fresh mint

●

Connecticut

•

Finalmente Trattoria, Westport

165 Post Rd. East, Westport, CT 06880

(203) 226-8500 • www.finalmentetrattoria.com

Andre Iodice's dream of opening a family-owned and operated regional Italian restaurant is alive with Finalmente Trattoria! Located in downtown Westport, CT just blocks away from the Westport Playhouse—it's the perfect place for an intimate dinner before or after the show.

While growing up in in Isola Di Ponza, Italy, off the coast of southern Lazio, south of Rome, Andre learned about food and culture by watching his family members in the kitchen concocting and tasting family recipes. Ponza is an island retreat of influential Romans who want to escape without the "see and be seen" aspect and crowds of Capri.

Surrounded by pristine Mediterranean waters, the island is naturally known for exceptional seafood! This is where Andrea's passion for the culinary arts was born. Andre came to New York in 1970 and worked at a butcher shop, and later in restaurants, including as a *pizzaiolo* or pizza maker in Greenwich before he and his wife, Mary, opened Finalmente in 2006. Andre is honored to share his life's passion for authentic Italian cuisine and warm, genuine "family-style" hospitality with his "family" of guests who come to enjoy Finalmente and the hospitality of the Iodice family, who have created an Italian gem in Westport. A true Italian-American success story—his dream has come true!

Recipe courtesy of Chef Andre Iodice.

. . . .

"Squaletto Isolano"
(Halibut with Sun-dried Tomatoes, Artichokes, Capers, Olives, & Prosecco)

Entrée • All Phases • Serves 1

INGREDIENTS

1 8-ounce fillet of Halibut

2 Tbsp. olive oil for sauté

2 Marinated artichoke hearts

3 Sun-dried tomatoes

1 Tbsp. capers

1 Tbsp. Gaeta olives

¼ cup fish broth

½ cup Prosecco

Pinch of salt and pepper

Italian parsley to garnish

INSTRUCTIONS

- Start with 2 Tbsp. olive oil and salt and pepper in a sauté pan. Brown the halibut fillet on both sides, discard excess oil.

- Add ½ cup Prosecco wine, capers, olives, artichokes and sun-dried tomatoes and sautée 5–7 minutes. At the end, add fish broth and bake in the oven for 10 minutes.

- Finish with minced Italian parsley to garnish.

NOTE

You can also use other fish, such as flounder, grouper, snapper, sole, swordfish, and Chilean sea bass. This is a preparation Chef Andre especially recommends for Christmas Eve dinner, which is typically a seafood event, called the *Vigilia di Natale*.

Nutrition Facts (per serving)
Calories: **493** • Calories from fat: **23%** • Fat: **13g**
Saturated fat: **2g** • Cholesterol: **72mg** • Carbohydrates: **29g**
Protein: **56g** • Sodium: **1,419mg** • Fiber: **12g**

●

Homestead Inn/Thomas Henkelmann, a Relais & Châteaux Luxury Resort and Restaurant,
Greenwich

420 Field Point Rd., Greenwich, CT 06830
(203) 869-7500 • www.homesteadinn.com

Thomas and Theresa Henkelmann have owned and operated the exquisite, luxurious hotel and renowned restaurant since 1997 in the exclusive Belle Haven section of Greenwich. The exclusive Relais & Châteaux property is an "architectural masterpiece with a luxury hotel and world-renowned French restaurant...an impressive modern showcase of elegance, warmth, and sophistication," says Theresa Henkelmann. Chef Henkelmann grew up working in his family's restaurant in the beautiful Black Forest region of Germany, close to the border of Alsace, France, trained at some of the top restaurants and hotels in Europe before coming to the U.S. He is also a proud recipient of the coveted titles: Relais & Châteaux—Grand Chef, Tradition et Qualité—Les Grandes Tables du Monde, and has received a 4-star rating by the New York Times. Thomas Henkelmann Restaurant offers contemporary French cuisine, seasonal specialties, and many signatures dishes for which he has become famous.

Chef Henkelmann calls his philosophy of creating edible art *gemütlichkeit*. I call it art on a plate! Homestead Inn and Thomas Henkelmann restaurant have long been considered one the country's finest dining and lodging destinations, and is considered the top restaurant in the state of Connecticut, located within an hour of Midtown Manhattan. After getting to know Fred and being featured together in a *Venu Magazine* article titled "Living Gourmet the Fred Bollaci Way," (Fall 2014), Theresa Henkelmann so generously referred to Fred Bollaci as "The Robert Parker of healthy gourmet food and travel"—indeed a major compliment! Thomas Henkelmann and Homestead Inn are a perfect destination for an award-winning dining and lodging experience: come for dinner and stay for the weekend!

Recipe courtesy of Chef Thomas Henkelmann.

Oven Baked Loin of Rabbit with Foie Gras

Entrée • Phases Two–Four • Serves 4

INGREDIENTS

1 pound rabbit saddle[2]

2½ ounces Hudson Valley duck
   foie gras

1 baby bok choy

2 medium-sized artichokes

1 shallot, sliced

1 ounce dry white wine

1 bouquet garni (tied bouquet of fresh
   herbs, see Note)

½ ounce dried raisins

½ ounce pine nuts

¼ ounce capers

1 ounce extra-virgin olive oil

¼ ounce balsamic vinegar

¼ ounce unsalted butter

salt and pepper, to taste

INSTRUCTIONS

Artichoke Purée[3]:

- Using a small pot, sweat the sliced shallot in ¼ ounce of olive oil until tender (not colored).

- Add the artichoke hearts and dry white wine.

- Add the bok choy.

- For the bouquet garni, either purchase one that is already assembled at a market, or make your own by tying fresh herbs together. Typically, they include thyme, Bay Leaf, parsley, basil, burnet, chervil, rosemary, peppercorns, and tarragon, among others, but assemble a mixture of fresh herbs—from the garden or store—and tie together with butcher string.

- Cover the pot and steam the artichokes and the bouquet garni.

- Season with a little salt and freshly ground pepper and cook until the artichokes and bok choy are each tender.

- Remove each from liquid when tender.

- Place bok choy into an ice bath (bowl with ice and water) for several seconds, and set aside to dry (you will use it to garnish the plates).

---

2   Have your butcher prepare the rabbit with the loins attached to the tenderloin.

3   This should be made in advance, before you begin searing the rabbit.

- Steam-dry the artichokes in a warm place for a few minutes.
- Clean the artichoke by trimming and removing outer leaves and the very bottom of the stem, peeling back with a paring knife until you have the heart. For home preparation, you may purchase artichoke hearts that have already been cleaned.
- Purée the artichoke hearts in a food processor until smooth, and then push through a sieve.

Rabbit:

- Remove the 2 loins and 2 tenderloins from the rabbit saddle with the flanks attached.
- Trim the flanks approximately 2½ inches in length.
- Cut the foie gras in 2 strips matching the loin of rabbit.
- Sear the foie gras in a very hot frying pan for 3–4 seconds, seasoned with salt and freshly ground pepper.
- Set foie gras in a cool place, spread out the loins of rabbit with flanks attached.
- Set the tenderloins of rabbit on top of the smaller part of the rabbit loin and the seared cooled foie gras slightly next to the loin.
- Wrap the flank around the loin and secure with butcher string.
- Heat a frying pan with ¼ ounce of olive oil, sear the rabbit quickly on 3 sides, and turn onto un-seared side.
- Place frying pan into pre-heated oven at 400 degrees Fahrenheit for 8–10 minutes.

Artichoke Chips (optional):

- Thinly slice 4 artichoke bottoms using a mandoline.
- Fry in vegetable oil until crisp.
- Drain on a paper towel and salt lightly.

Vinaigrette:

- Toast the pine nuts in a dry sauté pan, then deglaze and lightly reduce with the balsamic vinegar.
- Whisk the olive oil into the balsamic vinegar reduction to emulsify.
- Season to taste with salt and pepper.
- Add the raisins and capers.

- Keep warm.

Assembly:

- For each plate, form a small circle on the plate with a slice of the cooked bok choy.
- Slice the rabbit roulade into 3 even pieces and arrange the pieces evenly around the bok choy.
- Create 3 teaspoon-size quenelles of artichoke purée and arrange them between the rabbit slices.
- Place one artichoke chip on each quenelle like a sail.
- Spoon a small amount of the vinaigrette around the outer edge of the rabbit and artichoke.

Nutrition Facts (per serving)
Calories: **466** • Calories from fat: **51%** • Fat: **26.5g**
Saturated fat: **7g** • Cholesterol: **122mg** • Carbohydrates: **17g**
Protein: **41g** • Sodium: **500mg** • Fiber: **6g**

. . . .

Salmon in Brick with Russian Ossetra

Entrée • Phases Two–Four • Serves 6

INGREDIENTS

Salmon:

6 4-ounce center-cut fillets of salmon

6 feuille de brick[4]

6 ounces Ossetra caviar

1½ ounces extra-virgin olive oil

juice of ½ lemon

salt and pepper

4 ounces sour cream

1 ounce salmon roe

Sauce Diable[5]:

1 shallot minced

15 black peppercorns

2 ounces Champagne vinegar

---

4   This is the type of very thin pastry dough that may be purchased at a gourmet market or ordered online.

5   Yields about 2 cups.

3 ounces brown veal stock (or
   beef stock)

2 cups tomato juice
salt, cayenne pepper to taste

INSTRUCTIONS

Salmon:

- Core the salmon fillets in the center and fill each with ½ ounce of caviar.
- Season the fillets with lemon juice, salt, and pepper.
- Cut the *feuille* of brick the width of the salmon fillet and brush with olive oil.
- Set the salmon fillet on top of the *feuille* of brick and wrap tightly.
- Pre-heat oven to 420 degrees Fahrenheit.
- Use the remaining olive oil in a pre-heated non-stick fry pan.
- Sear each side of the wrapped-salmon fillets quickly until lightly golden.
- Place pan with salmon in pre-heated oven until rare (several minutes).
- Remove from oven and let rest in a warm place for 3–5 minutes.

Sauce Diable:

- Simmer the shallot and peppercorns in the champagne vinegar until it is reduced by half.
- Add the veal stock and tomato juice.
- Simmer for about 20 minutes.
- Strain and season to taste.
- Use the sauce to arrange on the plate with the salmon (as pictured).

Assembly:

- Arrange 2 pieces of cooked salmon fillets around the bok choy. Add a ring of Sauce Diable, and dollops of sour cream

NOTE

For weight-loss purposes, you may omit or use light sour cream, and add salmon roe, as shown.

Nutrition Facts (per serving)
Calories: **451** • Calories from fat: **41%** • Fat: **21g**
Saturated fat: **4.5g** • Cholesterol: **76mg** • Carbohydrates: **36g**
Protein: **33g** • Sodium: **646mg** • Fiber: **2g**

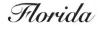

Florida

•

Abe and Louie's,
Boca Raton and Boston, MA

See recipe for Roasted Beet, Poached Pear, and Goat Cheese Salad, and recipe for Beef and Mushroom Barley Soup in Boston, MA.

•

Addison Reserve Country Club,
Delray Beach—Chef de Cuisine, Zach Bell

A private, member-owned equity club community
7201 Addison Reserve Blvd., Delray Beach, FL 33446
(561) 637-4004 • www.addisonreserve.cc

Addison Reserve Country Club features delicious cuisine prepared by Chef Zach Bell of Café Boulud fame in Palm Beach. Chef Bell, a four-time James Beard finalist, worked for Daniel Boulud in New York since 1999 at Café Boulud and was named the head chef at Palm Beach's Café Boulud from its inception in 2003 through 2011, when he came to join Addison. Addison, a private member-owned club, has been recognized as one of the top country club communities in the United States and designated a Platinum Club of America by *Boardroom Magazine*.

Recipes courtesy of Chef Zach Bell and Addison Reserve Country Club.

. . . .

Chilled Curry Cauliflower Soup

Soup • All Phases • Serves 8

INGREDIENTS

Soup base:

½ cup extra-virgin olive oil

7 cloves garlic, peeled and thinly sliced

2 leeks, white and light green
  parts only, halved, thinly sliced,
  and washed

1 medium onion, thinly sliced

a pinch of salt and pepper, to taste

2 Tbsp. madras curry powder

2 small Yukon gold potatoes, peeled
  and thinly sliced

5 pounds cauliflower, roughly cut

½ cup white wine

Garnish:

1 cup diced granny smith apple (diced
  small; without skin),

2 kiwis (diced small; without skin),

3 sprigs each mint, cilantro, and basil,
  washed and chopped

2 Tbsp. extra-virgin olive oil

INSTRUCTIONS

Soup:

- Heat the olive oil in a heavy-bottomed casserole over low heat.

- Add the garlic, leeks, and onion, season with salt and pepper, and cover
  with a lid.

- Sweat the garlic, leeks, and onion until tender and translucent, about
  5 minutes.

- Add the curry powder and sweat another minute. (Lower the heat
  if needed.)

- Add the potatoes and continue to cook, covered, for 5 minutes.

- Add the cauliflower and white wine and cook, covered, until all of the
  vegetables are tender, about 15 minutes.

- Taste and season with more salt and pepper if needed.

- Transfer the vegetables to a blender and whir until smooth, adding spring
  water if the mixture is too thick.

- Pour the soup into a container, cover, and refrigerate until cold. (The soup
  may be prepared one day in advance and kept covered in the refrigerator.)

Garnish:

- Gently combine and stir all of the ingredients together in a small mixing bowl. Set aside until needed.

Assembly:

- Re-taste the soup and freshly season if needed. If too thick, thin to desired consistency with spring water. Divide and spoon the soup among 8 chilled soup bowls. Put a spoonful of the garnish in the center of each soup and serve immediately.

NOTE

This is a great soup to enjoy in hot weather, and is a good alternative to *Vichyssoise*.

Nutrition Facts (per serving)
Calories: **270**• Calories from fat:**33%** • Fat: **18g**
Saturated fat: **2g** • Cholesterol: **omg** • Carbohydrates: **24g**
Protein: **5g** • Sodium: **106mg** • Fiber: **7g**

•

The Beach Bistro,
Holmes Beach (Anna Maria Island)

6600 Gulf Drive, Holmes Beach, FL 34217
(941) 778-6444 • www.beachbistro.com

Beach Bistro on Anna Maria Island, from inception, was created with the attempt to achieve perfection. One of the owner's, Sean Murphy, a Nova Scotia native, favorite maxims is, "If you pursue perfection you will achieve a high degree of excellence a good part of the time." Beach Bistro was opened by Sean Murphy and his wife Susan Timmins in the fall of 1985, following a hurricane that pounded the windows of the Bistro's waterfront location for three days. Sean, Susan, friends and family bailed and sand-bagged until exhausted, and only then could they return their attention to opening the restaurant in time for the start of "season"—November 1st. When Sean was asked why he was doggedly determined to open on schedule, he replied "We had spent all our money and were overdrawn by $800...opening night, we took in $848." The rest is history. The Bistro endeavors to procure the very best American food product and serve it at its best. The Bistro serves only fresh grouper, USDA Prime American beef, domestic lamb, and what owners call the "best smoked salmon in the free world." The Bistro's relentless pursuit of excellence in food and service earned substantial acclaim both locally and nationally and has been consistently awarded the highest *Zagat* rating in Florida for years.

Recipe courtesy of Sean Murphy.

. . . .

Beach Bistro's Famous Bouillabaisse

Entrée • All Phases • Serves 8 (6–8 at the restaurant)

INGREDIENTS

6 Tbsp. extra-virgin olive oil

2 cloves garlic, minced

½ cup finely chopped onion

1 cup finely chopped celery

1 leek, white parts only, finely chopped

2 Tbsp. shrimp or crab base

1 Tbsp. dried tarragon

1 Tbsp. fennel seed

2 cups white wine

¼ cup Pernod

1 quart seafood stock (can substitute
    clam juice)

2 cups tomato juice

1 Tbsp. tomato purée

1 dash Tabasco

3 medium tomatoes peeled, seeded,
    and roughly chopped

1 pinch of saffron

3 pounds firm-fleshed fish (ask
    your fishmonger to make
    a recommendation)

16 jumbo shrimp

2 lobster tails

2 dozen mussels, bearded and cleaned

2 dozen little neck or sweet clams,
    well cleaned

8 ounces cleaned, sliced calamari
    tubes and tentacles

INSTRUCTIONS

• Heat a heavy-bottom stockpot over high heat.

• Add oil and garlic.

• Sauté the garlic for 5 minutes and then add the onion, leek, and celery.

• Stir the vegetables well to prevent burning and allow to cook for an additional 3–4 minutes, or until translucent.

- Next add the shrimp or crab base, dried herbs, white wine, and Pernod, bring to a simmer and allow to reduce for 5 minutes.
- Add seafood stock (can substitute clam juice), tomato juice, tomato purée, Tabasco, tomatoes, and saffron and bring to a boil, reduce heat and simmer for 10 minutes.
- Add all the seafood and cook for 6 minutes, or until the shells have opened. Discard any shells that do not open.
- Taste and adjust seasoning.
- Serve with a dollop of aioli and toasted French bread (optional—omit for weight-loss purposes.

Nutrition Facts (per serving)
Calories: **498** • Calories from fat: **28%** • Fat: **15g**
Saturated fat: **2g** • Cholesterol: **195mg** • Carbohydrates: **14g**
Protein: **60g** • Sodium: **778mg** • Fiber: **2g**

•

Ben's Kosher Deli,
Boca Raton and New York locations

See recipe for Ben's Israeli Salad in New York.

•

Bern's Steakhouse, Tampa

1208 South Howard Avenue, Tampa, FL 33629
(813) 251-2421 • www.bernssteakhouse.com

Bern's Steakhouse in Tampa is an area landmark and dining institution, one of America's most highly regarded steakhouses. Founded over fifty years ago by Bern and Gert Laxer and currently owned by son David, Bern's honors their traditions with an outstanding selection of top-quality, dry-aged USDA Prime beef, cooked to exacting standards (you can specify the thickness and the exact cooking time); top-quality seafood; farm-fresh vegetables; their famous tableside Caesar salad; the largest wine cellar in the world; and the incredible Harry Waugh Dessert Room upstairs. Dining at Bern's is truly an event. Plan to spend several hours and save time to tour the kitchen and wine cellar and to enjoy the Harry Waugh Room. For the ultimate experience, book a stay at Bern's' Epicurean Hotel across the street and visit sister restaurants Élevage and rooftop bar, Edge (in the hotel) and Haven, also in Tampa.

Recipe courtesy of Brooke Palmer, Public Relations Director, Bern's Steakhouse and SideBern's, and Chef Habteab Hamde, Bern's Steakhouse.

. . . .
Grilled Wild King Salmon with Asparagus & Lobster Vinaigrette

Entrée • Phases Two–Four • Serves 2

INGREDIENTS

Salmon and asparagus:

1 pound wild king salmon
(2 8-ounce portions)
1 Tbsp. olive oil
1 tsp. sea salt

½ tsp. freshly ground white pepper
½ pound asparagus, cleaned and
steamed (trim off bottom, peel
the stalk)

Lobster Vinaigrette:

2 Tbsp. diced shallots
1 tsp. chopped garlic
1 tsp. Dijon mustard
1 Tbsp. tomatoes concasse (tomato
peeled, seeded, and chopped)
2 Tbsp. lobster glace (may substitute
lobster bisque)
2 Tbsp. red wine vinegar
¼ cup canola oil (reduced from ½ cup
for weight-loss purposes)
½ tsp. fresh chopped chervil
½ tsp. fresh chopped tarragon
½ tsp. fresh chopped parsley

½ tsp. fresh chopped chives
sea salt and white pepper, to taste

INSTRUCTIONS

Salmon and asparagus:

• Rub salmon with olive oil, season with sea salt and white pepper. Grill salmon over lump hardwood charcoal (or you may grill on a gas grill at home).

Lobster Vinaigrette:

• In a blender mix together the shallots, garlic, Dijon, tomatoes, lobster glace, and red wine vinegar and blend. Add canola oil slowly and blend to emulsify ingredients. Whisk in the chervil, tarragon, parsley, chives, and salt and pepper.

Assembly:

• Serve salmon with spears of steamed asparagus and lobster vinaigrette.

NOTE

For weight-loss purposes, I recommend using a 6-ounce portion of fish.

Nutrition Facts (per serving)
Calories: **647** • Calories from fat: **68%** • Fat: **49g**
Saturated fat: **5g** • Cholesterol: **101mg** • Carbohydrates: **8g**
Protein: **47g** • Sodium: **1,495mg** • Fiber: **3g**

●

Bice Ristorante,
Palm Beach, Naples, and Orlando
(with locations worldwide)

313 ½ Worth Avenue, Palm Beach, FL 33480
(561) 835-1600 • www.palmbeach.bicegroup.com
300 5th Avenue South, Naples, FL 34102
(239) 262-4044 • www.bice-naples.com
5601 Universal Blvd., Orlando, FL 32819
(407) 503-1415 • www.bice-orlando.com

With locations worldwide: www.bicegroup.com
Also visit their Caffé' Milano in Naples, Florida
www.caffemilanonaples.com

Bice began in fashionable Milan, Italy, in 1926 as the vision of Beatrice Ruggeri, who was known to her family and friends for her extraordinary hospitality and excellent cuisine. For years, those closest to her tried to persuade Beatrice to open a restaurant. In 1926, she reluctantly agreed and opened a neighborhood trattoria or "friendly gathering place," calling it il Ristorante Da Gino e Bice, which later became known as simply "Bice." It was a family affair, with Beatrice in the kitchen and her brothers and sisters serving in the dining room. Bice quickly became known as one of the top Milanese restaurants and Beatrice's sons Remo and Roberto expanded the original concept around the world. Today, Bice is overseen by grandson Raffaele and is consistently known across the globe for excellent Italian cuisine, inspired by the original in Milano. The group also owns fashionable Caffé Milano in downtown Naples.

Recipes courtesy of Raffaele Ruggeri and Bice Group.

. . . .

Branzino alla Griglia
con Vegetali Misti e Salmoriglio
(Mediterranean Sea Bass with Mixed Vegetables and Lemon-Olive Oil Dressing)

Entrée • All Phases • Serves 6

INGREDIENTS

3 whole European sea bass
(approximately 2 pounds each)[6]

1 large vine-ripened tomato, peeled
(use the pulp only), cut julienne
for garnish

6 ounces pumpkin flesh, diced

½ pound baby zucchini, diced

1 cup finely diced fresh hearts of palm

2 stems or leaves of fresh sage

1 pound jumbo lump crab meat

6 romaine hearts, chopped

8 ounces baby arugula

1 ounce diagonally sliced celery heart

juice of 2 lemons

¼ cup extra-virgin olive oil

salt and pepper, to taste

INSTRUCTIONS

• Bring a saucepan filled with water to a boil.

• Make cross incisions on the button of the tomatoes, set in boiling water for 15 seconds, remove to ice-water bath to shock, then peel. Cut into 6 wedges and remove and discard the heart. Use the fillet knife and cut each wedge in 3 and set aside for garnish.

• Peel and cut pumpkin into ½-inch cubes, heat a sauté pan on medium-high heat and pan roast the diced pumpkin, season with salt and pepper, to taste, along with the sage for aroma. Pan roast until softened, remove and let cool before serving.

• Heat a grill or oven to broil.

• Lightly season the fish with salt and pepper, brush a little olive oil on the fillets.

• Grill or broil with the skin side down for 6–7 minutes, or so the skin is crispy and the flesh is moist and flaky.

• Place each sea bass fillet on a dinner plate.

---

6 Filleted and deboned, or you may opt to buy fish already cleaned, leaving the skin on one side (approximately 6 8-ounce fillets).

- In a shallow salad bowl, toss together the zucchini, hearts of palm, and sage. Add the crab meat, romaine, arugula, and celery. Add the diced roasted pumpkin, pour in the lemon juice and olive oil, and toss with salt and pepper, to taste.

- Arrange the salad over and around the fish. Set 3 tomato fillets around each plate for color and serve immediately.

Nutrition Facts (per serving)
Calories: **464** • Calories from fat: **27%** • Fat: **14g**
Saturated fat: **2g** • Cholesterol: **151mg** • Carbohydrates: **7g**
Protein: **74g** • Sodium: **633mg** • Fiber:**2g**

. . . .

Minestrone di Verdure alla Casareccia (Minestrone Soup)

Soup • All Phases • Serves 6

INGREDIENTS

2 Tbsp. olive oil

3-ounce rind of prosciutto

2 large white onions, diced

1 Bay Leaf

12 ounces diced carrots

12 ounces diced celery

12 ounces diced zucchini

12 cups chicken broth

10 ounces green cabbage

1 pound diced potatoes

12 ounces green beans

8 ounces spinach

1 cup frozen peas

salt and pepper, to taste

INSTRUCTIONS

- Heat olive oil in a 6-quart saucepan over medium-high heat.

- Add the prosciutto rind and sauté until brown.

- Add and sauté the diced onion for 2 minutes, then add Bay Leaf, carrots, and celery; sauté another 2 minutes.

- Add the zucchini and chicken broth, bring to a boil, then add cabbage, potatoes, and green beans.

- When potatoes are tender, take 2 cups of the vegetables from the pot and purée in a blender, then pour back into the soup to thicken, stirring everything.

- Just prior to serving, add the spinach and peas and let cook for 1 minute.
- Add salt and pepper, to taste.
- Remove rind and Bay Leaf before serving.

> **Nutrition Facts (per serving)**
> Calories: **183** • Calories from fat: **33%** • Fat: **7g**
> Saturated fat: **3g** • Cholesterol: **13mg** • Carbohydrates: **27g**
> Protein: **7.5g** • Sodium: **2,168mg** • Fiber: **6g**

●

The Bijou Café

1287 First Street, Sarasota, FL 34236 • (941) 366-8111 • www.bijoucafe.net

Sarasota's Bijou Café has been a local landmark for fine Continental dining in the heart of Sarasota's theater and arts district since 1986. Chef Jean-Pierre Knaggs and his wife, Shay, have owned and operated the Bijou since its inception, overseeing every detail from the excellent cuisine (duck and rack of lamb are two signature dishes) to the quaint, yet modern setting with French windows and doors, fresh flowers, and soft candlelight. The cuisine reflects Jean-Pierre's French and South African heritage, and many of his recipes were developed and refined as he traveled the world as chef aboard a luxurious private yacht. Bijou is extremely popular for pre-theater dinner, and serves lunch weekdays.

Recipes courtesy of J. P. Knaggs, Bijou Café.

. . . .

Chilled Tomato-Tarragon Soup

Soup • Phases Two–Four (see Note) • Serves 6

INGREDIENTS

1 medium onion, finely diced
2½ Tbsp. unsalted butter
zest of 1 very ripe orange

4 cups peeled, seeded, and chopped
 fresh tomatoes (or good-
 quality canned)
1 cup good-quality tomato juice

4 cups freshly squeezed orange juice (or good-quality not-from-concentrate)

1 Tbsp. chopped fresh tarragon or 1 tsp. dried tarragon

salt and white pepper, to taste

orange slices and tarragon sprigs for garnish

INSTRUCTIONS

- Sauté the onion lightly in the butter; do not allow it to brown.

- Add the orange zest and stir well.

- In a large non-aluminum pot or stockpot, combine the remaining ingredients and stir well.

- Bring almost to a boil, lower the heat, and simmer for 15 minutes.

- Purée with an immersion blender or let cool and purée in batches in a blender. Chill for several hours before serving.

- Garnish with fresh sprigs of tarragon and very thin slices of unpeeled orange.

NOTE

This is a great soup in Phases Two–Four, but not Phase One, because of the butter (which can be reduced), and the fruit juice (natural sugars).

Nutrition Facts (per serving)
Calories: **167** • Calories from fat: **28%** • Fat: **5g**
Saturated fat: **3g** • Cholesterol: **13mg** • Carbohydrates: **29g**
Protein: **3g** • Sodium: **49mg** • Fiber: **3g**

. . . .

Mixed Greens and Goat Cheese Salad with Confit Tomatoes and Sherry Vinaigrette

Salad • Phases Two–Four • Serves 4

INGREDIENTS

Salad:

6 cups mixed greens

Sherry Vinaigrette

4 ounces goat cheese, cut into pieces

Tomato Confit

Tomato Confit:

2 Tbsp. extra-virgin olive oil

2 cloves garlic, peeled and finely sliced

8 leaves fresh basil, chopped roughly

3 sprigs thyme, leaves only

6 ripe plum tomatoes

½ tsp. granulated sugar (may use
   Splenda for dietary purposes)

salt and pepper, to taste

Sherry Vinaigrette:

2 Tbsp. Dijon mustard

1½ Tbsp. sherry vinegar

2 Tbsp. honey

4 Tbsp. canola oil

freshly ground pepper

INSTRUCTIONS

Tomato Confit:

- Pre-heat oven to 200 degrees Fahrenheit.
- Line a baking sheet with aluminum foil, drizzle with 1 tablespoon of the olive oil, and spread with pastry brush.
- Sprinkle with garlic and half of the herbs. Cut tomatoes in half and lay cut side down.
- Drizzle with remaining olive oil, herbs, sugar, and salt and pepper to taste.
- Place the pan in the middle rack of the oven and bake for 45 minutes.
- Remove from the oven and let cool to room temperature.

Vinaigrette:

- Combine the mustard, vinegar, and honey in a small bowl and slowly whisk in the oil. Season with pepper and reserve at room temperature.

Assembly:

- In a large bowl, drizzle the vinaigrette over the mixed greens and toss.
- Add the goat cheese and toss lightly to coat the cheese with the vinaigrette.
- Divide the greens and goat cheese among 4 plates, top with tomato confit, and serve.

Nutrition Facts (per serving)
Calories: **375** • Calories from fat: **73%** • Fat: **31g**
Saturated fat: **10g** • Cholesterol: **30mg** • Carbohydrates: **17g**
Protein: **11g** • Sodium: **203mg** • Fiber: **2g**

•

Bistro Chez Jean-Pierre,
Palm Beach

132 North County Road, Palm Beach, FL 33480

(561) 833-1171 • www.chezjean-pierre.com

Chef and owner Jean-Pierre Leverrier and his wife, Nicole, opened Chez Jean-Pierre in 1991. A true family affair, their younger son, Guillaume, cooks with his father, while their older son, David, runs the dining room with his mother. Jean-Pierre is a beautiful, elegant establishment. The Leverrier family comes from Normandy, France, and the menu is classic northern French. Jean-Pierre is an authentic French bistro with hearty portions and elegant, yet simple presentations and an extensive wine list. Jean-Pierre features a lovely, warm, and elegant décor that makes diners feel at home. Jean-Pierre has been among the highest *Zagat* rated restaurants in Palm Beach County since opening.

Recipe courtesy of Jean-Pierre Leverrier.

. . . .

Snapper with Herb Sauce and Ratatouille

Entrée • Phases Two–Four • Serves 4

INGREDIENTS

Snapper and Ratatouille:

2 whole snappers[7]	2 medium carrots, chopped
¼ cup olive oil	1 large onion, chopped
½ tsp. fennel seeds	1 leek, chopped

Keep 4 fillets, approximately 8 ounces each, for cooking; keep bodies for fish juice.

2 Tbsp. tomato paste

½ Tbsp. chopped fresh garlic

2 snapper bodies, gills removed,
cleaned thoroughly in cold water

2 tomatoes, chopped

1 large pinch of salt

Herb Butter (optional; see below)

Herb Butter (optional):

3 Tbsp. butter at room temperature

1 Tbsp. chopped Italian parsley

1 Tbsp. chopped chervil

½ Tbsp. chopped tarragon

pinch of salt

INSTRUCTIONS

Snapper:

- Heat ¼ cup olive oil on medium heat.
- Sauté snapper fillets until lightly golden brown (3–4 minutes per side)
- Reduce 1½ cups of fish juice by half, add 3 Tbsp. of Herb Butter and mix together with a whisk.

Ratatouille:

- Heat the olive oil on medium heat.
- Add the fennel seeds and stir 30 seconds.
- Add the carrots, onion, and leek and sweat for 5 minutes.
- Add the tomato paste and garlic and cook 1 minute.
- Add the fish carcasses and tomatoes, top with enough water to cover the fish bodies.
- Add the salt and bring to a boil. Lower the heat to a simmer, and let simmer for 45 minutes.
- Strain through a fine mesh sieve and reserve.

Herb Butter:

- Combine all ingredients and mix thoroughly. Set aside.

Assembly:

- Place a spoonful of ratatouille in the middle of your plate, place the snapper fillet on top of it, spoon sauce around.
- Serve immediately.

Nutrition Facts (per serving)
Calories: **464** • Calories from fat: **48%** • Fat: **25g**
Saturated fat: **8g** • Cholesterol: **104mg** • Carbohydrates: **12g**
Protein: **46g** • Sodium: **818mg** • Fiber: **3g**
Note: without butter, 387 calories per serving.

. . . .

Sautéed Pink Key West Shrimp with Citrus Sauce and Endive Salad

Entrée • All Phases (see Note) • Serves 6

INGREDIENTS

Sauce:

2 ounces lime juice
2 ounces orange juice
2 ounces lemon juice
1 Tbsp. Dijon mustard
salt, to taste
½ cup blended oil (25 percent olive, 75 percent vegetable; reduced for weight-loss purposes)

1 shallot, minced
1 Tbsp. orange zest
1 Tbsp. lemon zest
1 Tbsp. lime zest
2 Tbsp. chopped cilantro
½ cup diced tomato
2 Tbsp. chopped cilantro

Salad:

5 endives, chopped finely
1 cup vinaigrette (mix together ¼ cup sherry vinegar and ¾ cup olive oil)
3 Tbsp. orange juice

2 Tbsp. chopped chives
1 shallot minced
pinch of salt

Shrimp:

24 pink U-10 shrimp (10 per pound) (peeled, deveined, tail on)

1 Tbsp. canola oil

INSTRUCTIONS

• For the sauce, combine the lime juice, orange juice, lemon juice, mustard, and salt in a bowl and whisk together.

- Slowly whisk in the oil; add the shallot, zests, diced tomato, and cilantro. Reserve this mixture and set aside.

- To prepare shrimp, heat a non-stick sauté pan until hot but not smoking, add the canola oil, then add the shrimp being careful not to overcrowd the pan.

- Sear for 2 minutes on one side without disturbing, turn the shrimp over, and cook for 2 more minutes.

- Season with a little salt, turn the heat off, and add the citrus sauce.

- For salad, combine all the salad ingredients in a bowl and toss to mix well.

- Set a little mound of endive salad in the middle of each of 6 plates. Arrange four shrimp on each plate, and spoon the citrus sauce over them.

- Serve.

NOTE

I suggest reducing the amount of oil as much as possible to cut the calories, and this may be made for 8 people, (3 shrimp each), and would thus make it a suitable meal for all Phases.

Nutrition Facts (per serving)
Calories: **538** • Calories from fat: **79%** • Fat: **48g**
Saturated fat: **7g** • Cholesterol: **43mg** • Carbohydrates: **21g**
Protein: **12g** • Sodium: **210mg** • Fiber: **14 g**

•

Bleu Provence, Naples

1234 8th Street S., Naples, FL 34102 • (239) 261-8239 • www.bleuprovencenaples.com

Jacques and Lysielle Cariot opened Bleu Provence, French restaurant, as a labor of love in 1999 after retiring to Naples, Florida, from Provence, France. The couple considers their patrons welcome guests more than customers. Bleu Provence is home to old-world-style European hospitality, reflected in the wine selection and menu, as well as in the level of service and quality of the cuisine.

Lunch offers an array of lighter fares, many excellent sandwiches, salads, featured soups, as well as organic and healthy options. Jacques gladly will make wine suggestions based upon your meal. Traveling to different wineries around the world each year, Jacques returns with the best possible wine selection and the history of each one to share with interested patrons. The Cave is home to more than 20,000 bottles, representing more than 1,700 different wines, including some great finds that are surprisingly inexpensive. Bleu Provence was recently awarded the *Wine Spectator Grand Award* (one of only four establishments in Florida)—all are Golden Palate Partners, including The Breakers/HMF (Palm Beach), Marcello's La Sirena (West Palm Beach), and Bern's Steakhouse (Tampa). Jacques and Lysielle take pride in selecting the ingredients for the restaurant's menu. Fresh fruits and vegetables are delivered daily from local sources, and the couple sample meats, cheeses, olives, herbs, mushrooms, and a host of other ingredients from every source available to find and procure the finest quality.

Recipe courtesy of Jacques and Lysielle Cariot, Bleu Provence.

. . . .

Chilled Vegetable Salad with Honey Key Lime Dressing and Eggplant Caviar (Salad)

Entrée • All Phases • Serves 4

INGREDIENTS

Parmesan Tuile:
¾ cup fresh Parmesan, shredded

Eggplant Caviar:

2 Eggplants	1 tsp. cumin
10 chives	1 tsp. Piment d'Espelette
4 tsp. extra-virgin olive oil	5 large basil leaves
2 lemons (juiced)	

Key Lime Wild Honey Dressing:
3 Tbsp. wild honey
3 Key limes
1½ cups olive oil
2 kumquats
1 Madagascar vanilla bean

Chilled Vegetable Salad:

1 red onion

2 green asparagus

2 white asparagus

2 purple asparagus

2 baby carrots

1 red endive

1 Chioggia (red and white candy-
striped beet)

3 cups, arugula

1 Key Lime

2 kumquats

INSTRUCTIONS

Eggplant Caviar:

- Pre-heat oven to 350 degrees Fahrenheit.
- Cut eggplant vertically down the center and score the interior flesh in 1-inch intervals.
- Brush with Olive Oil and season with salt and pepper.
- Place on a baking sheet and bake for one hour, then let cool.
- Scrape the flesh and chop it. Combine eggplant flesh with lemon juice, cumin, Piment d'Espelette, salt and pepper.
- Chop chives and basil and combine them with eggplant.
- Refrigerate.

Dressing:

- Juice 3 Key limes. Zest 2 kumquats. Add the wild honey to the key lime juice and kumquat zest. Scrape out all of the vanilla bean seeds and drizzle all the ingredients with 1.5 cups of olive oil, season with salt and pepper. Refrigerate.

Chilled Vegetable Salad:

- Peel and shave the asparagus, baby carrots and Chioggia and combine in a mixing bowl.
- Fill with ice and a little cool water and set aside for 1 hour. Then, mix them with honey lime dressing and set aside.
- Thinly slice the red onion, kumquats, and the key lime.
- Wash the arugula and endives leaves.

Parmesan Tuile:

- Pre-heat oven to 350°F.

- Shred the fresh Parmesan.
- Place the silpat liner or parchment paper on the baking sheet.
- Divide the shredded Parmesan into 4 equal thin circles.
- Bake until golden brown, 5–6 minutes. Let cool.

Assembly:

- Place eggplant caviar in the center of the plate.
- Place a ball of arugula and red onion mix with wild honey dressing in the center of the eggplant caviar, trying to achieve as much height as possible.
- Dress all the vegetables and endives on top of the caviar and arugula, arranging them vertically.
- Garnish with Parmesan tuile, slice of kumquat and key lime and an edible flower.

NOTE

For weight-loss purposes, you may omit the Parmesan tuile, which will save approximately 20 calories per serving. This is also fabulous to accompany anything from grilled meat, lamb chops, and grilled or pan-seared seafood, such as salmon or tuna, for a complete meal!

Nutrition Facts (per serving)
Calories: **319** • Calories from fat: **43%** • Fat: **15g**
Saturated fat: **5g** • Cholesterol: **17mg** • Carbohydrates: **41g**
Protein: **12g** • Sodium: **323mg** • Fiber: **13g**

Boca Raton Resort & Club, by Waldorf-Astoria, Boca Raton[8]

501 East Camino Real, Boca Raton, FL 33432 • (561) 447-3000 • www.bocaresort.com

The landmark Boca Raton Resort was originally designed by renowned architect Addison Mizner. The Cloister Building opened in 1926, overlooking Lake Boca Raton. The resort grew over the years, adding the iconic twenty-seven-story tower, a beautiful new golf clubhouse, a tennis and state-of-the-art fitness center, a convention center, and a yacht club, in addition to the beautiful newly renovated beach club overlooking the Atlantic Ocean. There are numerous options for casual and gourmet dining, as well as many cocktail lounges.

Recipes courtesy of Carole Boucard, Director of Public Relations and Marketing, and Executive Chef Andrew Roenbeck, Boca Raton Resort & Club. Made by Boca Raton Resort & Club's Chef Adam Pile at Lucca Restaurant

. . . .

Preserved Lemon and Spinach Risotto

Entrée • Phases Three–Four • Serves 6

INGREDIENTS

¼ cup olive oil

1 large onion, diced

1 Tbsp. chopped garlic

6 bay leaves

1 Tbsp. chopped fresh thyme

2 cups vialone nano risotto or superfine aborio risotto from Italy

25 ounces (750 ml) dry white wine

1 cup hot chicken broth or stock (may also use fish stock if you wish to add seafood or water)

4 Tbsp. sweet butter

2 cups triple-washed fresh baby spinach, chiffonade

1 preserved lemon, chopped fine

freshly grated Parmesan cheese, to taste (see Note)

sea salt and white pepper, to taste

---

8 Boca Raton Resort & Club is a private resort, open to hotel guests and Premier Club Members and their guests only.

INSTRUCTIONS

- Heat oil in heavy-bottomed stainless-steel stockpot. Add onions and garlic and cook for 5 minutes over medium heat until the onions are translucent.

- Add bay leaves, thyme and risotto and stir thru to coat risotto well; cook over medium heat till risotto seals and starts to become sticky.

- Add wine and stir until all wine evaporates or is absorbed into rice.

- Then slowly begin to add chicken stock, water, or fish stock, and continue stirring the whole time until risotto is creamy and cooked to *al dente*. You should have 3 parts liquid to 1 part rice.

- To finish risotto, stir in butter, all the spinach, and ½ of the preserved chopped lemon; stir to mix together well off the heat.

- Taste and add salt and pepper, to taste; add more lemon if needed.

- Serve with optional garnish of 1 teaspoon Basil Blaze and freshly grated Parmesan cheese, to taste.

NOTE

For home/weight-loss preparation, the olive oil has been reduced from ½ cup and the butter has been reduced from 8 ounces. Imported Parmesan from Italy contains approximately 111 calories per ounce in solid form. When grated, the result is approximately 22 calories per teaspoon.

> **Nutrition Facts (per serving)**
> Calories: **461** • Calories from fat: **33%** • Fat: **17g**
> Saturated fat: **6g** • Cholesterol: **20mg** • Carbohydrates: **64g**
> Protein: **6g** • Sodium: **793mg** • Fiber: **3g**

· · · · · · · · · ·

Basil Blaze

Yields approximately 12 ounces

INGREDIENTS

1 cup extra-virgin olive oil
1 cup basil leaves
2 cloves garlic
salt and pepper, to taste

INSTRUCTIONS

Purée in a blender until smooth. This can also be used to accompany meat, poultry, and seafood dishes.

Nutrition Facts (per serving)
Calories: **81** • Calories from fat: **99%** • Fat: **9g**
Saturated fat: **1g** • Cholesterol: **10mg** • Carbohydrates: **0g**
Protein: **0g** • Sodium: **7mg** • Fiber: **0g**

· ·

Summer Sun Watermelon Salad

Salad • All Phases • Serves 6

INGREDIENTS

6 2-inch slices of sweet seedless
  red watermelon
1 cup feta cheese or goat cheese,
  crumbled
¼ cup aged white balsamic vinegar
1 Tbsp. lemon zest

1 Tbsp. orange zest
1 bunch fresh basil, fine chiffonade
  (finely sliced)
½ bunch fresh mint, fine chiffonade
¼ tsp. freshly ground black pepper
1 Tbsp. extra-virgin olive oil

INSTRUCTIONS

• Slice melon, remove rind, and cut into 2 by 2-inch cubes (you should end up with 24 cubes).

• Using a small melon scoop, scoop out a small hole in the top of each melon cube.

• Fill each hole with feta or goat cheese.

• Place a small drop of white balsamic vinegar on top of each piece.

• Sprinkle each piece with just a touch of all other ingredients, except the oil.

• Select a large white platter and stack all seasoned watermelon cubes to create a pyramid.

• Sprinkle the remaining zest and herbs over the top and drizzle olive oil over the stack and serve at room temperature with freshly ground pepper.

NOTE

This is an excellent light, healthy, and tasty salad for summer, which is perfect for entertaining when watermelon is fresh and local! It is ideal for having at your barbeque along with grilled seafood or meat. To make a larger salad, several cups of arugula make a nice addition, though you can add anything you like, such as sweet seedless grapes, fresh figs, mandarin oranges, etc.

Nutrition Facts (per serving)
Calories:**105** • Calories from fat: **67%** • Fat: **7g**
Saturated fat: **4g** • Cholesterol: **22mg** • Carbohydrates: **5g**
Protein: **4g** • Sodium: **282mg** • Fiber: **1g**

•

The Breakers, Palm Beach

One South County Road, Palm Beach, FL 33480
(888) 273-2537 • www.thebreakers.com

For over a century, The Breakers has lured generations of discerning travelers to this spectacular, oceanfront, Italian Renaissance style setting. Originally developed by Standard Oil magnate and railroad tycoon Henry Flagler, who was instrumental in establishing Palm Beach as the world's premier resort destination, the hotel we enjoy today was completed in 1927 and modeled after the Villa Medici in Rome. The Breakers is regarded as one of the most lavish resorts in North America, situated in the heart of Palm Beach, America's number-one winter playground of the elite. The magnificent resort overlooks the turquoise Atlantic Ocean, boasts an impeccably manicured golf course, world-class service, elegantly appointed rooms with modern amenities, a wonderful spa and fitness center, lovely boutiques, and an exciting array of gourmet dining venues.

Recipes courtesy of Ann Margo Peart, Public Relations Manager at The Breakers.

. . . .

Grilled Vegetable Salad with Lemon–Tomato Vinaigrette from The Flagler Steakhouse

Salad/Entrée • All Phases • Serves one

INGREDIENTS

Lemon-Tomato Vinaigrette[9]:

4 medium-sized ripe beefsteak
   tomatoes, washed

1 ounce white balsamic vinegar

1 tsp. chopped garlic

½ cup fresh lemon juice

¾ cup olive oil

salt and pepper, to taste

Grilled Vegetable Salad:

2 jumbo asparagus, cut in half

¼ cup heirloom tomatoes, chopped

¼ cup red peppers, square cut (cut into
   ¾ by ¾-inch squares)

¾ cup olive oil

a pinch of sea salt

¼ tsp. lemon zest

½ tsp. chives, cut in 1-inch sticks

1½ Tbsp. Lemon-Tomato Vinaigrette

1½ cups frisée lettuce

INSTRUCTIONS

Lemon-Tomato Vinaigrette:

• In a high-speed blender purée the tomatoes until smooth. Next, add the white balsamic vinegar, chopped garlic, and lemon juice to the blender. Once well incorporated, turn the blender on high and stream in the oil to create an emulsion. Season, to taste, with salt and pepper.

Grilling Vegetables:

• Toss asparagus, tomatoes, and red pepper with olive oil and season with salt and pepper. Place all vegetables on hot grill. Sear well on all sides. Cool for service.

Assembly:

• Mix together the grilled vegetables, the lemon zest, chives, and the vinaigrette dressing in a mixing bowl, reserving some dressing for garnish.

---

9 Yields 3½ cups.

- Place frisée in center of the plate with rest of the ingredients placed on top. Drizzle additional dressing around plate for garnish.

> **Nutrition Facts (per serving/one Tbsp.)**
> **for the Lemon-Tomato Vinaigrette**
> Calories: **28** • Calories from fat: **91%** • Fat: **3g**
> Saturated fat: **0g** • Cholesterol: **1mg** • Carbohydrates: **0g**
> Protein: **4g** • Sodium: **4mg** • Fiber: **1g**
>
> **Nutrition Facts (per serving) for the Grilled Vegetable Salad**
> Calories: **385** • Calories from fat: **70%** • Fat: **27g**
> Saturated fat: **5g** • Cholesterol: **242mg** • Carbohydrates: **15g**
> Protein: **25g** • Sodium: **1,581mg** • Fiber: **4g**

. . . .

Three-Minute Sicilian Calamari from the Italian Restaurant

Starter/Entrée • All Phases (see Note) • Serves 2

INGREDIENTS

2 Tbsp. extra-virgin olive oil

2 tsp. currants

1 tsp. large caper berries, cut in thirds

1 tsp. red pepper flakes

1 Tbsp. garlic, slivered

salt and pepper, to taste

3 Tbsp. white wine

4 ounces tomato sauce or
  crushed tomatoes

1 tsp. lemon juice

⅓ cup Israeli couscous

5 ounces calamari rings and tentacles

1 tsp. unsalted butter (optional at
  home for weight-loss purposes)

2 tsp. pine nuts

1 tsp. Italian parsley, chopped

INSTRUCTIONS

- In a sauté pan, mix together 1 Tbsp. of the olive oil, the currants, caper berries, pepper flakes, and garlic, and season with salt and pepper.

- Sauté for about one minute until fragrant.

- Add the wine, tomato sauce, and lemon juice.

- Bring to a boil and add couscous, calamari, and butter.

- Cook for about 2 minutes until calamari is cooked through then transfer to a plate for service.

- Garnish with pine nuts, remaining olive oil, and parsley.

NOTE

This is a great dish, especially given how quickly it comes together! The secret to calamari is not to overcook it. If you prefer, let your fishmonger cut and clean for you. For Phase One, omit the butter. You may also want to omit the couscous for dietary purposes and instead increase the amount of calamari in the dish.

Nutrition Facts (per serving)
Calories: **319** • Calories from fat: **63%** • Fat: **23g**
Saturated fat: **4g** • Cholesterol: **173mg** • Carbohydrates: **15g**
Protein: **14g** • Sodium: **381mg** • Fiber: **1g**

•

Buccan, Palm Beach

350 South County Road, Palm Beach, FL 33480
(561) 833-3450 • www.buccanpalmbeach.com

Chef Clay Conley has taken Palm Beach by storm with his trendy, modern American-Caribbean masterpiece, Buccan, and has recently expanded next door to open a second, Asian-inspired venue, Imoto, which means "little sister." Conley, a recent nominee for James Beard's Best Chef South, started his restaurant career at age thirteen as a dishwasher, growing up in Maine, where he was surrounded by excellent fresh seafood and farm-fresh produce. He worked his way up under the mentorship of Todd English, working in Boston, Washington, D.C., Las Vegas, and Tokyo for English, to eventually become the culinary director for English's Olives Group. After that tenure, Chef Clay assumed the role of head chef at Azul in Miami's Mandarin Oriental, then moved north to Palm Beach, where he opened Buccan in 2010. The name Buccan refers to a wood-frame grill common in the Caribbean, so as one would expect, many of Conley's signature dishes are grilled over a wood-fired grill and oven. Conley's latest ventures include Grato "grateful," his popular Italian-style gastro pub in West Palm Beach, and The Sandwich Shop, which serves lunch, also next to Buccan.

Recipes courtesy of Chef Clay Conley and Buccan.

. . . .

Grilled Shrimp Scampi with Mango Salsa

Entrée • All Phases • Serves 2

INGREDIENTS

Shrimp:

8 colossal (U-8) shrimp (8 per pound)

salt and pepper, to taste

2 Tbsp. extra-virgin olive oil

2 Tbsp. unsalted butter (reduced from 4 for home and weight-loss purposes)

2 shallots, minced

8 cloves garlic, minced

1 tsp. chili flakes

¼ cup white wine

juice of 2 lemons

¼ cup chicken stock

1 large ripe tomato, seeded and diced

2 Tbsp. chopped parsley

1 cup arugula

3 Tbsp. lemon vinaigrette

Lemon vinaigrette:

1 Tbsp. extra-virgin olive oil

juice of ½ lemon

INSTRUCTIONS

Shrimp:

- Build a wood-and-charcoal fire and allow to burn until only embers remain.
- Season shrimp with salt and pepper and a touch of olive oil.
- Place shrimp over hot part of the grill and char on both sides; remove from grill and keep warm.
- While shrimp is cooking, over medium heat, melt 1 Tbsp. butter with shallots, garlic, and chili.
- Cook until translucent.
- Deglaze pan with wine and lemon and reduce until dry.
- Add chicken stock and bring to a boil and reduce.

- Turn heat to low and whisk in additional Tbsp. butter.
- Add tomato, parsley and shrimp and cook until shrimp are cooked through. Set aside.
- Toss the arugula in lemon vinaigrette.
- Place a nest of arugula on each plate; place the shrimp on top and add sauce.

Lemon vinaigrette:

- Blend together oil and lemon juice. Set aside.

NOTE

At the restaurant, this is served with a toasted baguette. For home cooking and weight-loss purposes, it was omitted.

Nutrition Facts (per serving)
Calories: **336** • Calories from fat: **68%** • Fat: **26g**
Saturated fat: **9g** • Cholesterol: **94mg** • Carbohydrates: **16g**
Protein: **11g** • Sodium: **395mg** • Fiber: **2g**

. . . .

Mango Salsa

Snack/Accompaniment • All Phases • Makes a great garnish
for 2 servings of meat or fish

INGREDIENTS

1 ripe mango, diced small

2 Tbsp. red onion, minced

1 tsp. jalapeño, minced

2 Tbsp. chopped cilantro

1 Tbsp. red pepper, minced

juice of one lime

INSTRUCTIONS

Mix all ingredients and let sit for flavors to meld.

Nutrition Facts (per serving)
Calories: **83** • Calories from fat: **4%** • Fat: **0g**
Saturated fat: **0g** • Cholesterol: **0mg** • Carbohydrates: **22g**
Protein: **1g** • Sodium: **9mg** • Fiber: **2g**

•

The Café at Books & Books

265 Aragon Ave., Coral Gables, FL 33134 • (305) 448-9599
South Beach
927 Lincoln Road, Miami Beach, FL 33139 • (305) 695-8898
At the Adrienne Arsht Center
1300 Biscayne Boulevard, Miami, FL 33132 • (786) 405-1745
www.booksandbooks.com • www.thecafeatbooksandbooks.com

The internationally renowned Books & Books was founded in 1982 by Mitchell Kaplan, a former law student and trendsetter in the book world. "From the very start of law school, I pretty much knew I had a problem," Kaplan begins. "I found myself in local bookstores more than the law library. My moment of Zen came one day when I was in a Wills & Trusts class and was asked by the professor just what my strategy would be to solve a particularly thorny legal issue. The first thing that came to mind and the first thing I unfortunately blurted out was, 'I'd hire a lawyer,' and when it dawned on me that that might just be me, I realized it was time to go and I was forced to reassess just what my life's calling would be." The bookstore early on developed a very strong following for its vast collection of books on art, architecture, and photography, as well as the finest poetry, fiction and essays from the small and university presses. Now, over 30 years later, when you step foot into any Books & Books, you're still walking into your neighborhood bookstore, whether you find yourself in bustling Miami International Airport or on a Caribbean island.

Books & Books is the epitome of what a bookstore should be—a convivial place to mingle and browse an impressive literary collection in a beautiful setting, paired with gourmet cuisine and libations, a place that feels like home. Now housed in an exquisite 1927 building listed in the Coral Gables Register of Historic Places, across the street from the original store, Books & Books in Coral Gables is the central store, hosting over sixty author events a month, featuring presidents and Nobel prizes winners, athletes and artists, celebrities and poets and a variety of other community-based events. "This a golden time for bookselling," Mitchell says. "Writers are writing wonderful books and there is a vibrant group of readers wanting to read them, and as baby boomers age, they will have even more free time for books." Books & Books also has bookstore locations at the prestigious Bal Harbour Shops, Miami International Airport, Suniland Shops, Key West, and Grand Cayman.

The Café at Books & Books is a neighborhood Café-Bookstore (with three unique Miami area locations) that features a sustainable, healthy and hearty menu focusing on locally-grown produce, combined with a diverse selection of books and a vibrant, friendly gathering place. Dine surrounded by walls of books inside or in the historic, open-air courtyard at the original Coral Gables location (lunch and dinner seven days a week, from 9:00 a.m. until 11:00 p.m.). Acclaimed Chef Allen Susser oversees the menu, which includes bistro-style sandwiches, home-made soups, and healthy salads for lunch as well as coffee and freshly baked pastries throughout the day. The Café's Wine Bar, located at features craft beer and wines from around the world offered by the glass or by the bottle. A free, live music series showcases musicians of all types and genres, including Jazz, African, Latin, Caribbean and World Beat every Friday and Saturday beginning at 7:00 pm. Many of our visiting authors choose to organize pre- and post-reading receptions as part of their presentations at Books & Books.

The Café can prepare special menus for events, as well as for school visits, luncheons, private receptions, cocktail parties and private dinners. In South Beach, The Café's fun, fresh, and healthy take on contemporary and comfort food keeps locals and visitors coming back to the comfortable breezeway setting on Lincoln Road. The menu is as eclectic and flavorful as South Beach itself, using only the finest quality, all-natural ingredients. Bold flavors, friendly service, generous portions, and affordable prices are reasons to put The Café at Books & Books on Lincoln Road on your must-read list. The Café at the Arsht Center features delightful outdoor seating, table service, and specialty coffee bar. This Café is home to Chef Allen's Monday evening all-vegetarian, five course Farm-to-Table dinners featuring produce from Miami's local farmers and growers accompanied by live music.

Recipe courtesy of Chef Allen Susser.

· ·

Café Shrimp Mango Mojo

Entrée • All Phases • Serves 4

The natural sweetness of ripe mango will glaze and brown whatever you roast. This mojo is especially good for shrimp. Serve this with red quinoa & kale salad or salad greens of your choice.

INGREDIENTS

¼ cup olive oil

1 small onion, cut into ¼-inch dice

2 cloves garlic, minced

1 tsp. ground cumin

1 tsp. dried oregano

1 tsp. kosher salt

1 tsp. freshly ground black pepper

1½ cups freshly squeezed orange juice

½ cup dry white wine

¼ cup freshly squeezed lime juice

1 large ripe mango, peeled and cut into
    ¼-inch dice

1 pound jumbo shrimp

INSTRUCTIONS

Mojo:

- In a medium saucepan over medium heat, the olive oil and cook the onion for about 5 minutes, or until soft.
- Add the garlic and sauté for 1 minute.
- Add the cumin, oregano, salt, and pepper, and sauté for 2 minutes more.
- Add the orange juice, white wine, lime juice, and the mango.
- Bring the mixture to a simmer and cook for 15 minutes.
- Cool for 10 minutes then transfer to a blender and purée until smooth.

Jumbo Shrimp:

- Split open the shrimp, leaving the shell on, and marinate them in the mojo for 10 minutes.
- Pre-heat the grill very hot.
- Grill the tails approximately 2–3 minutes on each side until cooked rosy red.
- Baste each of the tails with the Mango Mojo, grilling for another minute.

NOTE

Bob's Red Mill Organic Whole-Grain Quinoa has 170 calories per ½ cup cooked serving (4 ounces) (which is ¼ cup dry), a reasonable amount per person with the shrimp and greens. There are 36 calories in 1 cup of raw kale. The best way to serve raw kale is to take a little olive oil and massage the kale with the oil, using your hands before plating.

Nutrition Facts (per serving)
Calories: **350** • Calories from fat: **41%** • Fat: **16g**
Saturated fat: **2g** • Cholesterol: **172mg** • Carbohydrates: **23g**
Protein: **25g** • Sodium: **653mg** • Fiber: **2g**

•

Café Chardonnay,
Palm Beach Gardens

4533 PGA Boulevard, Palm Beach Gardens, FL 33418
(561) 627-2662 • www.cafechardonnay.com

Since opening in 1986, Frank and Gigi Eucalitto's Café Chardonnay has been one of Palm Beach County's top restaurants, featuring fine dining in a casual, elegant atmosphere that is ideal for lunch, dinner, or a private party. The cuisine is American with Italian, French, tropical, and global influences. Chef Frank offers many creative, delicious specials in addition to the well-appointed menu. As one would expect, Café Chardonnay has a stellar wine list with many great selections by the glass or bottle.

Recipe Courtesy of Chef Frank Eucalitto, Café Chardonnay.

Jumbo Lump Crab Cakes with Mango, Hearts of Palm, and Local Heirloom Tomato Slaw

Entrée • All Phases • Yields 8 crab cakes

INGREDIENTS

Crab Cakes:

1 pound jumbo lump crabmeat

¼ cup red bell pepper, diced

2 scallions, thinly sliced

1 Tbsp. Dijon mustard

2 tsp. Old Bay seasoning

4 ounces mayonnaise (use Hellman's Light for weight-loss purposes)

1 egg white

¼ cup fine-ground plain breadcrumbs

juice of 1 lemon

salt and pepper, to taste

½ cup all-purpose flour, for dredging

4 Tbsp. vegetable oil, for sautéeing

Mango, Hearts of Palm, and Heirloom Tomato Slaw:

1 mango, firm but ripe

2 fresh hearts of palm, about 4 inches each

1 ripe heirloom tomato

2 ounces freshly squeezed orange juice

2 ounces passion fruit purée

2 ounces mango purée

1 Tbsp. rice wine vinegar

1 tsp. fresh cilantro, chopped

1 scallion, thinly sliced

½ tsp. finely minced fresh ginger

¼ tsp. kosher salt

INSTRUCTIONS

Crab Cakes:

• Pre-heat oven to 375 degrees Fahrenheit.

• Place all ingredients—except the crabmeat, vegetable oil, and flour—in a mixing bowl and mix together.

• Gently fold the crabmeat into the mixture, being careful not to break up the crab lumps.

• Chill for 1 hour.

• Form into 2-inch cakes, about 2½ ounces each.

• Place on tray, cover, and keep chilled until needed.

• When ready to serve, heat 2 ounces of vegetable oil in a non-stick sauté pan over medium heat.

- Dredge both sides of crab cakes with flour, shake off excess, and place in pan with hot oil. Test to be sure the oil is hot by sprinkling a pinch of flour into the oil. It should sizzle.
- Sauté the crab cakes over medium heat for about 2 minutes on each side or until golden brown.
- Place the cakes on a sheet tray and bake in oven for 4–5 minutes.
- Serve over a spoonful of the mango slaw.

Mango, Hearts of Palm, and Heirloom Tomato Slaw:

- Peel the mango and slice into julienne strips on a mandoline.
- Thinly slice the hearts of palm.
- Slice the tomato into thin slices and remove the seeds. Cut into julienne strips.
- Place mango, palm, and tomato in a stainless steel or glass bowl.
- Add the remaining ingredients, stir, and chill for 30 minutes.

NOTE

Per crab cake, the total with a serving of slaw is 216 calories. This recipe is all phases if using light mayonnaise.

Nutrition Facts (per serving) for the crab cakes:
Calories: **181** • Calories from fat: **59%** • Fat: **11g**
Saturated fat: **2g** • Cholesterol: **44mg** • Carbohydrates: **5g**
Protein: **11g** • Sodium: **324mg** • Fiber: **0g**

Nutrition Facts (per serving) for the slaw:
Calories: **35** • Calories from fat: **5%** • Fat: **0g**
Saturated fat: **0g** • Cholesterol: **0mg** • Carbohydrates: **8g**
Protein: **1g** • Sodium: **57mg** • Fiber: **1g**

Macadamia Nut-Crusted Yellowtail Snapper with Tropical Fruit Salsa

Entrée • Phases Three–Four • Serves 4

INGREDIENTS

Snapper:
½ cup crushed macadamia nuts

¼ cup flour

salt and white pepper, to taste

4 8-ounce yellowtail snapper fillets, skin and bones removed

½ cup milk (use skim milk for weight-loss purposes)

½ cup vegetable oil

¼ cup white wine

¼ cup freshly squeezed orange juice

1 tsp. chopped fresh chives

1½ cups Tropical Fruit Salsa (see below)

Tropical Fruit Salsa:
2 cups mixed diced fruit—choose from mango, papaya, kiwi, carambola, pineapple, blackberry, orange, watermelon, or any sweet tropical fruit.

Juice of 1 lime

¼ cup fresh squeezed orange juice

2 Tbsp. chopped fresh cilantro

1 tsp. sugar (may substitute agave nectar or omit for dietary reasons)

½ chili pepper, finely diced, seeds and membrane removed (Serrano or scotch bonnet)

½ small red bell pepper, finely diced

1 scallion, sliced into thin rounds

salt and pepper, to taste

INSTRUCTIONS

Snapper:

- Mix nuts with flour and salt and pepper.
- Dip fillets in milk then dredge in nut mixture.
- Heat oil or clarified butter in sauté pan over medium heat.
- Place fish, flesh side down, in pan and sauté until lightly browned. Turn fish and sauté for 2 more minutes.
- Remove oil from pan, reserving 2 tablespoons.
- Add wine and orange juice to pan. Reduce liquid by ½ and add chives with the fish in the pan.
- Remove fillets to a plate.

- Spoon 1 tablespoon wine-orange sauce over fish and top with 2 tablespoons of Tropical Fruit Salsa.

Tropical Fruit Salsa:

- Place fruit in a glass mixing bowl and add lime juice, orange juice, cilantro, sugar, peppers, and scallions. Mix well. Season with salt and pepper. Let sit for ½ hour before serving.

NOTE

This is a Phase Three–Four meal, as it is coated with flour and nuts and sautéed. For home preparation, you may use less oil for sautéing the fish and may wish to limit portion to 4–6 ounces per person. The Tropical Fruit Salsa is a fresh, tangy topping to grilled or pan-seared seafood, and poultry.

Nutrition Facts (per serving)
Calories: **620** • Calories from fat: **45%** • Fat: **32g**
Saturated fat: **5g** • Cholesterol: **84mg** • Carbohydrates: **31g**
Protein: **50g** • Sodium: **202mg** • Fiber: **4g**

●

Café L'Europe, Palm Beach

331 South County Road at Brazilian Avenue, Palm Beach, FL 33480
(561) 655-4030 • www.cafeleurope.com

For over thirty years, Café L'Europe has been considered one of Palm Beach's most elegant dining destinations. A favorite destination of the island's elite, Café L'Europe boasts a 2,000-bottle wine list, sumptuous Continental cuisine, and impeccable service in a lovely old-world setting with live piano music and fresh flowers.

Recipe courtesy of Café L'Europe, Palm Beach.

Peruvian Shrimp Ceviche with Guacamole

Starter/Entrée • All Phases • Serves 4

INGREDIENTS

2 Tbsp. olive oil

salt and pepper, to taste

4 large tomatoes, cut in half and seeds squeezed out

4 red peppers, halved and seeded

1 jalapeño, halved and seeded

2 whole peeled garlic cloves

12 ounces tomato juice

12 jumbo shrimp, deveined, cooked, and cut-up

½ large red onion, finely diced

1 red bell pepper, seeds removed, finely diced

1 yellow bell pepper, seeds removed, finely diced

1 cup chopped cilantro

lime juice, to taste

salt and pepper, to taste

Tabasco, to taste

guacamole

Taro chips

INSTRUCTIONS

- Place the tomatoes, peppers, and in a large bowl and toss with olive oil and salt and pepper. Drain vegetables of excess oil (should be lightly coated).

- Place the tomatoes, peppers, and jalapeño on a sheet pan, skin side up, and put under broiler until charred, but not burned.

- Allow to cool.

- Remove skin from tomatoes, peppers, and jalapeño.

- Place in blender with the garlic, blend until smooth.

- Add tomato juice.

- Pass through a strainer.

- Combine mixture with cut-up cooked shrimp, finely diced red onion, red and yellow pepper, and chopped cilantro.

- Add lime juice, salt, pepper, and Tabasco, to taste.

- Serve with guacamole and optional taro chips.

NOTE

Ceviche is a light, tangy, and delicious way to enjoy seafood. Experiment and try making it with sea scallops, calamari, lobster, or fresh, local white fish (snapper or flounder, etc.) of your choosing.

Nutrition Facts (per serving) without Guacamole or Taro Chips
Calories: **118** • Calories from fat: **9%** • Fat: **1g**
Saturated fat: **0.25g** • Cholesterol: **32mg** • Carbohydrates: **22g**
Protein: **8g** • Sodium: **149mg** • Fiber: **6g**

• • • • • • • • • •

Guacamole

All Phases • Yields 4 servings

INGREDIENTS

1 ripe avocado, diced

juice of one lime

½ large red onion, finely diced

¼ cup chopped cilantro

Tabasco, to taste

salt and pepper, to taste

INSTRUCTIONS

Combine all ingredients to desired consistency.

NOTE

Guacamole is delicious and healthy, and avocados are considered a "healthy" form of fat. You can enjoy guacamole on its own, or with crudités, raw vegetables.

Nutrition Facts (per serving)
Calories: **92** • Calories from fat: **68%** • Fat: **7g**
Saturated fat: **1g** • Cholesterol: **0mg** • Carbohydrates: **7g**
Protein: **1g** • Sodium: **53mg** • Fiber: **4g**

●

Café Martorano

3343 East Oakland Park Blvd., Fort Lauderdale, FL 33308 • (954) 561-2554
Seminole Hard Rock Casino in Hollywood, FL • (954) 584-4450
The Paris Las Vegas Rock Hotel & Casino in Las Vegas, NV • (702) 946-4656
Harrah's Atlantic City Resort & Casino, Atlantic City, NJ • (609) 441-5576
www.cafemartorano.com

Steve Martorano, native of South Philly has achieved the American dream, working his way up from humble beginnings spinning records as a DJ in the 70s, and having his own delivery sandwich shop in his apartment. Steve later expanded to his own restaurant, which featured pizza, sandwiches, pasta, and home-made water ice. During the recession in the early 1990s, Martorano lost everything and decided it was time for a change. He moved to Ft. Lauderdale with $40 to his name and opened Café Martorano, which has turned into a worldwide sensation! Today he is famous for excellent Italian-American comfort food, and a host of celebrity regulars. The restaurant was featured on the popular TV show *The Real Housewives of Miami*.

Recipe courtesy of Steve Martorano.

. . . .

Bucatini Amatriciana with Guanciale and Onions

Entrée • Phases Two–Four • Serves 4

This dish is adapted for home kitchens and weight-loss portions.

INGREDIENTS

1 pound bucatini (or perciatelli, straw-shaped pasta), or pasta of your choice, cooked to *al dente*
2 Tbsp. extra-virgin olive oil
2 cloves garlic, thinly sliced
4 slices guanciale[10], cut into thin dice

1 red onion, diced thin
crushed red pepper flakes, to taste
2 cups crushed San Marzano tomatoes
kosher salt and crushed black pepper, to taste
1 cup fresh basil leaves

---

10 Guanciale is cured pork jowl. It is available at some specialty markets or mail order sources. If not available, substitute pancetta or bacon.

4 Tbsp. freshly grated
   pecorino Romano

INSTRUCTIONS

- Heat a sautée pan with the olive oil and sautée the garlic and guanciale. When guanciale begins to render, add the onion and crushed red pepper flakes.
- Cook until the onions are soft.
- Add the tomatoes and season with kosher salt, pepper, and fresh basil.
- Simmer 10 to 15 minutes (while your pasta is boiling).
- When pasta is done, toss with the sauce and finish with 1 tablespoon Pecorino Romano per serving.

Nutrition Facts (per serving) without Guacamole or Taro Chips
Calories: **436** • Calories from fat: **26%** • Fat: **13g**
Saturated fat: **3g** • Cholesterol: **13mg** • Carbohydrates: **66g**
Protein: **16g** • Sodium: **774mg**

•

Café Sapori

205 Southern Blvd., West Palm Beach, FL 33405
(561) 805-7313 • www.cafesapori.com

Owned by Francesco Blanco and Chef Fabrizio Giorgi, Café Sapori features an extensive menu of modern and old-world delights from Northern and Southern Italy, expertly prepared and served in an upbeat, elegant dining room, a rich mahogany bar with illuminated onyx, or al fresco in the lovely courtyard.

Recipe courtesy of Fabrizio Giorgi, Café Sapori.

. . . .

Potato-Crusted Baked Orata (Mediterranean Sea Bream) with Taggiasche Olives

Entrée • Phases Two–Four (see Note) • Serves 2

INGREDIENTS

2 whole orata, 1½ pounds each, yielding approximately 2 8-ounce fillets (see Note)

3 Tbsp. olive oil[11]

salt and pepper, to taste

2 Tbsp. Italian parsley

3 sprigs fresh thyme

1 cup fish stock

½ cup Pinot Grigio

3 whole cloves garlic

½ cup Taggiasche olives (or Kalamata olives)

1 potato, peeled, pre-cooked, and sliced thin

2 additional Tbsp. chopped Italian parsley

juice of 1 lemon

INSTRUCTIONS

- Pre-heat oven to 450 degrees Fahrenheit.
- Debone the orata and season with salt, pepper, parsley, and thyme.
- Put the fish in a medium sauté pan with 2 tablespoons olive oil, fish stock, Pinot Grigio, garlic cloves, and olives.
- Cook for 9 minutes in a 450-degree oven.
- When the fish is cooked, take it out of the oven and remove the skin from the top of the fish.
- Coat the fish with the pre-cooked potato slices.
- Season with salt and pepper.
- Return fish to sauté pan and broil.
- Broil for 4 minutes or until the potatoes are crispy.
- Remove the fish from the sauté pan and set aside.
- Return the pan to the stovetop over medium-high heat.
- Add 1 remaining tablespoon olive oil and additional parsley and lemon juice to season.

---

11 Reduced from 5 for home/weight-loss purposes.

- Reduce the sauce by half.
- Pour the sauce over the fish, drizzle with 1 tablespoon olive oil and serve.

NOTE

Whole yellowtail snapper or branzino can be substituted for orata. For weight-loss purposes, I recommend sharing 1 fish between 2 diners. Also, if you eliminate the potato, the total calories would be 570 per serving, based on one fish per person. There are 119 calories in a tablespoon of oil (the original recipe had 818 calories per serving).

Nutrition Facts (per serving)
Calories: **699** • Calories from fat: **36%** • Fat: **28g**
Saturated fat: **4g** • Cholesterol: **107mg** • Carbohydrates: **40g**
Protein: **66g** • Sodium: **1,057mg** • Fiber: **4g**

●

Caffé Luna Rosa

34 South Ocean Blvd., Delray Beach, FL 33483
(561) 274-9404 • www.caffelunarosa.com

Situated directly across from the beach along breezy A1A in Delray Beach, Caffé Luna Rosa features an extensive menu of Italian-American and American favorites, serving breakfast, lunch, and dinner. With outdoor seating, it is a great spot to enjoy the ocean breeze and great food.

Recipes courtesy of Chef Ernesto De Blasi.

. . . .

Florida Yellowtail Ceviche

Starter • All Phases • Serves 4 (as an appetizer)

INGREDIENTS

1 pound very fresh skinless yellowtail snapper fillets, cut into ⅜-inch dice

½ cup fresh lime juice
½ cup fresh lemon juice

1 jalapeño, seeded and minced
½ cup finely diced red bell peppers
½ cup finely diced celery (hearts only)
¼ cup finely diced small red onion
1 small garlic clove, minced

pinch of ground cumin
salt, to taste
½ Tbsp. minced fresh cilantro
½ Tbsp. minced globe basil
1 Tbsp. extra-virgin olive oil

INSTRUCTIONS

- In a large bowl, toss the diced fish with the lime juice, lemon juice, jalapeño, red bell peppers, celery, red onion, garlic, and cumin. Season with salt to taste.

- Refrigerate the snapper ceviche for 30 minutes. Then stir in the cilantro, basil, and extra-virgin olive oil and serve. This can be served in a martini or margarita glass.

Nutrition Facts (per serving)
Calories: **203** • Calories from fat: **24%** • Fat: **5g**
Saturated fat: **1g** • Cholesterol: **53mg** • Carbohydrates: **9g**
Protein: **31g** • Sodium: **110mg** • Fiber: **1g**

. . . .

Dijon Mustard—Horseradish Aioli

Dip • All Phases[12] • Yields about 1 cup (6 servings as a dip)

Suggested with Florida Stone Crab Claws

INGREDIENTS

1 small garlic clove
a pinch of coarse salt
1 large egg yolk, room temperature
¾ tsp. grainy Dijon mustard
¼ cup canola oil
approximately 3 tsp. water, plus about
    2 at room temperature (see Note)
4 Tbsp. extra-virgin olive oil
1 tsp. fresh lemon juice
½ tsp. ground horseradish

2 dashes of Worcestershire sauce
dash of Tabasco
freshly cracked black pepper, to taste

---

12 Fresh Florida Stone Crabs, served with this dip are permitted in all Phases.

INSTRUCTIONS

- Using the side of a chef's knife, mash garlic and pinch of salt into a paste.

- Pulse egg yolk and mustard using a food processor or blender.

- With machine running, add enough canola oil, drop by drop, until mixture begins to emulsify (about ⅓ of the canola oil).

- Add remaining canola oil in a very thin, steady stream; as mixture thickens, add 1 teaspoon water.

- Continue blending, add olive oil, and as much water as needed to create a smooth, light consistency.

- Transfer to a bowl. Stir in horseradish, Worcestershire, Tabasco, and pepper.

- Aioli can be refrigerated, covered, up to one day.

NOTE

Add room temperature water if a thinner sauce is desired. Stone crab nutritional information from the Florida Bureau of Seafood and Aquaculture Marketing (www.fl-seafood.com).

Nutrition Facts (per serving)
Calories: **250** • Calories from fat: **98%** • Fat: **28g**
Saturated fat: **4g** • Cholesterol: **35mg** • Carbohydrates: **1g**
Protein: **1g** • Sodium: **42mg** • Fiber: **0g**

-

Nutrition Facts (per serving) or stone crab claws: (for 3 ounces cooked edible portions, equivalent to 4 medium or 2 jumbo claws)
Calories: **60** • Calories from fat: **0%** • Fat: **0g**
Saturated fat: **0g** • Cholesterol: **45mg** • Carbohydrates: **0g**
Protein: **15g** • Sodium: **0mg** • Fiber: **0g**

•

Casa D'Angelo, Boca Raton, Ft. Lauderdale, FL, and Atlantis, Paradise Island, Bahamas

---

171 East Palmetto Park Road, Boca Raton, FL 33432 • (561) 996-1234
1201 N. Federal Highway, Ft. Lauderdale, FL 33304 • (954) 564-1234
www.casa-d-angelo.com

Chef Angelo Elia's amazing Casa D'Angelo, the top-rated Italian restaurant in *Zagat* for Broward County for years, also has locations in Boca Raton and at Atlantis Paradise Island in the Bahamas. Chef Angelo created Casa D'Angelo as a nod to his homeland. His philosophy is *"tutto su gli ingredienti,"* or "it's all in the ingredients"—the freshest, best quality available. Casa D'Angelo features authentic, delicious dishes, a vast array of specials, including many fresh seafood and veal dishes. Also in the Angelo family are a several casual Angelo Elia Pizza Wine Bar and Tapas restaurants in South Florida.

Recipes courtesy of Casa D'Angelo and Chef Ricky Piper.

. . . .

Pan-Seared Sea Scallops with Endive, Orange, and Mint Salad

Starter/Entrée • All Phases • Serves 4

INGREDIENTS

½ cup all-purpose flour

2 tsp. seasoning salt (such as Lawry's)

1 tsp. chopped fresh oregano

1 tsp. chopped fresh thyme

½ tsp. kosher salt

2 Tbsp. lemon pepper

16 U-10 (10 per pound) sea scallops, rinsed and drained

2 Tbsp. olive oil

4 Tbsp. chopped fresh parsley

4 tsp. orange juice

2 tsp. sliced fresh mint

2 Belgian endive, shaved

INSTRUCTIONS

- In a large bowl, mix together flour, seasoning salt, oregano, thyme, kosher salt, and lemon pepper.
- Roll scallops in flour mixture until lightly coated on all sides.
- Heat olive oil in a skillet or frying pan over high heat.
- Add scallops to the pan and sear on all sides (about 2 minutes for each side).
- Toss with parsley, orange juice, fresh mint, and the shaved endive.

Nutrition Facts (per serving)
Calories: **220** • Calories from fat: **32%** • Fat: **8g**
Saturated fat: **1g** • Cholesterol: **20mg** • Carbohydrates: **23g**
Protein: **15g** • Sodium: **1,610mg** • Fiber: **9g**

•

Charley's Crab,
Palm Beach, FL, and Grand Rapids, MI

456 South Ocean Blvd., Palm Beach, FL 33480 • (561) 659-1500
63 Market Avenue, S.W., Grand Rapids, MI 49503 • (616) 459-2500
www.muer.com • www.landrysinc.com

Charley's Crab, overlooking the turquoise waters of the Atlantic Ocean in Palm Beach is one of Palm Beach's most popular dining destinations, serving up spectacular views and excellent food. Charley's Crab, the crown jewel of restaurants in the Landry's restaurant group features waterfront locations in Palm Beach and Grand Rapids, Michigan. Check out Landry's other restaurants, which include the popular Chart House, Morton's of Chicago, among many other popular establishments nationwide.

Recipe courtesy of Charley's Crab/Landry's.

Chilled Gazpacho with Charley's Crab's Fat-Free Italian Vinaigrette Dressing

Soup/Entrée • All Phases • Serves 8

INGREDIENTS

1 large cucumber, peeled, seeded, and finely diced (¼-inch cubes)

½ green pepper, finely diced

1 piece pimento, finely diced

½ large onion, finely diced

3 Tbsp. finely chopped Italian parsley

2 Tbsp. finely chopped fresh basil

1 large clove garlic, finely chopped

1 cup fat-free Italian Vinaigrette Dressing (see recipe below)

6 large tomatoes, peeled and seeded, or a 14-ounce can of plum tomatoes

1 cup tomato juice

salt and pepper, to taste

INSTRUCTIONS

Combine all ingredients in a container and refrigerate. Serve chilled and garnish with optional low-fat sour cream, watercress, cucumber, and/or cilantro, as examples.

Charley's Crab Fat-Free Italian Vinaigrette Dressing

Yields approximately one cup[13]
May be used to dress salads as well (1 Tbsp. per salad serving)

INGREDIENTS

½ cup olive oil

¼ cup plus 2 Tbsp. vegetable oil

3 Tbsp. white vinegar

¼ tsp. dried basil

¼ tsp. dried oregano

¼ tsp. minced garlic

1 Tbsp. sugar (may omit for weight-loss/dietary purposes)

dash of ground cumin

INSTRUCTIONS

Combine all ingredients by whisking together briskly. May store in a sealed container in the refrigerator and shake vigorously prior to use.

---

13 The dressing contains approximately 105 calories per Tbsp.

NOTE

Gazpacho is a summertime favorite. Make it more substantial by adding some cooked, chilled, and diced shrimp or lobster tail in when serving.

Nutrition Facts (per serving)
Calories: **289** • Calories from fat: **84%** • Fat: **27g**
Saturated fat: **4g** • Cholesterol: **0mg** • Carbohydrates: **11g**
Protein: **2g** • Sodium: **52mg** • Fiber: **3g**
Note: total calories include the sugar. (Sugar is 48 calories per Tbsp.; thus, omitting it would reduce the calories by 6 per serving. However, there are other reasons to omit sugar, such as diabetes.) You may want to consider substituting agave nectar instead.

•

Chop's Lobster Bar

---

101 Plaza Real South, Boca Raton, FL 33432 • (561) 395-2675
70 West Paces Ferry Road, Atlanta, GA 30305 • (404) 262-2675
www.chopslobsterbar.com

Chop's Lobster Bar has been called "The Tiffany of Steakhouses" by *Esquire* magazine, having earned a reputation as one of the finest steakhouses in the country. Part of Pano Karatassos's incredibly successful Buckhead Life Restaurant Group based in Atlanta, which owns ten top establishments in Atlanta and two in Boca Raton, Chop's combines classic steakhouse fare, including prime beef and chops, excellent soups, salads, sides, and service, with outstanding seafood, especially lobster.

Recipe courtesy of Tricia Jefferson and Sara Lett, Buckhead Life Restaurant Group Marketing Department.

· ·

Chop's Lobster Bar's Spinach Salad with Creamy Basil Dressing

Salad/Entrée • Phases Three–Four (see Note) • Serves 6

INGREDIENTS

Marinated mushrooms:

¼ cup sugar (you may substitute Splenda or omit for dietary purposes)

½ cup water
1 cup cremini mushrooms, stems removed

Salad:

1 pound baby spinach, washed and dried
3 strips bacon, cooked, drained, cooled, and chopped
1 Tbsp. toasted pine nuts

1 tsp. brown sugar (optional)
1 cup Creamy Basil Dressing
dash of Tabasco
dash of Worcestershire sauce

INSTRUCTIONS

- Stir together water with sugar (or Splenda) in a medium saucepan.

- Add mushroom caps and bring to a simmer, cooking for about 90 seconds. Remove from stove and let cool; leave mushrooms in sugar syrup.

- Prepare salad by washing spinach and discarding any long stems. Dry in a towel or salad spinner. Place in a large bowl. Set aside.

- Cook bacon until crisp in skillet over medium heat. Remove bacon and drain; wipe pan. Cool bacon and chop into bits. Return bacon to pan. Add pine nuts and stir. Cook over medium heat until nuts are lightly toasted, about 5 minutes. Add brown sugar.

- Drain marinated mushrooms and add to the pan. Cook until mushrooms begin to color, about 3 minutes. Add 1 cup of the Creamy Basil Dressing and a dash of Tabasco and Worcestershire. Turn off heat and stir well. Pour warm mixture over spinach leaves in bowl and toss well to coat. Serve immediately.

Nutrition Facts (per serving) without dressing
Calories: **86** • Calories from fat: **30%** • Fat: **3g**
Saturated fat: **1g** • Cholesterol: **4mg** • Carbohydrates: **12g**
Protein: **4g**

. . . .

Creamy Basil Dressing

Yields 2 cups or 12 servings

INGREDIENTS

2 Tbsp. red wine vinegar

1½ tsp. fresh lemon juice

½ cup tightly packed Italian parsley, minced

1 cup packed fresh basil leaves, stems removed

1 clove garlic, peeled

1½ tsp. Dijon mustard

½ tsp. salt

½ tsp. freshly ground white peppercorns

1¼ cups Hellman's Light Mayonnaise[14]

½ cup mixed olive oil and vegetable oil

INSTRUCTIONS

- Place all ingredients except mayonnaise and the mixed oils in the bowl of a food processor fitted with a steel blade.

- Process until pureed; open food processor and scrape down sides.

- Add mayonnaise and close processor.

- Pulse briefly just to blend mayonnaise.

- With processor running continuously, add oil mixture, pouring slowly through feed tube.

- Process until well blended.

- Dressing may be kept in the refrigerator for up to 3 weeks.

NOTE

Calorie count per serving with one serving of the dressing using Hellman's Light Mayonnaise: 86 calories in the spinach salad plus 162 calories in the dressing—248 calories total. Using regular mayonnaise (90 calories per

---

14 The restaurant uses regular mayonnaise; for home/weight-loss purposes, I have modified the recipe to use Hellman's Light Mayonnaise instead of regular mayonnaise.

tablespoon vs. 35 for Hellman's Light), there would be 750 more calories in the 2 cups of dressing, which works out to 63 additional calories per serving). This is suitable for Phases Three–Four, because of possible sugar, bacon, and mayonnaise. However, you can make the above substitutions for lower fat and calorie content at home.

Nutrition Facts (per serving)
Calories: **162** • Calories from fat: **94%** • Fat: **17g**
Saturated fat: **2g** • Cholesterol: **0mg** • Carbohydrates: **2g**
Protein: **2g** • Sodium: **281mg**

•

City Fish Market, Boca Raton and Atlanta Fish Market, Atlanta, GA

City Fish Market: 7940 Glades Road, Boca Raton, FL 33434 • (561) 487-1600
Atlanta Fish Market: 265 Pharr Road, NE, Atlanta, GA 30305 • (404) 262-3165
www.buckheadrestaurants.com

Atlanta Fish Market, owned by Pano Karatassos of the renowned Buckhead Life Restaurant Group (also owner of the Chops Lobster Bar) has been Atlanta's destination for the largest selection of the freshest seafood available. The menus are printed according to what is fresh, and feature selections from all over the world in a casual, family-friendly atmosphere. Pano has expanded this award-winning concept to Boca Raton, where City Fish Market features a similar selection of fresh seafood with an extensive menu that also includes prime beef, poultry, salads, and more! The Hong Kong-style fish is one of the most popular items in both locations. When in Atlanta, be sure to check out Pano's other outstanding establishments, including Bistro Niko, The Buckhead Diner, the Corner Café at Buckhead Bread, Chop's Lobster Bar (Atlanta and Boca Raton), Lobster Bar Sea Grille (Ft. Lauderdale and South Beach), Kyma, Nava, Pricci, and Veni Vidi Vici. Pano introduced Atlanta to fine dining in 1979 when he opened Pano's & Paul's, and his tradition of excellence continues today with his collection of restaurants featuring flavors from around the country and the world.

Recipe courtesy of Tricia Jefferson and Sara Lett, Buckhead Life Restaurant Group Marketing Department.

. . . .

Hong Kong-Style Fish

Entrée • Phases Two–Four (see Note) • Serves 4

INGREDIENTS

½ cup low-sodium soy sauce

¼ cup water

3 ounces dry sherry

2 Tbsp. granulated sugar[15]

2 Tbsp. sesame oil

2 Tbsp. olive oil

2 pounds spinach, fresh, washed, and stemmed

salt and freshly ground black pepper, to taste

4 6-ounce fillets of white fish (grouper, snapper, mahi, Chilean sea bass, and so forth; the dish is also featured with salmon at the restaurant)

2 Tbsp. fresh ginger, finely julienned

2 Tbsp. green onions, finely julienned

INSTRUCTIONS

- In a saucepan, combine soy sauce, water, sherry, and sugar and bring to a boil.
- Reduce heat to low to keep warm.
- In a large skillet, heat sesame and olive oils. Add spinach and toss until wilted. Season with salt and pepper and set aside.
- Steam or lightly sauté fish until just done. Do not overcook.
- To assemble, place a bed of spinach in a large soup bowl. Rest the fish on top of the spinach and garnish with ginger and green onions. Pour soy broth over fish and serve.

NOTE

For home and weight-loss preparation, we made double the amount of fish and spinach and kept the rest of the proportions the same as at the restaurant. This is a Phase Two–Four meal, because of the sherry and potential sugar.

---

15 For dietary purposes, you may wish to substitute Splenda, or simply omit.

Nutrition Facts (per serving)
Calories: **503** • Calories from fat: **37%** • Fat: **31g**
Saturated fat: **4g** • Cholesterol: **115mg** • Carbohydrates: **36g**
Protein: **42g** • Sodium: **2,442mg**

•

Columbia Restaurant

2117 East 7th Avenue, Tampa, FL 33605
(813) 248-4961 • www.columbiarestaurant.com

Founded in 1905 in Tampa, Columbia is Florida's oldest and perhaps most famous Spanish/Cuban restaurant. The original location, in Tampa's historic Ybor City, features live Flamenco dancing. Today, Columbia also has restaurants in Sarasota, on fashionable St. Armand's Circle, Clearwater Beach, St. Petersburg, St. Augustine, and Celebration.

Recipe courtesy of Angela Geml, Marketing and Public Relations Manager for the Columbia Restaurant.

Columbia's Original "1905" Salad™

Entrée • Phases Two–Four • Serves 4 (for weight-loss purposes[16])

The Columbia's Original "1905" Salad was selected as "One of America's Top 10 Best Salads" by *USA Today*.

INGREDIENTS

Salad:

4 cups chopped iceberg lettuce (broken into 1½ by 1½-inch pieces)

1 ripe tomato, cut into eighths

½ cup julienned baked ham (2 by ⅛-inch pieces); may substitute turkey, shrimp, or lobster tail

½ cup julienned Swiss cheese (2 by ⅛-inch pieces)

½ cup pimiento-stuffed green Spanish olives

2 cups "1905" Dressing (see recipe below)

16 At the restaurant, serves 2 as entrée, 4 as a starter.

½ cup grated Romano cheese

2 Tbsp. Lea & Perrins
   Worcestershire Sauce

juice from 1 lemon

"1905" Dressing:

½ cup extra-virgin Spanish olive oil

4 garlic cloves, minced

2 tsp. dried oregano

⅛ cup white wine vinegar

salt and pepper, to taste

INSTRUCTIONS

Salad:

- Combine lettuce, tomato, ham, Swiss cheese, and olives in a large salad bowl.
- Before serving, add "1905" dressing, Romano cheese, Worcestershire, and the juice of 1 lemon.
- Toss well and serve immediately.

"1905" Dressing:

- Mix olive oil, garlic, and oregano in a bowl with a wire whisk.
- Stir in vinegar, gradually beating to form an emulsion, and then season with salt and pepper.
- For best results, prepare 1–2 days in advance and refrigerate.

NOTE

For home preparation and weight-loss purposes, you may substitute reduced-fat Swiss cheese.

Nutrition Facts (per serving)
Calories: **483** • Calories from fat: **77%** • Fat: **42g**
Saturated fat: **12g** • Cholesterol: **53mg** • Carbohydrates: **11g**
Protein: **17g** • Sodium: **830mg** • Fiber: **2g**

Cucina dell'Arte, Palm Beach

257 Royal Poinciana Way, Palm Beach, FL 33480
(561) 655-0770 • www.cucinadellarte.com

Cucina dell'Arte (affectionately shortened by locals as "Cucina") is a Palm Beach island favorite, serving breakfast, lunch, and dinner daily, 365 days a year. It is a local's "home away from home" which is always friendly, the food always fresh and good, and the atmosphere upbeat, with outdoor seating overlooking Royal Poinciana Way. Cucina is open late for dancing (3AM), though the kitchen closes earlier. The Snapper is one of the most popular dishes on their extensive Italian-American influenced menu, and one of the best renditions I've had! For a lively and delicious taste of Palm Beach, visit Cucina!

Recipe courtesy of Nick Coniglio and John Kent Thurston III.

. . . .

Snapper Livornese

Entrée • Phases Two–Four • Serves 1

INGREDIENTS

1 fresh, local yellowtail snapper fillet (6 ounces) with the bloodline removed completely

½ cup Wondra flour (to lightly coat fish)

1 Tbsp. capers

1 tsp. fresh minced shallot

½ diced Roma tomato

blended fresh tomato

½ cup Pinot Grigio

4 fresh basil leaves

4 imported Italian black olives

salt and pepper to taste

4 Tbsp. olive oil to sauté

optional pad of European butter or drizzle of high-quality extra-virgin olive oil

INSTRUCTIONS

• While heating the olive oil over medium heat in a pan, pat the fish dry, lightly season and dust with Wondra flour, shake it off.

• Place the fish—presentation side down—in the hot olive oil and cook until it's lightly browned, then flip it over and drain some of the oil

- Add the white wine, shallots, tomatoes, capers, and let simmer lightly for about 2 minutes.

- Add optional pad of butter (or drizzle of olive oil), basil and black olives and serve hot right away.

NOTE

This recipe is Phases Two–Four due to butter and flower.

Nutrition Facts (per serving)
Calories: **634** • Calories from fat: **47%** • Fat: **33g**
Saturated fat: **5g** • Cholesterol: **80mg** • Carbohydrates: **19g**
Protein: **48g** • Sodium: **1,036mg** • Fiber: **2g**

•

CUT 432, Delray Beach

---

432 East Atlantic Avenue, Delray Beach, FL 33483 • (561) 272-9897 • www.cut432.com

---

Cut 432 is the trendy Delray Beach version of a prime steakhouse, specializing in USDA Prime beef, Japanese A5 Kobe, top-quality seafood, and an eclectic mix of innovative starters, salads, and sides in a hip, modern space along trendy Atlantic Avenue. Owned by bar-managers turned restaurateurs Brandon Belluscio and Brian Albe, along with Chef Anthony Pizzo, a three-time Florida Golden Spoon Award-winner, Cut 432 brings a refreshing, contemporary take to great steaks, sides, and cocktails.

Recipe courtesy of Cut 432.

. . . .

USDA Prime Steak Tartare

Starter/Entrée • All Phases • Serves 1

INGREDIENTS

3.5 ounces USDA Prime beef
  tenderloin, diced into small cubes

½ tsp. cracked black peppercorn
½ tsp. finely diced lemon peel

½ tsp. finely chopped Italian parsley

½ tsp. minced capers

½ tsp. finely diced cornichons

½ red onion, finely diced

1 tsp. stone-ground mustard seed

1 tsp. extra-virgin olive oil

Pinch of ground sea salt (the
    restaurant uses Maldon sea salt)

1 quail egg yolk

INSTRUCTIONS

Dice the beef into small pieces and mix with all the remaining ingredients—except quail egg. Chill. Placed quail egg yolk on top of tartare and serve ice cold!

Nutrition Facts (per serving)
Calories: **312** • Calories from fat: **48%** • Fat: **17g**
Saturated fat: **5g** • Cholesterol: **159mg** • Carbohydrates: **10g**
Protein: **30g** • Sodium: **400mg** • Fiber: **1g**

●

Donatello, Tampa

232 N. Dale Mabry Highway, Tampa, FL 33607
(813) 875-6660 • www.donatellotampa.com

For over thirty years, Donatello has been my favorite destination for fine Italian cuisine in the Tampa Bay area. Once you step inside, you feel as though you are in a Venetian villa and could have just as easily stepped off a gondola after a ride on the Grand Canal. Owner Guido Tiozzo brings years of training at the finest hotels and restaurants in Europe to Donatello. His Old-World-style, class, and elegance are unmistakable. Donatello is a family affair, where Guido, along with son Gino and wife, Alessandra, attend to every detail, from freshly made pastas to tableside preparation, and the long-stem roses for the ladies to ensure every experience will be memorable. With soft pink lighting, a beautiful piano bar, tuxedoed waiters with Italian accents, delectable food, and a great wine list, Donatello is the perfect place for a romantic evening, a family celebration, or to seal any deal, and has been a personal favorite for over twenty years.

Recipe courtesy of Guido, Alessandra, and Gino Tiozzo, Donatello Restaurant.

. . . .

Ossobuco alla Milanese (Braised Veal Shank)

Entrée • Phases Two–Four • Serves 4

The Ossobuco has been a signature dish at Donatello since opening in 1984.

INGREDIENTS

4 veal shanks with marrow bone (12 ounces each)

salt, pepper, and flour to lightly coat shanks

2 Tbsp. olive oil, to coat pan

1 large carrot, chopped fine

1 onion, chopped fine

3 stalks celery, chopped fine

8 ounces dry white wine

24 ounces whole Italian plum tomatoes, peeled and chopped

½ bunch sage, chopped very fine

½ bunch rosemary, chopped and mixed with the sage

1 lemon rind

1 orange rind

INSTRUCTIONS

• Season shanks and dredge lightly in flour.

• Sear on all sides in a skillet with pre-heated hot oil over medium-high heat.

• Add the carrot, onion, and celery and sauté a few minutes, then add white wine.

• When mixture has reduced about ⅓ add the tomatoes, herbs, and lemon and orange rinds.

• Cover and simmer either on a slow flame or in a 400-degree oven.

• Cook until fork tender, at least 1½ to 2 hours.

NOTE

For weight-loss purposes, I suggest having this with a side of vegetables or a salad. The restaurant traditionally serves it with saffron risotto "alla Milanese." Also, to incorporate your serving of vegetables, I sometimes add in several additional cups of larger slices of carrots and celery. I also suggest getting a spiralizer and making "zucchini noodles" or "zoodles" which go very nicely with the braising juices and vegetables and will save you calories over pasta or risotto.

Nutrition Facts (per serving)
Calories: **569** • Calories from fat: **30%** • Fat: **19g**
Saturated fat: **5g** • Cholesterol: **256mg** • Carbohydrates: **25g**
Protein: **69g** • Sodium: **758mg** • Fiber: **4g**

. . . .

Vitello Dolce Vita
(Veal with Ham, Sage, and Mushrooms)

Entrée • Phases Two–Four • Serves 2

INGREDIENTS

12 ounces veal scaloppini (2 6-ounce cutlets)
all-purpose flour to coat veal
2 Tbsp. olive oil
1 Tbsp. chopped shallots
2 ounces julienned prosciutto cotto (Italian cooked prosciutto)

2 ounces julienned Portobello mushrooms
4 fresh sage leaves
2 ounces white wine
1 tsp. black truffle shaving
¾ cup brown veal stock
1 ounce chilled butter

INSTRUCTIONS

• Dust veal scaloppini with flour.

• Heat the olive oil in a large skillet.

• Add veal and cook for one minute each side.

• Remove veal and keep it warm.

• In the same skillet, add shallots and cook for 2 minutes until transparent.

• Add prosciutto and cook more.

• Add mushrooms and sage. Cook for 2 minutes.

• Add wine and let reduce by half.

• Add truffle and veal stock.

• Place veal in the sauce with the chilled butter. Cook for 2 minutes. (For weight-loss purposes, may omit or reduce the amount of butter.)

- Place veal on 2 plates and cover with sauce.

Nutrition Facts (per serving)
Calories: **447** • Calories from fat: **44%** • Fat: **22g**
Saturated fat: **6g** • Cholesterol: **146mg** • Carbohydrates: **17g**
Protein: **42g** • Sodium: **586mg** • Fiber: **1g**

•

Euphemia Haye, Longboat Key

5540 Gulf of Mexico Drive, Longboat Key, FL 34228
(941) 383-3633 • www.euphemiahaye.com

For over thirty years, Chef Raymond Arpke and wife, D'Arcy, have owned this renowned restaurant on beautiful Longboat Key. Euphemia Haye offers a wide array of delicious foods, which showcase a combination of international and contemporary dishes. Chef Ray grew up in Wisconsin, where he was raised on the grounds of a mental institution where his father worked as a superintendent. The hospital had its own farm, dairy, and orchard and grew much of their own fruits and vegetables during the summer months. Ray experienced "farm-to-table" before it became trendy and learned by watching the culinary staff create everything from scratch. Fresh, quality, local ingredients became an important part of Chef Ray's philosophy. Ray went on to culinary school and worked at some of Sarasota's best restaurants before purchasing Euphemia Haye in 1980 and making it one of the Gulf Coast's top restaurants. Chef Ray also hosts cooking classes, and in addition to many decadent treats, features a number of dishes that are healthy and delicious!

Recipes courtesy of Chef Raymond Arpke, Euphemia Haye.

. . . .

Faux Fettuccini[17]

Side Dish or Entrée • All Phases • Serves 8

INGREDIENTS

2½ pounds zucchini (washed, ends removed)

4 Tbsp. extra-virgin olive oil

salt and pepper, to taste

2 cups marinara sauce (see **Fred's San Marzano Sauce**, or I recommend Rao's Marinara)

freshly grated Parmesan cheese, to taste

INSTRUCTIONS

- Slice the zucchini in $\frac{1}{16}$-inch-thick strips down the length of the vegetable. (This is most easily done with a mandoline, but can be done with a knife or vegetable peeler.)

- Cut the zucchini strips into ¼-inch-wide strips to emulate fettuccine. (This will be approximately 10 cups, but considerately less once it is cooked.)

- Heat a thin layer of olive oil in a large non-stick skillet until it just begins to smoke.

- Add a thin layer of the sliced zucchini.

- Season with salt and pepper, to taste. Sautée ingredients, stirring the whole while, until done (about 1 minute). You may need to do this in several batches depending on the size of your skillet.

- Portion the Faux Fettuccine in the center of 8 decorative bowls. Place a few generous spoonfuls of marinara sauce on top and sprinkle with freshly grated Parmesan cheese.

NOTE

This is a nice option for diners concerned about carbs, gluten, or calories, and is delicious. You should feel free to substitute zucchini "noodles" in place of pasta for a healthier, lower-calorie meal.

---

17 Made with zucchini

Nutrition Facts (per serving)
Calories: **72** • Calories from fat: **84%** • Fat: **7g**
Saturated fat: **1g** • Cholesterol: **0mg** • Carbohydrates: **3g**
Protein: **1g** • Sodium: **27mg** • Fiber: **1g**
Note: compare to pasta, which has approximately 100 calories per ounce.

· · · · · · · · · · · · · · · · ·

Cauliflower Mash

Side •.Phases Two–Four • Serves 6 as a side dish

Substitute Mashed Potatoes for this side.

INGREDIENTS

1 head cauliflower (2 pounds)

4 cloves garlic

¼ cup olive oil

¾ cup freshly grated Parmesan

salt, to taste

white pepper, to taste

INSTRUCTIONS

- Pre-heat oven to 350 degrees Fahrenheit.

- Remove the leaves and bottoms of the stem from the cauliflower.

- Score the core of the cauliflower all the way to the center 5 or 6 times.

- Steam the cauliflower until completely soft (about 15–20 minutes).

- Allow the cauliflower to cool without covering it (you want it to dry out), or you may pat it dry with paper towels.

- In a saucepan submerge the garlic in the olive oil and cook over a low flame until cooked through and slightly browned.

- Remove cauliflower and dice into smaller pieces.

- Purée cauliflower in a food processor with the garlic and oil until completely smooth.

- Add Parmesan, salt, and pepper, to taste, and run food processor until completely mixed.

- Place mixture in an oiled dish and bake at 350 degrees Fahrenheit until heated through and slightly browned (about 20 minutes).

- Serve in place of mashed potatoes.

NOTE

An excellent choice in place of mashed potatoes, which are high in carbs and are often loaded with butter.

Nutrition Facts (per serving)
Calories: **156** • Calories from fat: **73%** • Fat: **13g**
Saturated fat: **3g** • Cholesterol: **11mg** • Carbohydrates: **5g**
Protein: **6g** • Sodium: **392mg** • Fiber: **2g**

•

The French Brasserie Rustique

366 5th Avenue S., Naples, FL 34102 • (239) 315-4019 • www.thefrenchnaples.com

Award-winning Chef Vincenzo Betulia of Osteria Tulia and Bar Tulia fame has a third jewel in his crown of wonderful, authentic dining destinations in downtown Naples. Betulia opened his fabulous Parisian-style Brasserie in early 2017 to much acclaim, featuring a combination of French comfort food and fresh, light, delicious seafood, oysters, salads, and more! For more information, visit Osteria Tulia's website.

Recipe courtesy of Chef Vincenzo Betulia.

. . . .

Salade Niçoise

Entrée • All Phases (omit potatoes Phase One–Three) • Serves 1

INGREDIENTS

Vinaigrette:
2 cups olive oil
¼ cup rice wine vinegar
¼ cup white balsamic vinegar
1½ Tbsp. Dijon mustard
1 Tbsp. fresh Tarragon
salt and pepper to taste
1 large shallot, finely minced.

Salad:

3 Butter Lettuce leaves

2 hard-boiled eggs, quartered

1½ Roma tomatoes, wedged

½ cup Haricots verts (green beans), blanched

1 cup Red potatoes, boiled and quartered

3 salt packed anchovies, filleted in halves

12 Niçoise olives

1 4-ounce Yellowfin or Ahi Tuna Steak

INSTRUCTIONS

Vinaigrette:

- Mix all vinaigrette ingredients to make the vinaigrette and set aside.

Salad:

- Arrange Butter lettuce on a plate and top with vegetables, anchovies, olives and tuna.
- Pour some of the vinaigrette atop the tuna and salad.

NOTE

For nutritional purposes, the vinaigrette is assumed to yield 16 servings. There is enough vinaigrette for several servings; you can store this in a mason jar in your refrigerator and shake it anytime you want to use. About 3–4 Tbsp. of the vinaigrette is enough to make it delicious!

Nutrition Facts (per serving) for the Vinaigrette:
Calories: **245** • Calories from fat: **99%** • Fat: **27g**
Saturated fat: **3.6g** • Cholesterol: **0mg** • Carbohydrates: **1g**
Protein: **0g** • Sodium: **447mg** • Fiber: **0g**

Nutrition Facts (per serving) for the Salad:
Calories: **515** • Calories from fat: **32%** • Fat: **18.5g**
Saturated fat: **3.6g** • Cholesterol: **442mg** • Carbohydrates: **43g**
Protein: **46g** • Sodium: **862mg** • Fiber: **8g**

Henry's, Delray Beach

16850 Jog Road, Delray Beach, FL 33446

(561) 638-1949 • www.henrysofbocaraton.com

Henry's, named for the owner's beloved Cavalier King Charles Spaniel, is a local favorite on "Country Club Mile" in West Boca-Delray, known for its signature gourmet California-American cuisine since opening in 2000. Veteran restaurateur Burt Rapoport has several other popular local restaurants, including Deck 84 on the Intracoastal Waterway in Delray, and is partnered with Dennis Max at Burt & Max's in West Delray.

Recipe courtesy of Burt Rapoport.

• •

Turkey Burger with Cranberry Relish and a Cup of "Magical" Split Pea Soup

Soup/Entrée • All Phases • Serves 4

INGREDIENTS

Burger:

2 pounds coarsely ground turkey
   thigh meat
⅛ cup minced yellow or white onion
⅛ cup minced red onion

1 Tbsp. finely diced red bell pepper
   (optional)
salt and pepper, to taste

Cranberry Relish:

2 Tbsp. olive oil
1 cup cranberries
½ cup rice wine vinegar
1½ cups cranberry juice
½ cup honey
1 Tbsp. salt
¼ Tbsp. black pepper

INSTRUCTIONS

Burger:

• Mix together turkey, onions, and pepper; portion into 4½-pound patties. Grill patties until cooked through.

Cranberry Relish:

• Sauté cranberries in olive oil until soft. Deglaze pan with vinegar, add the remaining ingredients, and bring to a simmer.

• Reduce liquid until a syrupy consistency is achieved.

• Chill the relish.

• Place grilled turkey patty on whole-wheat bun (optional), top with chilled cranberry relish.

> **Nutrition Facts (per serving) for the Turkey Patties:**
> Calories: **345** • Calories from fat: **48%** • Fat: **22g**
> Saturated fat: **6g** • Cholesterol: **167mg** • Carbohydrates: **5g**
> Protein: **46g** • Sodium: **178mg** • Fiber: **2g**
>
> **Nutrition Facts (per serving) for Cranberry Relish:**
> Calories: **258** • Calories from fat: **24%** • Fat: **7g**
> Saturated fat: **1g** • Cholesterol: **0mg** • Carbohydrates: **53g**
> Protein: **0g** • Sodium: **1,749mg**
> Note: may substitute sugar-free cranberry juice

. . . .

Magical Low-Fat Split Pea Soup

All Phases • Serves 8

INGREDIENTS

¼ cup olive oil

2½ white onions, diced

12 ounces of carrot, diced

12 ounces of celery, diced

1 Tbsp. of minced garlic

2 scallions (ends removed), chopped

2 pounds split peas

1½ gallons water

4 ounces vegetable broth or stock

1 ounce chicken broth or stock

½ bunch fresh Italian parsley, chopped

salt and pepper, to taste

INSTRUCTIONS

- In a large stock pot, sauté onions, carrots, celery, and garlic in olive oil until soft.
- Add scallions and sauté one minute.
- Add split peas and water and bring to a roiling boil.
- Add the vegetable and chicken broths.
- Cook until the peas are very tender. Keep in mind it can take one hour or more to cook un-soaked peas. You may wish to soak the peas in water overnight at room temperature, to reduce the cooking time.
- Add parsley and mix until very smooth.
- Season with salt and pepper, to taste.

NOTE

The Split Pea Soup and Turkey Burger make a great go-to, healthy, complete meal in all Phases, either at the restaurants or at home—tasty and satisfying!

Nutrition Facts (per serving)
Calories: **212** • Calories from fat: **30%** • Fat: **7g**
Saturated fat: **1g** • Cholesterol: **0mg** • Carbohydrates: **29g**
Protein: **0g** • Sodium: **96mg** • Fiber: **10g**

•

Jack Dusty at The Ritz-Carlton, Sarasota

1111 Ritz Carlton Drive, Sarasota, FL 34236 • (941) 309-2000 • www.ritzcarlton.com

The Ritz-Carlton, Sarasota, is an elegant hotel and resort, overlooking Sarasota Bay in downtown Sarasota and convenient close to the arts and theater district. In 2012, the hotel opened trendy new Jack Dusty, featuring fresh seafood, prime steaks, and showcasing local produce and artisan products with a regional, nautical theme. The Ritz-Carlton, Sarasota, also features a lovely spa, conference center, beautiful beach club overlooking the Gulf on nearby Lido Key, and golf club located east of Sarasota, and is a great place to enjoy the good life on Florida's west coast.

Recipe courtesy of Caleb Taylor, Chef de Cuisine at Jack Dusty.

. . . .

Jack Dusty's Signature Cornmeal Blinis and Lemon Crème Fraiche, Served with Mote Marine Sustainable Sturgeon Caviar Raised in Sarasota

Appetizer • Phases Two–Four • Yields 4 servings of 3 blinis (12 blinis total[18])

INGREDIENTS

Blinis:

½ cup cornmeal

½ cup all-purpose flour

1 tsp. baking powder

1 tsp. kosher salt

2 Tbsp. local wildflower honey

1 large free-range egg, beaten

½ cup and 2 Tbsp. of organic whole milk (may substitute skim for dietary reasons)

1 Tbsp. melted butter (may substitute with nonfat cooking spray for dietary reasons)

Lemon crème fraiche[19]:

1 cup crème fraiche (for dietary reasons, you may substitute with low-fat sour cream)

zest of 1 lemon

INSTRUCTIONS

Blinis:

- Combine cornmeal, flour, baking powder, and salt.

- Mix egg, milk, and honey then stir into dry ingredients.

- Slowly add whole butter to melt in a non-stick pan.

---

18 Use 1 ounce of caviar per blini.

19 Prepare in advance

- Once butter is melted, start spooning half dollar sized dollops of the blinis into the pan, do not overcrowd.
- Cook on medium heat until very lightly golden, turn over, allowing the other side to cook until very lightly golden.
- Once cooked, place blinis on paper towels to absorb grease.

Lemon crème fraiche:

- Mix well, and set aside. Serve immediately or chill.

Assembly:

- Jack Dusty arranges 3 blinis on a plate per appetizer order with a dollop of the crème fraiche and spoonful of Mote Marine Sturgeon Caviar on top.

NOTE

This is a delicious and easy appetizer and is great for impressive entertaining. Using low-fat sour cream reduces calories to 297 per serving. Using skim milk and cooking spray instead of butter further reduces calories to 264. I suggest enjoying 2 per person at home (you will want more than one). This is great with a glass of champagne (average of 85 calories per 4-ounce glass). When entertaining at home, I sometimes prepare a platter of these for my guests, along with some lighter bites, like jumbo shrimp with cocktail sauce, and crudité of vegetables. Mote Marine Caviar is available online and in specialty markets, including Whole Foods stores in Florida.

**Nutrition Facts (per serving) 3 blinis,
topped with lemon crème fraiche and caviar**
Calories: **339** • Calories from fat: **48%** • Fat: **18g**
Saturated fat: **10.5g** • Cholesterol: **78mg** • Carbohydrates: **37g**
Protein: **8g** • Sodium: **670mg** • Fiber: **2g**

Joe's Stone Crab

11 Washington Avenue, Miami Beach, FL 33139

(305) 673-0365 • www.joesstonecrab.com

In 1913, Joe Weiss, his wife Jennie, and son Jesse moved to Miami from New York City. Joe moved on the advice of his doctor that a change in climate would be beneficial for his asthma. Immigrants from Hungary, Joe had worked as a waiter, and Jennie cooked in restaurants. In 1918, Joe and Jennie bought a bungalow across the street and opened a restaurant, with seven or eight tables, and a patio. They served breakfast, lunch, and dinner and became very popular. In 1921, a customer brought Joe a bag of stone crabs from Biscayne Bay, which was loaded with them. People were unaware they were edible. Joe threw them in a pot of boiling water, and the rest is history! Over the years, Joe's Stone Crab became an icon.

Recipes courtesy of Joe's Stone Crab.

. . . .

Joe's Crab Cakes

All Phases (omit sugar) • Yields 8 crab cakes

INGREDIENTS

1 pound jumbo lump crabmeat, picked over

½ red bell pepper, seeds and stem removed, chopped

4 scallions, trimmed and chopped

¼ cup chopped fresh Italian parsley

1 garlic clove, minced

1 egg, lightly beaten

2 Tbsp. Dijon mustard

2 Tbsp. fresh lemon juice

½ tsp. Worcestershire sauce

½ tsp. Tabasco sauce

¾ cup fine dry bread crumbs

2 Tbsp. vegetable oil for sauté

lime or lemon wedges, for garnish

INSTRUCTIONS

• In a large mixing bowl, combine the crabmeat, red pepper, scallions, parsley, and garlic.

- In a small bowl, stir together the egg, mustard, lemon juice, Worcestershire, and Tabasco.
- Gently fold egg mixture into the crabmeat mixture, then add ¼ cup of bread crumbs, mixing gently until combined.
- Form 8 patties, using ½ cup of the crabmeat mixture for each. The patties should be made in ovals about ½-inch thick and 3½-inches long. Coat the patties with the remaining bread crumbs and place them on a wax paper-lined baking sheet. Refrigerate until set, at least 1 hour.
- Heat the vegetable oil in a large skillet, preferably non-stick, over medium heat.
- Add 4 of the crab cakes at a time.
- Cook until golden on first side, about 5 minutes.
- Adjust the heat so the oil remains a steady, gentle sizzle.
- Gently flip the crab cakes with a spatula and cook other side until golden, about 5 minutes.
- Serve hot, garnished with lemon or lime wedges.

NOTE

This is a light and flavorful rendition of crab cakes that works in all Phases, and is nice with a salad of mixed greens, hearts of palm, avocado, chopped red onion, and mandarin oranges—very Miami!

Nutrition Facts (per serving)
Calories: **140** • Calories from fat: **35%** • Fat: **5g**
Saturated fat: **1g** • Cholesterol: **71mg** • Carbohydrates: **10g**
Protein: **13g** • Sodium: **285mg** • Fiber: **1g**

. . . .

Joe's Vinaigrette

All Phases[20] • Yields enough to dress 24 salads (24 1-Tbsp. servings)

INGREDIENTS

¼ cup chopped onion or scallion
3 Tbsp. minced fresh Italian parsley

2 Tbsp. chopped pimento peppers

---

20 Without the sugar.

1½ tsp. sugar (may substitute with agave nectar for home preparation).

1 tsp. salt

½ tsp. cayenne pepper

½ tsp. drained capers (optional)

⅓ cup wine or cider vinegar

¾ cup olive oil

INSTRUCTIONS

Whisk together all ingredients. Serve by tossing with salad and approximately 1 Tbsp. dressing per person. May be stored in the refrigerator.

Nutrition Facts (per serving)
Calories: **62** • Calories from fat: **96%** • Fat: **7g**
Saturated fat: **1g** • Cholesterol: **0mg** • Carbohydrates: **1g**
Protein: **0g** • Sodium: **100mg** • Fiber: **0g**

•

Kathy's Gazebo Café, Boca Raton

4199 N. Federal Highway, Boca Raton, FL 33431

(561) 395-6033 • www.kathysgazebo.com

Setting the standard for fine dining in a friendly, Old-World atmosphere, Kathy's Gazebo Café features excellent French and Continental fare, expertly prepared and served by a professional, accommodating, knowledgeable staff led by gracious hosts Gerard and Claudio. While there are many excellent dishes, perhaps the most popular is the Gazebo's famous Dover Sole, which is flown in fresh from Holland and is delicately prepared and deboned tableside. It is the best around!

Recipe courtesy of Claudio Pedron and Kathy's Gazebo Café.

. . . .

Dover Sole Meunière

Entrée • Phases Two–Four (see Note) • Serves 1

INGREDIENTS

1 fresh whole Dover sole, skin and
  guts removed
salt and pepper, to taste
flour for dusting
2 Tbsp. olive oil

1 tsp. unsalted butter
2 ounces white wine
2 Tbsp. lemon juice
½ lemon for garnish

INSTRUCTIONS

- Pre-heat oven to 400 degrees Fahrenheit.
- Season Dover sole with salt and pepper.
- Cover both sides with flour; shake off excess.
- In a 12-inch sauté pan bring olive oil to high heat.
- Put sole in the pan and cook on one side for 5 minutes until brown.
- Remove pan from stove, discard oil, and turn over the sole.
- Place butter[21] on top of sole, add lemon juice and wine to pan, and continue cooking in oven for 6–7 minutes.
- Garnish with lemon.

NOTE

Suitable for Phases Two–Four, because of butter and breading. You could typically share a Dover sole (or eat half) and order it with vegetables and a salad; I suggest one whole fish to serve 2 diners.

> ### Nutrition Facts (per serving)
> Calories: **693** • Calories from fat: **45%** • Fat: **37g**
> Saturated fat: **8g** • Cholesterol: **169mg** • Carbohydrates: **25g**
> Protein: **57g** • Sodium: **399mg** • Fiber: **1g**

---

21 The standard recipe calls for 2 Tbsp. butter on top, but for weight-loss purposes, cut it down to 1 teaspoon. It's always wise to ask restaurants to go light on oil, butter, and so forth.

. . . .

Salmon Tartare

Starter or Entrée • All Phases • Serves 5

INGREDIENTS

1 pound of diced fresh salmon
½ pound jumbo lump crabmeat
juice of 1 lemon
4 ounces of caviar of your choice
2 Tbsp. capers
2 shallots, minced

1 ripe avocado, diced
1 ounce olive oil
Tabasco, to taste
½ cup minced Italian parsley
salt and pepper, to taste

INSTRUCTIONS

- In a large bowl, marinate the salmon and crabmeat in lemon juice for 10 minutes.
- Add the capers, shallots, avocado, olive oil, Tabasco, and parsley.
- Add salt and pepper, to taste and mix all ingredients.
- Fill 5 3½-inch ring molds each equivalent and top with caviar.
- Refrigerate, remove molds and serve chilled.

Nutrition Facts (per serving)
Calories: **308** • Calories from fat: **49%** • Fat: **17g**
Saturated fat: **3g** • Cholesterol: **210mg** • Carbohydrates: **7g**
Protein: **33g** • Sodium: **660mg** • Fiber: **3g**

●

Limoncello Ristorante

2000 PGA Blvd., Palm Beach Gardens, FL 33408
(561) 622-7200 • www.limoncellorestaurant.com

Limoncello, a charming Italian restaurant in Palm Beach Gardens, is owned by renowned chef and restaurateur Mario Ghini, proprietor of the famed Pappagallo in Glen Head, Long Island. Today, Mario has brought a taste of his native Emilia-Romagna (its capital—Bologna—is home to the richest cuisine in all of Italy) to South Florida with excellent freshly made pastas, seafood, veal, and other specialties.

Recipe courtesy of Mario Ghini.

. . . .

Stuffed Artichokes

Starter/Entrée • All Phases • Serves 4

Ingredients

2 large artichokes[22]

1 quart water

¼ cup extra-virgin olive oil, plus extra oil to drizzle over the artichoke tops (optional)

1 clove garlic, minced

½ cup plain breadcrumbs

½ cup Parmigiano-Reggiano, diced into small cubes

1 cup chicken or beef broth or stock

INSTRUCTIONS

- To prepare the artichokes: clean, remove the middle "choke," trim the stem off the bottom, and snip the sharp points off the leaves

- Place the artichokes in a stockpot with the water and cook upside down over low heat for 45 minutes.

- To prepare filling: mix together the ¼ cup olive oil, garlic, breadcrumbs, and diced cheese.

- Carefully flip the artichokes right side up and stuff them with filling while they are in the pot.

- Add the broth or stock to pot and optional drizzle of oil over filling, and cover the pot.

- Simmer over low heat at least 20–30 minutes, or until cooked (taste the leaves to be sure). You should be able to scrape some soft flesh of the artichoke from the underside of the leaves with your teeth. Serve hot in large bowls.

---

22 These artichokes are great for sharing family-style.

Nutrition Facts (per serving)
Calories: **266** • Calories from fat: **60%** • Fat: **18g**
Saturated fat: **4g** • Cholesterol: **11mg** • Carbohydrates: **19g**
Protein: **9g** • Sodium: **484mg** • Fiber: **5g**

· ·

Chicken Pappagallo—Boneless Chicken Breast with Agrodolce (Sweet and Sour) Sauce with Grapes and Olives

Entrée • Phases Two–Four • Serves 4

INGREDIENTS

4 8-ounce chicken breasts

salt and pepper, to taste

1 Tbsp. extra-virgin olive oil (for sauté
version, see Note)

1 cup red wine vinegar

1 cup imported black or green olives

2 cups seedless grapes

juice of 2 lemons

1 cup freshly squeezed orange juice

1 Tbsp. honey

INSTRUCTIONS

• Season the chicken with salt and pepper, to taste.

• Prepare the chicken by either grilling or pan sautéing in extra-virgin olive oil until thoroughly cooked.

• In a large saucepot, heat the red wine vinegar over medium-high heat until simmering; add the olives, grapes, lemon juice, orange juice, and honey and allow to reduce for several minutes.

• Place the chicken in the sauce to simmer for a minute and remove to serve.

• Plate the chicken, and spoon sauce with olives and grapes over the chicken.

NOTE

This is a delicious, light preparation, ideal for Phases Two–Four due to sugar content in the orange juice, which should be limited or avoided in Phase One.

•

Louis Pappas Fresh Greek

2560 Mc Mullen Booth Road, Clearwater, FL 33761
(727) 797-3700 • www.louispappas.com • (also in Tampa and Lakeland, FL)

The Pappas family is known throughout Tampa Bay and beyond for having excellent Greek food. The family, which came from Sparta, Greece originally opened their Tarpon Springs landmark restaurant in 1925. The restaurant remained one of the area's most popular until 2002, when the Pappas' decided to launch their new market and café concept, which has grown into a mini-chain of fast, casual, quality Greek restaurants that are ideal for a quick and delicious Greek salad or bite.

Recipe courtesy of Louis L. Pappas, Louis Pappas Market Café.

. . . .

Louis Pappas Famous Greek Salad™

Salad or Entrée • Phases Two-Four (with potato salad,
Phases Three–Four) • Serves 1

INGREDIENTS

Salad:

5 ounces romaine lettuce, torn

1 large tomato, sliced lengthwise

4 Kalamata olives

2 pepperoncini

2 radishes

4 slices cucumber

6 spinach leaves

1 ounce crumbled feta

1 ring green bell pepper, sliced widthwise

1 beet

1 jumbo shrimp

1 anchovy

1 scallion

Potato Salad:

Serves 4

6 potatoes

1 to 2 Tbsp. red wine vinegar

salt to taste

¼ cup fresh parsley, finely chopped

½ cup green onions, thinly sliced

½ cup mayonnaise (I suggest this with Hellman's Light or Fat-Free Mayonnaise, or you may wish to try Greek yogurt instead.)

Dressing:

1½ Tbsp. extra-virgin olive oil

¼ cup red wine vinegar

salt, pepper, and oregano, to taste

INSTRUCTIONS

Arrange the ingredients in individual salad bowls, or if preferred, you may chop the salad ingredients and dress.

NOTE

This salad is typically served atop home-made potato salad, which is omitted here for weight-loss purposes.

Nutrition Facts (per serving) for the salad without dressing:
Calories: **166** • Calories from fat: **43%** • Fat: **8g**
Saturated fat: **5g** • Cholesterol: **34mg** • Carbohydrates: **17g**
Protein: **10g** • Sodium: **747mg** • Fiber: **5g**

-

Nutrition Facts (per serving) for the dressing:
Calories: **186** • Calories from fat: **96%** • Fat: **20g**
Saturated fat: **3g** • Cholesterol: **0mg** • Carbohydrates: **3g**
Protein: **0g** • Sodium: **156mg** • Fiber: **0g**

Marcello's La Sirena,
West Palm Beach

6316 S. Dixie Highway, West Palm Beach, FL 33405

(561) 585-3128 • www.lasirenaonline.com

Marcello's has been a favorite in the Palm Beaches since opening in 1986, and has held the top Italian rating in *Zagat* in Palm Beach County for many years. A lot has to do with the expert skill and passion of Chef/Owner Marcello Fiorentino and wife Diane who attend to every detail in creating an elegant, Old-World environment with excellent, authentic Italian cuisine and friendly, attentive service. They are hands-on owners who meet and greet guests as though they are family. Their extensive menu and award-winning wine list—one of only four *Wine Spectator* Grand Award winners in the entire state of Florida—are sure to please even the most discriminating diner.

Recipe courtesy of Marcello Fiorentino.

. . . .

Scaloppine di Vitello Sciue

Entrée • Phases Two–Four (see Note) • Serves 2

INGREDIENTS

8 ounces veal escalopes or cutlet(s) (2 4-ounce cutlets)

all-purpose flour, to coat veal

1 Tbsp. extra-virgin olive oil for sauté

½ cup grape tomatoes

1 tsp. capers

5 Gaeta olives

3 slices fresh mozzarella (3 ounces)

pinch of oregano

1 fresh basil leaf, julienned

INSTRUCTIONS

- Lightly dust the veal with flour.

- Coat the bottom of a sauté pan with olive oil and heat.

- Add veal. After the veal is lightly browned on one side, turn over.

- Add the grape tomatoes, capers, and olives and turn down the heat.

- Slowly cook the dish until the tomatoes become soft. Remove from heat.

- Remove veal from sauce and arrange veal on plate.
  - Top with the slices of mozzarella.
  - Add the basil and oregano to the sauce and stir.
  - Top the mozzarella slices with the sauce and serve.

NOTE

In the restaurant, this recipe serves one. For weight-loss purposes, I suggest sharing this with a dining companion or eating half and enjoying a salad and some vegetables as well for your meal. The reduced quantity is suitable for Phases Two–Four, along with other similar veal and chicken dishes, such as Parmigiana, Saltimbocca, and Marsala (not in Phase One, because of flour and cheese).

Nutrition Facts (per serving)
Calories: **394** • Calories from fat: **47%** • Fat: **21g**
Saturated fat: **8g** • Cholesterol: **122mg** • Carbohydrates: **15g**
Protein: **35g** • Sodium: **478mg** • Fiber: **1g**

●

Mario's Osteria, Boca Raton

1400 Glades Road, Boca Raton, FL 33431 • (561) 239-7000 • www.mariosofboca.com

Since 1985, "Bocanites" have been fortunate to have Mario's, a "go-to" for casual, sophisticated Southern Italian cuisine. The all-day Happy Hour in both the indoor and covered outdoor lounge areas with a dazzling array of discounted small plates is one of the best deals in town!

Recipe courtesy of Tony and Laurie Bova.

. . . .

Snapper Vesuvio

Entrée • Phases Two–Four (see Note) • Serves 4

INGREDIENTS

Artichokes:

8 baby artichokes

2 whole garlic cloves, peeled

2 sprigs fresh rosemary

¼ cup lemon juice

Peppers:

2 red bell peppers

vegetable oil to coat peppers

salt, to taste

Snapper:

4 red snapper fillets, 5 ounces each

1 tsp. salt

½ tsp. black pepper

 cup flour

2 large eggs

¼ cup canola oil

½ cup white wine

juice of 1 lemon

1½ cups clam juice

1 Tbsp. capers

1 Tbsp. unsalted butter (may use less
  for weight-loss purposes)

1 bunch flat-leaf Italian parsley,
  chopped

INSTRUCTIONS

Artichokes:

• Peel outer leaves off artichokes and place cleaned artichokes in a medium saucepan.

• Cover with water and add garlic cloves, rosemary, and lemon juice.

• Bring to a boil over medium-high heat.

• Once the pot boils, remove pot from heat and cover; let steep for about 10 minutes or until the artichokes are tender.

• Drain and cool the artichokes.

• Cut in half lengthways and reserve.

Peppers:

• Pre-heat oven to 500 degrees Fahrenheit.

- Rub peppers with oil and sprinkle lightly with salt.
- Place peppers on oven rack and roast until the skin is well charred; turn halfway through roasting.
- Place in a small bowl and cover tightly with plastic wrap for 15 minutes to loosen skins.
- Remove plastic wrap and cool peppers.
- Slip skins off and cut in half. Remove seeds and stems. Cut into ¾-inch pieces. Set aside.

Snapper and Assembly:

- Season snapper fillets with salt and pepper.
- Place flour into a shallow pan and lightly coat fish with flour.
- Lightly beat eggs in shallow bowl.
- Dip fillets in beaten egg.
- Heat large skillet over medium heat and when hot, add oil.
- Add fillets, and cook over medium heat until golden brown; turn and cook for approximately 2 more minutes.
- Remove pan from heat and add white wine and lemon juice.
- Return pan to medium-high heat and cook for about 1 minute with the fish remaining in the pan.
- Add clam juice and stir sauce.
- Add reserved artichokes and reserved red peppers; add capers.
- Add butter and parsley and serve at once.

NOTE

You can substitute sole, grouper, flounder, or other similar fish of your choice. This preparation is zesty and delicious; if you omit the butter, it is fine in Phase One.

Nutrition Facts (per serving)
Supplied by the restaurant.
Calories: **395** • Calories from fat: **50%** • Fat: **22g**
Saturated fat: **4g** • Cholesterol: **137mg** • Carbohydrates: **16g**
Protein: **35g** • Sodium: **254mg** • Fiber: **6g**

•

Matteo's

---

233 S. Federal Highway, Boca Raton, FL 33432

(561) 392-0773 • www.matteosristorante.com

Other locations in Hallandale, FL and Huntington and Roslyn, NY

Matteo's began twenty-five years ago when founder Salvatore Sorrentino and his two sons, Andrew and Matthew, opened their first location in New York. Since day one, Matteo's has been synonymous with large, delicious platters of Southern Italian comfort food, served "family-style." Dining at Matteo's is great with a large group, as the platters are ideal for sharing—a full order "Matteo's-style" can easily serve several guests. One of the most popular items is the Shrimp Wendy, which is served with their famous "Burned String Beans."

Recipe courtesy of Christina Ho, Public Relations for Matteo's.

. . . .

Shrimp alla Wendy with Burned String Beans

Entrée • All Phases •Serves 2

INGREDIENTS

Shrimp:

6 U-15 (15 per pound) fresh shrimp, cleaned, peeled, and deveined

½ tsp. Dijon mustard

1 Tbsp. fresh lemon juice

1 tsp. fresh garlic, finely chopped

salt and pepper, to taste

¼ cup all-purpose flour

1 Tbsp. olive oil

lemon wedges, to garnish

Dijon-Lemon side sauce:

½ tsp. Dijon

1 Tbsp. lemon juice

1 tsp. chopped fresh garlic

INSTRUCTIONS

Shrimp:

• In a bowl, combine the mustard, lemon juice, garlic, and salt and pepper, mixing thoroughly.

• Add the shrimp to bowl and coat with the mixture.

• Dust the shrimp in flour and shake off excess.

• Heat oil in a sauté pan, add shrimp, and sauté until cooked through (approximately several minutes).

• Serve with Burned String Beans (recipe below) or vegetable of your choice, Dijon-Lemon sauce on the side, and lemon wedges as garnish.

Dijon-Lemon side sauce:

• Mix together the mustard, lemon juice, and garlic. Set aside to serve with shrimp.

Nutrition Facts (per serving)
Calories: **147** • Calories from fat: **44%** • Fat: **7g**
Saturated fat: **1g** • Cholesterol: **27mg** • Carbohydrates: **15g**
Protein: **6g** • Sodium: **133mg** • Fiber: **1g**

. . . .

Burned String Beans

Vegetable/Side • All Phases • Serves 2 (an excellent side dish)

INGREDIENTS

12 ounces fresh string beans
3 cloves fresh garlic, sliced in half
3 tsp. olive oil

6 ounces chicken broth or stock
salt and pepper, to taste

INSTRUCTIONS

• Blanch the string beans for several minutes in boiling water. Remove and set aside.

• Heat an ovenproof sautée pan with olive oil and sauté garlic until golden brown.

- Add the blanched string beans, chicken stock, salt, and pepper and cook several minutes until heated through.

- Drain off liquid and place the whole pan in the oven under the broiler and cook until slightly burned or charred.

NOTE

Matteo's "burned Broccoli" is also excellent and can be prepared the same way.

Nutrition Facts (per serving)
Calories: **124** • Calories from fat: **74%** • Fat: **10g**
Saturated fat: **1g** • Cholesterol: **0mg** • Carbohydrates: **7g**
Protein: **2g** • Sodium: **268mg** • Fiber: **3g**

●

Mediterraneo, Sarasota

1970 Main Street, Sarasota, FL 34236 • (941) 365-4122 • www.mediterraneorest.com

Since opening in 1996, Mediterraneo has been a favorite spot for contemporary northern Italian cuisine in Sarasota. The restaurant features a wide variety of delicious salads, appetizers, pastas, veal, and seafood, drawing inspiration from all over Italy. The setting is chic and lively, with a wood burning pizza oven, and the walls are adorned with dozens of great photos of Italy. Their Veal Milanese is famous, and is one of the best renditions I have had anywhere.

Recipe courtesy of Daniele Baroni and Mediterraneo.

Veal Milanese with Arugula and Tomato Salad

Entrée • Phases Two–Four (see Note) • Serves 1

INGREDIENTS

2 large eggs, beaten
salt and pepper, to taste

1 Tbsp. chopped fresh Italian parsley
all-purpose flour, for dredging the veal

1 cup plain breadcrumbs

1 10-ounce bone-in Veal chop, pounded
   to ¼-inch thick[23]

½ cup extra-virgin olive oil, to coat pan

1 Roma tomato, cored and cubed

1 bunch arugula, coarse stems
   discarded and leaves washed well
   and spun dry

½ lemon, juiced

2 Tbsp. cup extra-virgin olive oil

salt and fresh ground black pepper,
   to taste

½ lemon, to garnish

INSTRUCTIONS

- Combine eggs, salt, pepper, and parsley in a shallow bowl.
- Place the flour in a second shallow bowl and the breadcrumbs in another shallow bowl.
- Dredge the veal in the flour, shake off excess.
- Dip into the egg mixture, then cover with breadcrumbs, shake off excess.
- Heat ½ cup olive oil in a sauté pan over medium heat.
- When oil is hot, fry the veal until golden brown, about 2 to 3 minutes per side.
- Remove from pan and place veal onto paper towels to absorb excess oil.

Assembly:

- In a salad bowl, toss tomatoes, arugula, lemon juice, oil, salt, and pepper.
- Plate veal and top with the salad.
- Serve with wedge of lemon.

NOTE

I recommend sharing the chop at the restaurant or at home, or preparing one 4-ounce cutlet per person, with the salad on top. This is suitable for Phase Two and up, being that it is breaded and fried. If making at home, blot the veal with paper towels to absorb oil. To compensate for the smaller portion of meat, just add additional tomato, arugula, and other salad items of your choice.

---

23 This also works with chicken, pork, and turkey cutlets.

Nutrition Facts (per serving)
Calories: **674** • Calories from fat: **56%** • Fat: **43g**
Saturated fat: **8g** • Cholesterol: **300mg** • Carbohydrates: **34g**
Protein: 36g • Sodium: **424mg** • Fiber: **3g**

•

Michael's on East, Sarasota

1212 East Avenue, Sarasota, FL 34239 • (941) 366-0007 • www.bestfood.com

Michael's on East has been recognized for excellence in dining since opening in 1987. To date, it is Sarasota's only AAA 4-Diamond restaurant. Owned by Michael Klauber and Phil Mancini, Michael's is Sarasota's version of a supper club. Enjoy excellent lunch and dinner options, including the popular "City Light Lunch Menu," featuring healthy gourmet options with calorie counts—in fact I was on local TV with Michael in 2012 to promote the delicious, wonderful concept! Michael's on East is also considered Sarasota's top caterer, and I have attended many fabulous events in the adjacent ballroom. The restaurant was among the first in the area to feature iPad wine lists, and is known for an excellent selection. Join the Gulf Coast Connoisseur Club, earn points, and consider traveling with Michael, as he takes a group of discerning patrons to top food and wine destinations for VIP tours all over the world, including South Africa, Australia, New Zealand, France, and Italy! Stop by Michael's wine cellar next door to find the perfect bottle of wine or bubbly to take home, and their café in nearby Marie Selby Botanical Gardens offers healthy dining options in a beautiful setting!

Recipe courtesy of Chef Jamil Pineda.

. . . .

Grilled Skirt Steak with Chimichurri, Grilled Red Onions & Roasted Roma Tomatoes

Entrée • All Phases • Serves 4

INGREDIENTS

Skirt Steak:

4 6-ounce skirt steaks

3 Tbsp. olive oil

salt and freshly ground black pepper

Chimichurri:

½ yellow onion, finely diced

½ bunch flat parsley, chopped finely

½ bunch curly parsley, chopped finely

½ bunch cilantro, chopped finely

¾ cup extra-virgin olive oil

1 tomato, crushed

½ jalapeño, seeded

4 cloves garlic

2 Bay leaves

2 limes, juiced

¼ cup rice wine vinegar

¼ cup distilled vinegar

Roasted Tomatoes:

6 Plum Tomatoes, halved

2-ounce Olive Oil

½ Tsp. Chopped Garlic

salt and fresh ground black pepper

Grilled Onions:

2 medium red onions, peeled and cut
   in 4 slices

2 Tbsp. olive oil

salt and fresh ground black pepper

INSTRUCTIONS

Skirt Steak:

• Coat each skirt steak with salt and pepper, then brush with olive oil. Over high heat, grill steaks to desired temperature. Immediately upon removing from grill, slice and then allow to rest.

Chimichurri:

• Place the first 6 ingredients in a bowl and mix well. In a blender, place all remaining ingredients and blend until smooth. Add blended ingredients to the ingredients in bowl and mix well.

Roasted Tomatoes:

- Pre-heat the oven to 350 degrees Fahrenheit. In a mixing bowl, add the tomatoes halves, oil and the garlic season with salt and pepper. Place on a sheet pan and roast for approximately 6 minutes.

Grilled Onions:

- In a small bowl, mix the onions with oil and salt and pepper. Over high heat, grill the onions on both sides.

Assembly:

- In a small mixing bowl, add the onions, tomato, potatoes and 1 Tbsp. of Chimichurri and mix well. Place a spoonful of the mixture in the middle of dinner plate, slice the skirt steak against the grain and place on top of the mixture. Top the steak with additional Chimichurri and serve!

NOTE

Chimichurri is a great marinade as well as sauce to accompany grilled or pan-seared seafood, meats, and poultry. I suggest using several spoonfuls of it, considerably less than one portion as indicated above; I would suggest a maximum of several spoonfuls of the Chimichurri for caloric purposes.

Nutrition Facts (per serving) for the Skirt Steak:
Calories: **450** • Calories from fat: **71%** • Fat: **35g**
Saturated fat: **14g** • Cholesterol: **105mg** • Carbohydrates: **0g**
Protein: **30g** • Sodium: **679mg** • Fiber: **0g**

Nutrition Facts (per serving) for the Chimichurri:
Calories: **395** • Calories from fat: **96%** • Fat: **42g**
Saturated fat: **6g** • Cholesterol: **0mg** • Carbohydrates: **0g**
Protein: **1.5g** • Sodium: **590mg** • Fiber: **2g**

Nutrition Facts (per serving) for the Roasted Tomatoes:
Calories: **59** • Calories from fat: **44%** • Fat: **3g**
Saturated fat: **0.4g** • Cholesterol: **0mg** • Carbohydrates: **9g**
Protein: **2g** • Sodium: **598mg** • Fiber: **2g**

Nutrition Facts (per serving) for the Grilled Onions:
Calories: **41** • Calories from fat: **50%** • Fat: **2g**
Saturated fat: **0.3g** • Cholesterol: **0mg** • Carbohydrates: **5g**
Protein: **1g** • Sodium: **583mg** • Fiber: **1g**

•

Mystic Fish, Palm Harbor

3253 Tampa Road, Palm Harbor, FL 34684
(727) 771-1800 • www.3bestchefs.com

Mystic Fish has been recognized as one of the top seafood destinations in Greater Tampa Bay since opening in 2001. Mystic is owned by veteran restaurateur Eugen Fuhrmann, who started the Lobster Pot restaurant in Bermuda (and later in Redington Shores, Florida) and Chef Doug Bebell, the chef from the Lobster Pot, which was a landmark in the area since 1978. Mystic has two sister restaurants—Guppy's on the Beach, a fun, casual seafood restaurant, and E&E Stakeout Grill in Belleair Bluffs.

Recipe courtesy of Doug Bebell, Mystic Fish.

. . . .

Bronzed Chilean Sea Bass with Hijiki Sauce

Entrée • All Phases[24] • Serves 4

INGREDIENTS

Sea Bass:

4 6-ounce Chilean sea bass fillets[25],
  1–2 inches thick
2 Tbsp. Cajun blackening seasoning[26]
  of your choice

2 Tbsp. canola oil, to coat pan
Hijiki Sauce (see below)
lemon wedges, to garnish

Hijiki Sauce (yields 4 servings):

1 tsp. dried hijiki seaweed (black or
  red)[27]

½ tsp. sake or white wine
1 tsp. sesame oil

---

24 Use light mayonnaise at home or sauce on the side.

25 Any white fish can be substituted, including flounder, snapper, sole, halibut, and striped bass.

26 Paul Prudhomme's is recommended.

27 Hijiki can be purchased at Asian markets. Nori sheets can be minced and substituted for hijiki.

½ tsp. rice vinegar

1 tsp. low-sodium soy sauce

a dash of sriracha sauce

½ tsp. minced garlic

1 tsp. finely minced pickled ginger

¾ cup Hellman's Light Mayonnaise (adapted here for weight-loss purposes; the restaurant uses regular mayonnaise)

INSTRUCTIONS

Sea Bass:

• Pre-heat oven to 375 degrees Fahrenheit.

• Coat one or both sides of fillets with Cajun blackening seasoning.[28]

• Heat large sauté pan over medium heat; coat pan with 2 Tbsp. canola oil.

• Place fillets in pan, brown on both sides, then transfer to pre-heated oven for approximately 5–8 minutes. Remove fillets to each of 4 plates.

• Spoon hijiki sauce over sea bass after plating. For weight-loss purposes, place sauce on the side.

• Garnish with lemon wedges and serve.

Hijiki Sauce:

• Place all ingredients but the mayonnaise in food processor and purée well. Add mixture to mayonnaise and mix well.

NOTE

Using Hellmann's Light Mayonnaise reduces the calories attributed to the mayonnaise from 1,080 down to 420 for ¾ cup. If using regular mayonnaise, don't use as much sauce with the fish.

Nutrition Facts (per serving) for the Chilean sea bass, without sauce:
Calories: **258** • Calories from fat: **46%** • Fat: **13g**
Saturated fat: **2g** • Cholesterol: **116mg** • Carbohydrates: **1g**
Protein: **32g** • Sodium: **419mg** • Fiber: **0g**

Nutrition Facts (per serving of 4 Tbsp.) for Hijiki Sauce:
Calories: **161** • Calories from fat: **90%** • Fat: **16g**
Saturated fat: **2g** • Cholesterol: **0mg** • Carbohydrates: **3g**
Protein: **0g** • Sodium: **386mg** • Fiber: **0g**

---

28 "Bronzed" is the same as lightly blackened. Use your favorite blackening seasoning, such as Paul Prudhomme's; Paul Prudhomme's seasoning is 0 calories.

. . . .

Bermuda Fish Chowder

Soup • Phases Two–Four • Serves 8

INGREDIENTS

Chowder:

1 Tbsp. olive oil

½ cup minced carrots

½ cup diced sweet onions

1 rib celery, minced

¼ cup minced fresh red peppers

1 Tbsp. chopped Italian parsley

2 Tbsp. chicken or vegetable bouillon

2 cups crushed Roma tomatoes

1 cup diced Roma tomatoes

½ tsp. sugar

¼ tsp. salt

¼ tsp. Old Bay Seasoning

¼ tsp. gumbo file

2 Tbsp. Worcestershire

¼ tsp. dried thyme

1 tsp. Paul Prudhomme's Blackened
   Fish Seasoning

8 ounces mild white fish (raw), such
   as snapper

½ tsp. granulated garlic

¼ cup dry sherry

1 quart water

Brown roux (see below)

Optional: add a shot of Myer's Dark
   Rum and/or hot sauce of your
   choice to top your cup of soup at
   the table.

Brown Roux:

2 ounces butter or vegetable oil (for
   weight-loss purposes at home, use
   oil; if avoiding flour, omit the roux)

½ cup flour

INSTRUCTIONS

Chowder:

- Using a large stock pot, sauté carrots, celery, and onion in oil until soft.
- Add all other ingredients.
- Bring to a boil, then let simmer for 20 minutes.
- Stir in roux and simmer an additional 15 minutes.
- Serve with optional drizzle of Myer's rum and optional hot sauce.

Brown Roux:

- Mix together butter or oil and flour in a sauce pan over very low heat.

- Cook and stir mixture until roux is golden brown and has a nutty smell, 25 to 30 minutes.

NOTE

The roux adds approximately 38 calories per serving. Myers rum contains 69 calories per ounce. Alcohol, other than wine should not be consumed during the first two Phases, and should be consumed in moderation thereafter.

Nutrition Facts (per serving) for Bermuda Fish Chowder, without the roux:
Calories: **88** • Calories from fat: **29%** • Fat: **3g**
Saturated fat: **0g** • Cholesterol: **13mg** • Carbohydrates: **5g**
Protein: **8g** • Sodium: **182mg** • Fiber: **1g**

. . . .
Kona-Seared Salmon with Pistachio-Dill Pesto

Entrée • All Phases • Serves 4

INGREDIENTS

Salmon:

4 6-ounce salmon fillets	2 Tbsp. vegetable oil, to coat pan

Kona spice rub:

½ tsp. granulated garlic	½ tsp. ancho chili powder
½ tsp. granulated onion	½ tsp. black peppercorns
½ tsp. fennel seed	1 Tbsp. espresso beans
½ tsp. kosher salt	1 Tbsp. cornstarch
½ tsp. paprika	

Pistachio-Dill Pesto (yields 8 servings):

1 ounce fresh dill, de-stemmed	½ tsp. Montreal seasoning
4 ounces pistachios, removed from shells	2 Tbsp. white wine
1 tsp. fresh garlic minced	¼ cup salad or soybean oil
1 ounce Parmesan, grated	

INSTRUCTIONS

Salmon:

- Heat sauté pan over medium heat. Coat bottom of pan with vegetable oil. Coat top of salmon fillet with Kona rub and place fillet in pan, Kona side down.
- Sear for 4 minutes on one side. Turn over and sear for approximately 4 minutes on other side, or to desired temperature.
- Transfer salmon to plate.
- Spoon pistachio-dill pesto over salmon after plating.

Kona Spice Rub:

- Grind all the Kona spice rub ingredients together in a spice grinder or coffee grinder. Set aside.

Pistachio-Dill Pesto:

- Purée all pesto ingredients in food processor. Use as needed. (Will keep in refrigerator for several weeks.)

NOTE

This preparation can be used with other types of fish as well, including swordfish, tuna, grouper, snapper, and others. A great dinner at Mystic Fish is either the Salmon or Sea Bass, the Bermuda Chowder, and either a side salad or vegetable.

Nutrition Facts (per serving) for the Kona-Seared Salmon without Pesto:
Calories: **406** • Calories from fat: **62%** • Fat: **25g**
Saturated fat: **4g** • Cholesterol: **100mg** • Carbohydrates: **0g**
Protein: **34g** • Sodium: **249mg**

Nutrition Facts (by serving) for the Pesto:
Calories: **146** • Calories from fat: **68%** • Fat: **23g**
Saturated fat: **4g** • Cholesterol: **6mg** • Carbohydrates: **16g**
Protein: **8g** • Sodium: **267mg** • Fiber: **2g**

Nino's of Delray

13900 S. Jog Road, Delray Beach, FL 33445 • (561) 499-3988 • www.ninosofdelray.com

For over twenty years, Nino's has been the go-to place in the Boca and Delray area for authentic Southern Italian fare and New York-style pizzas in a casual, family-friendly setting. Nino's features excellent fresh fish, amazing eggplant, and cuisine from Nino Tribunella's native Sicily, by way of New York. One of my favorite dishes at Nino's is their Flounder Francese, which is light and lemony. It pairs perfectly with fresh fish, chicken, shrimp, or veal—this is a simple and delicious winner.

Recipe courtesy of Nino Tribunella.

. . . .

Flounder Francese

Entrée • Phases Two–Four (see Note) • Serves 2

INGREDIENTS

2 8-ounce flounder fillets (or other similar seafood, such as sole, grouper, snapper, tilapia, shrimp, lobster tail, or chicken breasts or veal cutlets)

½ cup flour, for dredging

salt and pepper, to taste

2 eggs, beaten

1 Tbsp. canola oil to coat pan

1 tsp. butter[29] (reduced from 1 Tbsp. for weight-loss purposes)

½ cup white wine

1 cup chicken stock or broth

juice of 1 lemon, plus lemon wedges to garnish

1 Tbsp. finely minced Italian parsley to garnish

INSTRUCTIONS

• Rinse, pat dry, and dredge flounder fillets in flour and season with salt and pepper, to taste.

• Whisk 2 eggs in a bowl, dip the flounder in the egg mix, set aside.

---

29 Always ask the restaurant to reduce or limit butter if possible.

- Heat a sauté pan over medium-high heat with a drizzle of canola oil. When hot, add the fish and cook both sides until lightly golden brown.

- Remove fish and set aside.

- In a fresh sautée pan, heat butter over medium-high heat. Add the wine, chicken broth, and lemon juice, and allow to simmer for several minutes until thick and amalgamated.

- Add the fish back to the pan and finish in the simmering sauce for a minute or less.

- Serve immediately and garnish with minced Italian parsley and lemon wedges.

NOTE

Francese is a delicious preparation for seafood, chicken, and veal. If you omit the butter, it is suitable for Phase One.

Nutrition Facts (per serving)
Calories: **551** • Calories from fat: **30%** • Fat: **19g**
Saturated fat: **5g** • Cholesterol: **373mg** • Carbohydrates: **19g**
Protein: **64g** • Sodium: **637mg** • Fiber: **1g**

•

Ophelia's on the Bay

9105 Midnight Pass Road, Sarasota, FL 34242
(941) 349-2212 • www.opheliasonthebay.net

Ophelia's has been a Siesta Key favorite since 1988. Ophelia's is renowned for fresh seafood, beautiful views of the bay (watch dolphins splash while you dine), and has been a perennial people's-choice winner in Sarasota for best seafood, best waterfront restaurant, and most romantic restaurant. Arrive by car or boat, and in nice weather, dine *al fresco* overlooking the bay.

Recipe courtesy of Ophelia's on the Bay.

· ·

Seared Sea Scallops with Sesame Buckwheat Noodle Stir-Fry and Baby Bok Choy

Entrée • Phases Two–Four (see Note) • Serves 4

INGREDIENTS

1 pound U-10 (10 per pound)
sea scallops
2 Tbsp. peanut oil
¼ cup shredded carrot
¼ cup julienned red bell pepper
¼ cup chopped scallions
2 Tbsp. sesame oil

2 Tbsp. mirin
2 Tbsp. low-sodium soy sauce
¼ cup Mae Ploy Sweet Chili Sauce
6 ounces organic buckwheat Soba
noodles (or pasta/noodles of
your choice)
8 baby bok choy, washed and drained

INSTRUCTIONS

- For the dressing, in a large mixing bowl, stir together carrots, bell peppers, scallions, sesame oil, mirin, soy sauce, and sweet chili sauce.
- Cook Soba noodles according to package.
- When draining the Soba noodles, place them immediately in an ice bath to stop cooking.
- Once cold, drain them completely and add to bowl of dressing. Toss to coat and set aside.
- In a large sauté pan, heat peanut oil until hot but not smoking, over medium-high heat.
- Carefully place sea scallops in the pan and allow them to sit until completely caramelized on one side. Flip scallops and cook for an additional 2–3 minutes.
- Remove scallops from pan and reduce heat to medium.
- Add baby bok choy to pan and sauté just until wilted.
- Add dressed Soba noodles to bok choy stir-fry until just warm.
- Present caramelized scallops atop of the Soba noodle salad and baby bok choy.

NOTE

This preparation is fine in Phase One without the noodles, and is also nice with shrimp.

Nutrition Facts (per serving)
Calories: **542** • Calories from fat: **34%** • Fat: **16g**
Saturated fat: **3g** • Cholesterol: **37mg** • Carbohydrates: **43g**
Protein: **34g** • Sodium: **1384mg** • Fiber: **32g**

•

Osteria Tulia/Bar Tulia, Naples

466 5th Avenue S., Naples, FL 34102 • (239) 213-2073 • www.tulianaples.com

Osteria Tulia opened in January 2013 in downtown Naples and has quickly become known as Naples' hottest restaurant. Part of the buzz is due to Chef and Partner Vincenzo Betulia's passion and commitment to excellence and authenticity, where he has developed a huge following locally and worldwide, after thirteen years as a leading chef in Naples at Campiello, before opening his own restaurants. Since opening, savvy diners and critics have praised Osteria Tulia as on par with the hottest, chef-driven, rustic Italian restaurants in "foodie meccas" like New York and San Francisco; I concur.

Chef Vincenzo was born in Sicily and grew up in Milwaukee, Wisconsin, a Midwest hotbed of innovative chefs including Paul Bartolotta and Michael White (of the Altamarea Group). The three chefs worked together exploring the ancestral food traditions of Italy's diverse culinary regions. Betulia attended Kendall Culinary School in Chicago with Michael White, and the two chefs also worked together at the famed Spiaggia in Chicago. Diners can expect the highest quality from artisanal growers in Italy as well as America, home-made cheese, sausage and pasta, local produce, fresh seafood, and meat from farms that make the smallest eco-footprint possible. Tulia offers daily specials and a wine list with many great selections from Italy that pair perfectly with the cuisine.

Don't miss the popular Bar Tulia next door, Chef Vincenzo's Italian gastro pub, the leading spot for great craft cocktails in Naples, and be sure to visit his newest restaurant, The French Brasserie Rustique, located across the street on 5th Avenue South. The French pays homage to turn-of-the-century Parisian brasseries and features a wonderful blend of authentic French country cuisine as well as seafood specialties.

Recipe courtesy of Chef Vincenzo Betulia.

. . . .

Florida Black Grouper all' Acquapazza "Crazywater-style"

Entrée • All Phases • Serves 4

INGREDIENTS

3 Tbsp. grapeseed oil

4 6-ounce portions Florida
   black grouper

12 Florida Gulf shrimp (16/20 count),
   peeled and deveined

salt and pepper

3 cloves garlic, sliced

2 Bay Leaves

pinch of crushed red chili flakes

4 ounces white wine

12 ounces marinara sauce (use my
   recipe or substitute Rao's)

4 ounces fish broth or light
   chicken broth

INSTRUCTIONS

- Pre-heat the oven to 450 degrees Fahrenheit.

- In a large ovenproof sauté pan, heat the grapeseed oil over medium-high heat to nearly smoking.

- Meanwhile, season the grouper and shrimp with salt and pepper. Carefully place the grouper in the pan and sear over a medium-high heat to allow the fish to caramelize to a golden-brown color. Carefully flip the fish over and add the shrimp to the pan. Cook for about 1 minute, lower the heat and add the sliced garlic, Bay Leaves and chili flakes.

- Cook the garlic to a nice golden brown, for about 1 minute, then deglaze the pan with the white wine. Cook until the wine is reduced by half.

- Add the marinara and fish broth and cook until the sauce is slightly reduced, about 3 to 4 minutes.

- Transfer the pan to the oven and cook until the fish is fully cooked, about 8–10 minutes.

- Serve immediately.

NOTE

This goes great with 3–4 ounces of *al dente* pasta per person, such as linguini. Cook *al dente* while the fish is in the oven, remove the fish from the pan, add the pasta to the sauce with the shrimp, put back on the hot stove a minute and toss. Plate immediately with the fish atop the pasta. This also is great with sautéed spinach, escarole, broccolini, or broccoli rabe, *"aglio olio"* style with slices of fresh garlic, lightly golden brown in extra-virgin olive oil.

Nutrition Facts (per serving)
Calories: **327** • Calories from fat: **22%** • Fat: **8g**
Saturated fat: **2g** • Cholesterol: **107mg** • Carbohydrates: **9g**
Protein: **48g** • Sodium: **912mg** • Fiber: **2g**

•

Paradiso Ristorante

625 Lucerne Ave., Lake Worth, FL 33460 • (561) 547-2500 • www.paradisolakeworth.com

Angelo Romano, Chef/Owner of Paradiso Ristorante, has accumulated and honed his culinary skills by working at a wide range of luxurious resort towns including the Italian Riviera, island of Capri, Anacapri, the island of Bermuda and in Palm Beach. Through his experiences he learned to appeal to the most finicky of palates and please the fancies of vacationing diners venturing out to taste something extraordinary. Chef Angelo's culinary roots trace back to his early childhood, as he was born into a family of Italian olive oil and wine producers in Massa Lubrense (Sorrento), Italy. His background has influenced Angelo's desire to include only the freshest ingredients in his menu selections. He was only fourteen years old when he was chosen for a summer job at the restaurant Faraglioni, located on Capri, the island known for its mouthwatering Mediterranean cuisine. There he learned tricks of the trade from the best chefs of Northern Italy, France and Switzerland. Chef Angelo celebrates twenty years as one of the top Italian restaurants in the Palm Beaches in the heart of downtown Lake Worth, where he shares his passion for fresh, seasonal, ingredient driven Italian cuisine, paired with fine wine. "The first thought I have in the morning is about how I am going to make my restaurant better," says Chef Angelo.

This is a fall inspired dish with an array of complimenting flavors; perfect for a unique lunch or seasonal entertaining.

Recipe courtesy of Chef Angelo Romano.

. . . .

Fig & Chestnut Risotto

Entrée or side dish • Phases Two–Four • Serves 8

INGREDIENTS

4 cups imported Arborio rice

1 pound cooked chestnuts

½ pound fresh or dried figs

1 shallot

5 Tbsp. extra-virgin olive oil

2 Tbsp. unsalted butter

1 cup vegetable or chicken broth

5 Tbsp. freshly grated
    Parmesan cheese

INSTRUCTIONS

Broth:

- Bring the broth to boil and keep hot.

Risotto:

- Finely chop shallots.

- Braise until golden brown with virgin olive oil in risotto pan.

- Add the rice to the shallot and virgin olive oil in the risotto pan

- Slowly add broth, keeping broth just covering the rice.

- As the rice absorbs the broth, slowly add more. Repeat and continue until the rice has cooked for a total of 20 minutes.

Chestnuts & figs:

- To prepare, purée half of the chestnuts and figs. To incorporate, after 10 minutes into the rice cooking, stir in the pureed chestnuts and figs.

Parmesan, butter, and remaining chestnuts:

- Stir in the 3 Tbsp. of Parmesan, 1 Tbsp. of butter and ½ of the remaining whole chestnuts while rice is still over the heat

- The flavors are slowly released during 5 additional minutes of cooking

- Remove from the heat and add remaining butter and Parmesan cheese and chestnuts in what we call *mantecare*[30].

Assembly:

- If using fresh figs, decorate the risotto with the remaining figs.

Nutrition Facts (per serving)
Calories: **363** • Calories from fat: **35%** • Fat: **14g**
Saturated fat: **4g** • Cholesterol: **10mg** • Carbohydrates: **55g**
Protein: **6g** • Sodium: **192mg** • Fiber: **4g**

●

Renato's, Palm Beach

---

87 Via Mizner, Palm Beach, FL 33480
(561) 655-9752 • www.renatospalmbeach.com

For years, Renato's has been a Palm Beach favorite for elegant Italian dining in a beautiful, romantic setting with roses, candlelight, and live piano music. The food is expertly prepared and graciously served, under the watchful eye of dedicated owner Arlene Desiderio. Renato's beautiful private courtyard is ideal for dining al fresco and enjoying the ocean breezes. Adorned with flowers, colorful tablecloths and umbrellas, and surrounded by Mediterranean architecture, Renato's patio is reminiscent of al fresco dining in Italy. Their more casual Pizza al Fresco, located nearby, serves wonderful pizzas, salads, and seafood, as does the newest location at the Palm Beach Par 3 Golf Course on the Ocean.

Recipes courtesy of Renato's Manager, Brad Stapleton.

---

30 *Mantecare:* Italian word to describe the last process of making risotto to bind the butter and Parmesan, done while rice is removed off of the heat to avoid breaking the butter and creating the creamy texture.

. . . .

Costoletta di Vitello—Grilled Marinated Veal Chops

Phases Three–Four • Serves 4

INGREDIENTS

2 shallots, minced

2 Tbsp. butter (may reduce)

1½ cups red wine

1 quart veal stock

1½ cups marsala wine

8 ounces porcini mushrooms, sliced

salt and pepper, to taste

4 tsp. white truffle oil (optional)

4 14-ounce center-cut veal chops

1 Tbsp. chopped fresh herbs (basil, parsley, sage, or marjoram)

3 Tbsp. extra-virgin olive oil

INSTRUCTIONS

- Pre-heat oven to 450 degrees Fahrenheit.

- For the sauce, sautée the shallots until golden brown in the butter, then add red wine and cook until reduced by half.

- Proceed to add the veal stock and marsala, increase heat and when sauce starts to boil, add the porcini mushrooms and salt and pepper, to taste.

- Lower the heat and allow sauce to reduce by a fourth, and finally add the truffle oil.

- In a shallow dish, combine the herbs and olive oil, salt and pepper, to taste.

- Marinate the veal chops with olive oil mixture for several hours in the refrigerator. Remove from refrigerator and allow to reach room temperature before grilling.

- Sear both sides of the meat on either on a hot grill or in a sauté pan and proceed to cook in a pre-heated oven to desired degree; I suggest using a meat thermometer, and recommend medium-rare.

NOTE

For home/weight-loss preparation, butter was reduced from 4 Tbsp., olive oil was reduced from 6 Tbsp., and truffle oil was reduced from 4 Tbsp. to 4 tsp.. When dining out, if you are trying to be healthy, always ask your server if butter or oil content can be reduced; often it can. This is suitable for Phases Three–Four.

Nutrition Facts (per serving)
Calories: **574** • Calories from fat: **44%** • Fat: **29g**
Saturated fat: **8g** • Cholesterol: **206mg** • Carbohydrates: **15g**
Protein: **53g** • Sodium: **1756mg** • Fiber: **0g**

•

Simon's Coffee House, Sarasota

5900 S. Tamiami Trail, Sarasota, FL 34231 • (941) 926-7151 • www.simonstogo.com

Simon's, owned by Michelle and Simon Kirby, is Sarasota's destination for healthy, organic foods. Their offerings include excellent home-made soups, delicious salads, raw foods, healthy smoothies, sandwiches, wraps, paninis, and so much more! With a fun, friendly atmosphere and quality, healthy fare, it is no wonder Simon's is so popular! Michelle says, "Our raw food is never heated over 110 degrees, in order to keep all the enzymes alive, which are lost in many foods when prepared at high cooking temperatures. The benefits and flavors are incredible." In 2012, I appeared on Sarasota cable channel SNN6 with Chef Tyler Kirby, Michelle and Simon's son, to speak about Simon's unique, healthy, delicious cuisine. Also check out Gulf Coast Caviar, run by Tyler Kirby, specializing in locally sourced, sustainable Bottarga (dried, salted red mullet roe from Cortez Bay), a tasty, low-calorie addition to anything from pasta, eggs, or seafood.

Recipe courtesy of Michelle Kirby of Simon's Coffee House.

. . . .

Simon's Raw Beet Ravioli and Jicama Slaw

Entrée • All Phases • Serves 8

INGREDIENTS

Ravioli:

"Cashew Cheese" filling and
   beetroot ravioli
16 ounces cashews
1 Tbsp. organic miso

2 ounces fresh organic lemon juice
sea salt and black pepper, to taste
2 large red and/or gold beetroots

Sauce:

1 cup sun-dried tomatoes

2 large ripe tomatoes

2 cloves fresh garlic

½ cup extra-virgin olive oil

½ cup fresh basil

½ cup fresh Italian parsley

pinch of sea salt, to taste

INSTRUCTIONS

Filling:

- Overnight, soak 16 ounces cashew nuts in water. Drain and rinse in the morning.

- Place in a food processor along with the Tbsp. of miso, 2 ounces fresh organic lemon juice, and sea salt and black pepper, to taste.

Ravioli:

- Peel beetroots and slice very thin (on a meat slicer or mandoline). Make into circles approximately 2½ inches wide.

- Spoon the cashew cheese into the center of the beetroot circle and place another slice on top. Press the outside down to seal in the cashew cheese.

Sauce:

- Soak the cup of sun-dried tomatoes in water for 30 minutes to rehydrate.

- Remove core from raw tomatoes and dice.

- In a food processor, combine both types of tomatoes, the 2 cloves fresh garlic, ½-cup extra-virgin olive oil, ½-cup fresh basil and parsley, pinch of sea salt, to taste, and blend well. Spoon sauce over the ravioli.

Nutrition Facts (per serving) for the Beetroot Ravioli:
Calories: **327** • Calories from fat: **64%** • Fat: **25g**
Saturated fat: **4g** • Cholesterol: **0mg** • Carbohydrates: **20g**
Protein: **11g** • Sodium: **55mg** • Fiber: **3g**

Nutrition Facts (per serving) for the Sauce (yields 8 servings total):
Calories: **147** • Calories from fat: **83%** • Fat: **14g**
Saturated fat: **2g** • Cholesterol: **0mg** • Carbohydrates: **6g**
Protein: **2g** • Sodium: **164mg** • Fiber: **2g**

· · · · · · · · · · ·

Jicama Slaw

Side/Accompaniment • All Phases • Serves 8

INGREDIENTS

4 large jicamas, peeled, chopped, and marinated overnight (see below)

½ cup Braggs organic apple cider vinegar

4 Tbsp. grapeseed oil

sea salt, to taste

½ Napa cabbage, shredded

2 carrots, shredded

1 cucumber, diced

1 each red, green, yellow, and orange bell peppers, stems and seeds removed and finely dice

¼ cup dried cranberries

¼ cup chopped fresh cilantro

1 Tbsp. fresh lime juice

freshly ground black pepper, to taste

INSTRUCTIONS

• Peel and chop or slice the jicama. Place in large bowl.

• Add ½ cup Braggs organic apple cider vinegar, grapeseed oil, and sea salt, to taste, to jicama. Cover bowl, and let sit overnight.

• Add raw veggies for color and flavor, including dried cranberries, cabbage, carrots, cucumber, and assorted bell peppers. Add dried cranberries and cilantro. You may add other raw veggies if desired.

• Add squeeze of lime juice and freshly ground black pepper, to taste.

• Plate Jicama and place ravioli on top with the sauce over the ravioli.

NOTE

The Jicama Slaw can be served on its own, as can the ravioli. The slaw is also delicious with seafood, such as seared tuna and is excellent with added fruit, such as diced ripe mango.

Nutrition Facts (per serving)
Calories: **287** • Calories from fat: **4%** • Fat: **1g**
Saturated fat: **0g** • Cholesterol: **0mg** • Carbohydrates: **66g**
Protein: **6g** • Sodium: **63mg** • Fiber: **33g**

●

Ta-boo, Palm Beach

221 Worth Avenue, Palm Beach, FL 33480 • (561) 835-3500 • www.taboorestaurant.com

This Palm Beach landmark on Tony Worth Avenue has been a social hub for the many celebrities, affluent residents, and visitors to Palm Beach since 1941. Patrons included John F. Kennedy, Frank Sinatra, the Duke and Duchess of Windsor, among others. The restaurant is the place to see and be seen in the most fashionable winter resort town in America. It has been hailed as the best night spot in the country to "drink, laugh, and meet people," and is on everyone's to-do list when visiting Palm Beach.

Recipes courtesy of Mark Mariacher, Manager, Ta-boo Restaurant.

. . . .

Ta-boo Wellness Salad

Salad/Entrée • All Phases (see Note) • Serves 4

INGREDIENTS

Fat-free balsamic vinaigrette:

1 cup fat-free plain yogurt

1 tsp. Dijon mustard

1 tsp. minced fresh garlic

¼ cup balsamic vinegar

kosher salt, to taste

white pepper, to taste

Salad:

1 cup toasted walnuts, roughly chopped

1 cup sun-dried cranberries

1 red onion, chopped

1 cup cooked plain black beans (if canned, rinse and drain very well)

1 cup French green beans, blanched and cut in thirds

1 cup egg whites (from hard-boiled eggs), roughly chopped

1 cup mixed sweet red and yellow peppers, julienned

4 cups baby spinach, chopped

4 cups romaine lettuce, chopped[31]

---

31 Cut spinach and lettuce at last minute with a very sharp knife.

INSTRUCTIONS

Fat-free balsamic vinaigrette:

- Mix all dressing ingredients thoroughly, preferably with an immersion blender or a food processor. Prepare at least an hour in advance. Will keep well in the refrigerator if made with fresh yogurt

Salad:

- Combine all salad ingredients in a large bowl with the dressing (2 ounces per portion).
- Mix thoroughly; salad should be well-coated. At the restaurant, the salad may be ordered with optional poached salmon (133 calories per 4-ounce serving of poached or steamed salmon) and is also good with seared tuna, grilled chicken breast, turkey, or shrimp. If you are looking to reduce your calorie intake, divide the salad portion among two people and top it with a 4-ounce serving of salmon or other protein. It's a win-win!

Nutrition Facts (per serving)
Calories: **591** • Calories from fat: **30%** • Fat: **20g**
Saturated fat: **1g** • Cholesterol: **1mg** • Carbohydrates: **74g**
Protein: **31g** • Sodium: **254mg** • Fiber: **15g**

●

32 East

32 East Atlantic Avenue, Delray Beach, FL 33444 • (561) 276-7868 • www.32east.com

32 East was an instant success when it opened in 1996 at the site of a former auction house in historic downtown Delray, and has set the standard for over 20 years for fine dining in South Palm Beach County and helped transform a once sleepy downtown into a hip, happening destination for dining and nightlife. 32 East features a distinctive, approachable menu that is created daily, based on what is fresh and seasonal. Enjoy great food and wine in a sophisticated, upbeat setting.

Recipe courtesy of 32 East.

. . . .

American Lamb Loin with Wild Mushrooms, Asparagus, and White Wine

Entrée • All Phases • Serves 4

INGREDIENTS

1 tsp. fresh oregano, chopped

½ tsp. fresh garlic, chopped fine

1 Tbsp. white truffle oil (optional)

1 tsp. lemon zest, chopped fine

4 6-ounce lamb loins, trimmed of all fat
   and sinew

2 Tbsp. olive oil to sauté

8 ounces sliced wild mushrooms

1 shallot, thinly sliced

6 ounces white wine

8 ounces chicken stock

8 ounces asparagus, blanched
   and chopped

1 large ripe tomato, peeled and diced

1 Tbsp. herb mixture (finely chopped
   fresh Italian parsley, oregano,
   and chives)

salt and pepper, to taste

4 ounces micro greens

INSTRUCTIONS

- Prepare the marinade by combining the oregano, garlic, truffle oil, and lemon zest in a large bowl.

- Add the lamb, tossing carefully to distribute marinade evenly.

- Let rest overnight in the refrigerator or for at least 2 hours.

- In a heavy-bottomed sauté pan, heat 1 Tbsp. of olive oil until it just smokes.

- Place the lamb into the pan and sear on both sides. Cook until desired doneness, suggest using a meat thermometer and recommend medium-rare.

- Remove the lamb from the pan and let rest for 5 to 10 minutes.

- Toss out remaining oil. Using the same pan, add new Tbsp. of oil with the mushrooms and shallots and sauté.

- Deglaze the pan with white wine and reduce until almost dry.

- Add the chicken stock and reduce by half. Add the asparagus, tomato, herb mixture, and salt and pepper.

Assembly:

- Slice the lamb onto a large platter or on separate dinner plates, then spoon the mushroom sauce over the lamb and garnish with microgreens. I like to serve this with oven-roasted Brussel sprouts or steamed haricots verts with a pinch of sea salt and a drizzle of lemon juice and olive oil.

Nutrition Facts (per serving)
Calories: **511** • Calories from fat: **47%** • Fat: **27g**
Saturated fat: **7g** • Cholesterol: **162mg** • Carbohydrates: **5g**
Protein: **53g** • Sodium: **311mg** • Fiber: **2g**

●

Tramonti Ristorante

119 East Atlantic Avenue, Delray Beach, FL 33444
(561) 276-1944 • www.tramontidelray.com
Angelo's of Mulberry Street
146 Mulberry Street, New York, NY 10013
(212) 966-1277 • www.angelosofmulberryst.com

Delray Beach is fortunate to have the sister location of New York City's famous Angelo's of Mulberry Street, a New York landmark since opening in 1922. Angelo's and Tramonti feature excellent Southern Italian cuisine, with an emphasis on home-style Neapolitan specialties, including a rich tomato sauce, home-made *braciole* (braised, rolled, and stuffed flank steak), freshly made pastas, excellent seafood, and more!

Recipe courtesy of Tramonti Ristorante, Chef Alessandro Silvestri.

. . . .
Zucchini Flowers

Starter/Entrée • Phases Three–Four • Serves 2

INGREDIENTS

Blossoms:

1 cup ricotta (see Note)   ¼ cup fresh mozzarella, diced

3 salted anchovies, chopped

6 large zucchini flower blossoms
(see Note)

Batter:
2 light beers
1 cup all-purpose flour
pinch salt and pepper

½ cup soybean, canola, or olive oil,
for frying

Assembly:
2 cups baby arugula
2 lemon wedges
2 Tbsp. of tomato sauce

optional tsp. of toasted pine nuts
(sprinkle a few on each plate)

INSTRUCTIONS

- Combine ricotta, mozzarella, and anchovies in a bowl.
- Mix well and stuff each zucchini blossom to the top and slightly squeeze top so the flowers hold the filling in place.
- To prepare the batter, mix beer, flour, salt, and pepper until thick. If too thick, add water to thin it out.
- Pop each zucchini blossom in the batter, completely coating each, and allow excess to drip off. Set aside.
- Heat oil in a large pan. When hot, add the flowers and fry until they are lightly golden brown, turning once (about several minutes).
- Prepare a plate lined with paper towels to place cooked flowers on to absorb excess oil.

Assembly:

- Prepare 6 salad plates: Distribute baby arugula equally around the edges of each plate; place a tablespoon of tomato sauce in the middle of each plate. For tomato sauce, I suggest using my recipe, **Fred's San Marzano Tomato Sauce** (page 480). Place one zucchini flower on each plate (not in the sauce), and place lemon wedge on each plate. Serve immediately.

NOTE

This recipe is for large zucchini flowers, approximately 5 inches long. If large flowers are unavailable, substitute 12 smaller flowers. To prepare them the "Roman way," simply omit the ricotta and otherwise prepare as above. Zucchini flowers may also be stuffed with chopped up mixed seafood, such as shrimp and crabmeat, as well as an olive tapenade and may also be brushed with oil and lightly grilled for a lower-calorie alternative.

For home/weight-loss preparation, you may substitute part-skim ricotta, which lowers the calorie count to 574 per serving of 3 flowers. Considering they are both fried and contain cheese, these should be enjoyed in moderation. I recommend limiting them to Phases Three–Four, and limiting the quantity to 1 or 2 as a starter.

Nutrition Facts (per serving) for 3 blossoms:
Calories: **618** • Calories from fat: **60%** • Fat: **41g**
Saturated fat: **15g** • Cholesterol: **79mg** • Carbohydrates: **37g**
Protein: **24g** • Sodium: **532mg** • Fiber: **4g**

•

Trattoria Romana

499 E. Palmetto Park Rd., Boca Raton, FL 33432
(561)-393-6715 • www.trattoriaromanabocaraton.com

Since 1993, Trattoria Romana has been one of Boca Raton's most popular and delicious Italian restaurants. Owned and operated by the Gismondi family (also of Arturo's, The Cannoli Kitchen, and La Nouvelle Maison), this local favorite features an extensive menu with all your favorites such as sumptuous antipasto, amazing seafood, and desserts made from scratch. Don't miss the nightly specials board—favorites include Shrimp Saltimbocca and Langostinos. Also, don't miss adjacent Bar Sorana, with great cocktails and a well-appointed wine list in the heart of fashionable East Boca. The Eggplant Pie (recipe below) has been a house specialty since day one, and is a personal favorite. Although typically served as a starter, it is substantial enough to be an entrée, and is great with a nice salad, or Trattoria Romana's Bruschetta, made with ripe red tomatoes, fresh basil, and garlic.

Recipe courtesy of Guido Barisone, Trattoria Romana.

Trattoria Romana's Eggplant Pie

Starter to share or Entrée • Phases Two–Four •Serves 8

INGREDIENTS

6 large eggs

2 cups all-purpose flour

3 medium eggplant, peeled and sliced
⅛-inch thick

1½ quarts marinara sauce[32]

¾ cup grated Parmigiano-Reggiano

2 cups shredded mozzarella cheese

salt and black pepper, to taste

canola oil, for frying

INSTRUCTIONS

• Using a large, shallow bowl, whisk the eggs with salt and pepper, to taste.

• Using a large, shallow bowl, season flour with salt and pepper, to taste.

• Using a large saucepan, heat a ½-inch of oil to 350 degrees Fahrenheit.

• Line a baking sheet with paper towels, set aside.

• Dredge eggplant in flour, shaking off excess.

• Dip eggplant in egg wash.

• Working in batches, fry eggplant until golden brown, drain on prepared baking sheet, adding more oil as needed.

• Pre-heat the oven to 350 degrees Fahrenheit.

• Place a thin layer of marinara sauce in the bottom of a 9-inch pie plate.

• Cover with a thin overlapping layer of eggplant.

• Top with a thin layer of marinara and sprinkle with Parmigiano-Reggiano.

• Repeat the process with remaining eggplant.

• Cover with foil and bake 30 minutes. Remove foil, top with mozzarella and bake 5 minutes. To serve, cut into wedges.

Nutrition Facts (per serving)
Calories: **478** • Calories from fat: **41%** • Fat: **22g**
Saturated fat: **7g** • Cholesterol: **170mg** • Carbohydrates: **49g**
Protein: **23g** • Sodium: **1,186mg** • Fiber: **8g**

32 Use my recipe, or purchase a quality jarred sauce, such as Rao's Homemade.

•

Trevini, Palm Beach

290 Sunset Avenue, Palm Beach, FL 33480 • (561) 833-3883 • www.treviniristorante.com

Since opening in 2000 in Palm Beach, owners Gianni Minervini and Claudio Trevisan have been featuring a wonderful blend of Northern and Southern Italian cuisine, with Claudio being from Stresa in the north, and Gianni from Bari in the south. Trevini recently moved to a beautiful new location in the historic Bradley Park Hotel in Palm Beach, with a modern interior and a lovely, romantic, old-world courtyard, reminiscent of Italy. Gianni, who presides over the elegant, contemporary dining room is a gentleman, one of the nicest, most accommodating restaurant owners anywhere—please tell him I sent you!

Recipe courtesy of Gianni Minervini.

. . . .

Orecchiette con Polpa di Granchio e Asparagi (Ear-shaped Pasta with Crabmeat and Asparagus)

Entrée • Phases Two–Four • Serves 2

INGREDIENTS

1 Tbsp. olive oil

1 Tbsp. fresh garlic, minced

8 stalks asparagus, blanched and cut
    into small pieces

6 ounces lump crabmeat

12 cherry tomatoes, cut into quarters

½ ounce Pinot Grigio or dry white wine

1 ounce vegetable broth

salt and pepper, to taste

1 Tbsp. Italian parsley, chopped

4 basil leaves, torn

6 ounces orecchiette pasta, cooked

INSTRUCTIONS

• In a saucepan, heat olive oil and garlic until golden brown.

• Add the asparagus, crabmeat, and tomatoes and sauté for 2 minutes.

• Add the white wine and vegetable broth.

- Season with salt and pepper.
- Add parsley and basil.
- Cook the pasta *al dente*.
- Add sauce to pasta and serve.

Nutrition Facts (per serving)
Calories: **490** • Calories from fat: **17%** • Fat: **10g**
Saturated fat: **1g** • Cholesterol: **66mg** • Carbohydrates: **71g**
Protein: **29g** • Sodium: **599mg** • Fiber: **5g**

Georgia

•

Atlanta Fish Market

See recipe for Hong Kong-Style Fish at City Fish Market in Boca Raton, FL.

•

Buckhead Diner

3073 Piedmont Road, Atlanta, GA 30305
(404) 262-3336 • www.buckheadrestaurants.com

Buckhead Diner, owned by Pano Karatassos and the Buckhead Life Restaurant Group, behind Chop's Lobster Bar and City Fish Market in Boca Raton is truly a gourmet diner and an Atlanta staple. Featuring a fun, upscale atmosphere, skillful service, and an innovative menu, Buckhead Diner is one of many musts attributable to the Buckhead Life Restaurant Group on any Atlanta itinerary!

Recipe courtesy of Tricia Jefferson and Sara Lett, Buckhead Life Restaurant Group Marketing Department.

. . . .
Butternut Squash Soup

Soup • All Phases • Yields 20 cups

INGREDIENTS

2 Tbsp. olive oil

4 cups chopped onions (about 3
   medium onions)

2 cups diced carrots (about 5 medium)

4 cloves garlic

3 large butternut squash, peeled, cut
   in half, seeded, and diced (about 4½
   pounds yielding 12 cups chopped)

1 red Fresno pepper, stem and seeds
   removed, chopped

10 cups low-sodium chicken stock
   or broth

2 Tbsp. salt

5 sprigs thyme

1 sprig rosemary

1 stick cinnamon

1 Bay Leaf

½ tsp. black peppercorns

white pepper, to taste

honey to taste

Tabasco, to taste

INSTRUCTIONS

• In a large stockpot, heat olive oil over medium-high heat and add onions,
  carrots, and garlic.

• Sauté 5 minutes or until onion is translucent.

• Add squash and pepper and cook until vegetables just begin to soften,
  about 5 minutes.

• Add chicken stock and salt, and adjust heat so soup is simmering.

• Make a bouquet garni by wrapping thyme, rosemary, cinnamon, Bay
  Leaf, and peppercorns in a small square of cheesecloth. Drop into soup.
  Simmer soup for 1 hour. Remove bouquet garni.

• In the jar of a blender, or using an immersion blender, purée the soup,
  then strain through a sieve. Season, to taste, with white pepper, honey
  and Tabasco.

Nutrition Facts (per serving) provided by the restaurant:
Calories: **144** • Calories from fat: **22%** • Fat: **5g**
Saturated fat: **Trace** • Cholesterol: **0mg** • Carbohydrates: **26g**
Protein: **12g** • Sodium: **1,114mg**

•

Chop's Lobster Bar, Atlanta

See Chop's Lobster Bar's Spinach Salad with Creamy Basil Dressing in Boca Raton, FL.

•

Kyma

3085 Piedmont Road, Atlanta, GA 30305
(404) 262-0702 • www.buckheadrestaurants.com

Kyma is the Buckhead Life Restaurant Group's contemporary seafood taverna, showcasing an upscale, extensive Greek- and Mediterranean-inspired menu with many excellent choices, which are low in calories and high in flavor.

Recipe courtesy of Tricia Jefferson and Sara Lett, Buckhead Life Restaurant Group Marketing Department.

. . . .

Kyma's Slow-Cooked Eggplant Stew with Sweet Onions and Tomatoes

Soup/Entrée • All Phases (see Note) • Serves 6

INGREDIENTS

Stew:

5 Tbsp. olive oil, divided

5 medium sweet onions (about 6 cups), thinly sliced

1½ tsp. kosher salt, divided

3½ pounds Japanese eggplants, cut diagonally into 1-inch thick pieces

freshly ground black pepper

4 garlic cloves, halved

3 Tbsp. chopped fresh thyme

1¼ cups tomato sauce (see below)

⅓ cup chopped parsley

Tomato sauce:

1 onion, sliced

2 garlic cloves, sliced

1 28-ounce can puréed tomatoes

pinch of granulated sugar (omit
    in Phase One, optional for
    dietary reasons)

1 Bay Leaf

1 tsp. dried oregano

salt and pepper, to taste

INSTRUCTIONS

Stew:

- Pre-heat oven to 300 degrees Fahrenheit.

- In a large heavy saucepan over medium heat, add 2 Tbsp. oil.

- Add the onions and ½ teaspoon salt.

- Cook slowly, stirring occasionally, until golden brown and cooked down to about 1 cup, about 40 minutes. Set aside to cool.

- Meanwhile, in another large heavy saucepan over medium heat, add the remaining 3 Tbsp. oil.

- Add the eggplant, 1 teaspoon salt, and season with pepper.

- Cook for 15 minutes, stirring occasionally.

- Add garlic and thyme and continue cooking, stirring occasionally, until eggplant is golden brown and cooked down to about 6 cups, about 15–20 minutes.

- Season with salt and pepper, to taste, drain on paper towels and cool.

- In a 2-quart casserole, pour in enough tomato sauce to just cover the bottom.

- Spread a third of the onions and then top with a layer of eggplant, using about 2 cups.

- Season with pepper.

- Cover eggplant with half of remaining sauce, half of remaining onions, and another layer of eggplant.

- Season with pepper.

- Top with remaining sauce, remaining onions, and remaining eggplant, arranging slices decoratively.

- Season with pepper.

- Cover casserole and bake 20–30 minutes or until extremely hot. To serve, garnish with parsley.

Tomato Sauce:

- In a medium saucepan over high heat, add oil.
- Once oil is hot, add the onion and cook until translucent and golden.
- Add garlic and cook 2 minutes.
- Add tomatoes, sugar (omit in Phase One, optional for dietary reasons in other Phases), Bay Leaf, oregano, and season with salt and pepper, to taste.
- Bring to a simmer and cook for 45 minutes, stirring every 10 minutes.
- Remove Bay leaf and run sauce through a food mill or purée in a blender.

NOTE

For maximum efficiency, cook the sauce, onions and eggplant simultaneously in 3 separate pots. Serve leftovers over pasta with the unused tomato sauce.

Nutrition Facts (per serving)
Calories: **241** • Calories from fat: **42%** • Fat: **12g**
Saturated fat: **2g** • Cholesterol: **0mg** • Carbohydrates: **33g**
Protein: **5g** • Sodium: **323mg**

•

La Grotta Ristorante, Atlanta

2637 Peachtree Road, NE, Atlanta, GA 30305 • (404) 231-1368 • www.lagrottaatlanta.com

Since 1978, La Grotta has been offering fine northern Italian dining in a lovely, intimate setting overlooking a beautiful garden in the heart of upscale Buckhead. Owned by Chef Antonio Abizanda and Sergio Favalli, La Grotta offers one of the most interesting and innovative Italian menus in Atlanta and has held the prestigious AAA Four Diamond Award and been voted "Best Italian Restaurant" in *Atlanta* magazine for many years. Excellent food, a lovely atmosphere, and very cordial, accommodating owners and staff make La Grotta a perennial winner and a favorite of mine in Atlanta. The slightly more casual La Grotta Ravinia opened in 1993 and has also been awarded the AAA Four Diamond Award. La Grotta's chef is always willing to accommodate guests, whether it be to prepare a favorite dish not featured, or to prepare high-quality vegetarian, cholesterol-free, and grilled specialties, along with excellent pasta, meat, and seafood dishes.

Recipe courtesy of Chef Antonio Abizanda, La Grotta.

. . . .

Granchio con Avocado, Arancia, e Pompelmo (Lump Crabmeat with Grainy Mustard over Avocado, Orange, and Grapefruit Segments)

Starter/Entré • All Phases • Serves 4

INGREDIENTS

2 lightly packed cups jumbo lump crabmeat (about 8 ounces)

3 Tbsp. extra-virgin olive oil, divided

2 Tbsp. grainy mustard

salt and pepper, to taste

2 ripe Haas avocados, halved, seeded and cut into ¼-inch cubes

juice of one lime

1 large navel orange

1 large grapefruit

1 large ripe tomato, cut into 4 slices

½ cup of basil micro greens[33]

INSTRUCTIONS

- In a medium bowl, pick through crab, removing any bits of shell.
- Toss with 1 Tbsp. olive oil and mustard.
- Season lightly with salt and freshly ground pepper. Set aside.
- In a small bowl, toss avocado cubes with lime juice and 1 Tbsp. olive oil. Season, to taste, with salt and freshly ground pepper. Set aside.
- Cut colored peel and white membrane off orange and grapefruit.
- Over a plate, hold the orange in your hand and use a paring knife to slice next to one of the membranes that holds the segments together. Cut down to the core of the orange. Move your knife to the membrane on

---

33 Micro greens are sometimes available at local specialty and farmers markets; if unavailable, substitute with finely sliced fresh basil leaves.

the other side of that segment and slice down to the core. Remove the segment and put on a plate.

- Repeat for the remainder of the orange and then for the grapefruit.
- You can squeeze the juice left in the orange and grapefruit membranes and core and reserve for another use.
- Prepare 4 serving plates. Arrange a slice of tomato on each plate. Using a ring mold, top each tomato with ¼ of the prepared avocado.
- Top the avocado with ¼ of the prepared crab.
- Garnish crab with microgreens and divide orange and grapefruit segments (all fruit with no pith or membrane) between the plates.
- Drizzle with the remaining Tbsp. of olive oil and serve immediately.

Nutrition Facts (per serving)
Provided by the restaurant.
Calories: **352** • Calories from fat: **65%** • Fat: **27g**
Saturated fat: **4g** • Cholesterol: **44mg** • Carbohydrates: **19g**
Protein: **14g** • Sodium: **283mg**

•

Pricci

500 Pharr Road, NE, Atlanta, GA 30305
(404) 237-2941 • www.buckheadrestaurants.com

Pricci is a contemporary Italian restaurant owned by the Buckhead Life Restaurant Group, and is best known for its innovative menu, which includes classic Italian with a fun, modern twist.

Recipe courtesy of Tricia Jefferson and Sara Lett, Buckhead Life Restaurant Group Marketing Department.

· ·

Grilled Lamb Chops with Mushroom Funghetto

Entrée • Phases Two–Four (see Note) • Serves 3 (in the restaurant, this serves 2)

INGREDIENTS

1 cup crushed Italian tomatoes

¼ cup extra-virgin olive oil

2 Tbsp. fresh lemon juice

1 Tbsp. whole-grain mustard

1 ounce (about ¼ cup) fresh rosemary, roughly chopped

3 garlic cloves, minced

1 tsp. salt

½ tsp. ground black pepper

6 thick-cut Frenched rib lamb chops

1 Tbsp. butter

9 ounces wild mushrooms (see Note)

¼ cup veal jus (see Note)

INSTRUCTIONS

- In a 9-inch-square baking dish, combine the tomatoes, olive oil, lemon juice, mustard, rosemary, garlic, salt, and pepper and whisk until well combined. Marinate the lamb in tomato mixture in the refrigerator overnight.

- To cook, pre-heat the grill. In a sauté pan over medium-high heat, melt the butter and then add mushrooms and sauté until tender, 4–5 minutes. Wipe off the extra marinade from the chops and grill to desired doneness, about 3 minutes per side for medium-rare.

- Arrange half the mushrooms on each of 2 plates. Top with 3 chops each. Drizzle each with half the veal jus.

NOTE

Although Chef Piero Premoli uses a combination of beautiful wild mushrooms—shiitake, maitake and chanterelle—you can substitute any combination. For the veal jus, look for a high-quality concentrated stock available in grocery and specialty stores, then dilute according to package. The chef recommends pairing the lamb with a simply sautéed vegetable, such as kale or Swiss chard. Additionally, this should be a Phase Two or later meal, and should be 2 chops per person.

Nutrition Facts (per serving) Serves 3
Calories: **666** • Calories from fat: **39%** • Fat: **30g**
Saturated fat: **7g** • Cholesterol: **89mg** • Carbohydrates: **72g**
Protein: **35g** • Sodium: **1,111mg**

Maine

•

Balance Rock Inn

21 Albert Meadow, Bar Harbor, Maine 04609
(207) 288-2610 • www.balancerockinn.com

Originally built as a family "cottage" in 1903, when wealthy tycoons selected the most desirable locations along the rocky Maine coast for their summer mansions, the AAA Four Diamond Balance Rock Inn today is the preferred choice for secluded, romantic and luxury amenities reflecting a time gone by. The inn is set on a secluded tree-covered property with panoramic views of Frenchman's Bay and the ocean, and offers a tremendous sense of privacy and serenity, only steps away from downtown Bar Harbor. Enjoy comfortably appointed guest rooms or luxury suites, craft cocktails, and gourmet dining.

Recipe courtesy of chef/owner Aaron Miles.

Shrimp and Lobster Cakes, with Preserved Lemon Aioli & Lobster Oil

Entrée • All Phases • Serves 4

INGREDIENTS

Lobster Cakes:

½ pound raw shrimp peeled and
    deveined, tails off
1 Tbsp. chopped tarragon
zest and juice 1 lemon
zest 1 orange

1 clove garlic
1 tsp. ground coriander
2 tsp. kosher salt
1 1½ pound live Maine lobster
pot of water

Lobster Oil:

Reserved lobster shells crushed
1 cup canola oil

Aioli:

2 egg yolks	1 sprig tarragon
1 cup canola or olive oil	juice 1 lemon
1 clove garlic	1 preserved Meyer lemon

INSTRUCTIONS

Lobster Cakes:

- Boil water to kill lobster. Suggest placing the lobster in a large tray or dish and pour boiling water over the lobster. This makes it easier to clean while still keeping the meat raw.

- Clean lobster and chop meat reserving the shells.

- Put shrimp and all other ingredients in a food processor and blend to a paste.

- In a bowl fold in lobster meat.

- Line a baking sheet with parchment paper and fill ring molds with lobster mix. Bake at 300 degrees Fahrenheit until liquid forms at the top of each cake.

Lobster Oil:

- Cover shells in oil and simmer for 30 minutes, oil should be bright red.

- Strain through a coffee filter for the most clarity

Aioli:

- Clean the lemon of pith leaving only the rind, run the rind under cold water.

- Add the yolks garlic tarragon, lemon juice, and preserved lemon to a blender or food processor.

- With the mixer on high slowly add the oil to the mix, being sure to get a solid emulsification.

- Season with salt and pepper. If too thick, it can be thinned out with lemon juice or water to achieve the desired consistency.

- Plate the cakes. Drizzle the Lobster Oil and Aioli on each plate and serve with choice of greens optional.

NOTE

The Lobster Oil quantity has been scaled down from 2 cups oil to 1 cup for home use. It should be lightly drizzled on each plate, approximately 1 tablespoon (½ ounce) per serving (thus yields approximately 16 servings).

The Aioli should also be lightly drizzled on the plate, approximately 1 tablespoon per serving, so we will approximate 16 servings. This is great topped with a spicy salad. The hotel uses watercress, fennel, and red amaranth. You may wish to omit the Lobster Oil in Phase One.

Nutrition Facts (per serving)
Calories: **85** • Calories from fat: **13%** • Fat: **1g**
Saturated fat: **0.2g** • Cholesterol: **86mg** • Carbohydrates: **4.5g**
Protein: **12.2g** • Sodium: **1,353mg** • Fiber: **1.6g**

-

Nutrition Facts (per serving) for the Lobster Oil
Calories: **120** • Calories from fat: **100%** • Fat: **14g**
Saturated fat: **1g** • Cholesterol: **0mg** • Carbohydrates: **0g**
Protein: **0g** • Sodium: **Trace from lobster shell** • Fiber: **0g**

-

Nutrition Facts (per serving)
Calories: **130** • Calories from fat: **98%** • Fat: **14g**
Saturated fat: **1g** • Cholesterol: **23mg** • Carbohydrates: **1g**
Protein: **0.5g** • Sodium: **1mg** • Fiber: **0.3g**

•

Natalie's at Camden Harbour Inn

83 Bayview St., Camden, Maine 94843 • (207) 236-4200 • www.camdenharbourinn.com

Camden Harbour Inn features the ultimate luxurious accommodations, service, and attention to detail that Relais & Châteaux is synonymous with worldwide. The inn and Natalie's Restaurant boast sweeping panoramic views of Camden Harbor, the mountains, and Penobscot Bay and is an experience not to be missed. The AAA Four Diamond Natalie's combines impeccable European style with the welcoming spirit of New England and offers a modern take on New England cuisine inspired by the seasons and enhanced with global flavors to create a world-class dining experience. Natalie's uniquely blends a current sense of place and time with modern techniques and the bounty of Maine, sourcing ingredients from local fishermen and farmers. With the leadership of Executive Chefs Chris Long and Shelby Stevens, Natalie's has become one of the most awarded and exclusive culinary destinations in all of New England. Natalie's cocktails are as renowned as the food, and the wine list features over two hundred hand-picked bottles representing some of the world's best vineyards. Natalie's offers a seasonal 5-course Maine Lobster Tasting Menu, 3-course *Prix Fixe* as well as a bar menu.

Reservations at Natalie's are strongly encouraged, especially during the summer season, even for guests of the Inn. For the ultimate luxurious culinary escape, you will want to stay over and enjoy the charming towns of Camden, Rockport, and Rockland, where you will find more great restaurants, boutiques, recreational opportunities, and even a few wineries. Inn guests enjoy complimentary coffee, tea, and snacks all day and a complimentary gourmet à la *carte* champagne breakfast featuring freshly baked treats prepared by pastry chef Shelby, and extensive à la carte offerings. For the ultimate culinary escape to Maine, check out sister property The Danforth Inn in Portland, which is home to Tempo Dulu, modern Southeast Asian fine dining, and Opium, an exotic, sophisticated cocktail bar and lounge.

Recipe courtesy of Julienne Engelstad, Camden Harbour Inn Marketing.

. . . .

Black Bass with Gnocchi and Vegetables

Entrée • Phases Two–Four • Serves 4

INGREDIENTS

Black Bass:

2 12-ounce fillets of bass, cut in half to create 4 portions (skin left on one side)	1 Tbsp. butter 3 sprigs of thyme

Gnocchi:

1 russet potato	1 pinch of black pepper
1 egg yolk	¾ cup flour
½ tsp. kosher salt	½ cup salt for roasting

1 Tbsp. olive oil for drizzle at end

Vadouvan Butter Sauce:

1 Tbsp. minced shallots

1 Tbsp. canola oil

¼ cup dry white wine

¼ cup vegetable stock

3 Tbsp. butter

2 tsp. Vadovan powder

lemon juice to taste

salt to taste

Vegetables:

½ cup Morel Mushrooms

½ cup Chanterelle Mushrooms

½ cup of asparagus tips, blanched

1 tsp. chives, cut small

1 tsp. preserved lemon rind, minced

3 Tbsp. dry white wine

¼ cup vegetable stock

2 Tbsp. butter

sherry vinegar to taste

1 tsp. canola oil

salt to taste

INSTRUCTIONS

Black Bass:

- Season the fillets with salt and sear the Bass skin side down in a hot pan on medium-high heat keeping the skin flat against the bottom of the pan. Once the skin is crispy, turn the heat off the pan and flip the Bass over.

- Baste the fish with the butter and thyme sprigs. Allow the Bass to finish cooking from the residual heat of the pan. If you have a thicker fillet, place it in the oven to finish.

Gnocchi:

- Wash the russet potato and poke small holes in it with a knife.

- Place ¼ cup of salt on a small roasting pan then place the potato on top of the pile of salt and evenly pour the remaining ¼ cup of salt on top of the potato.

- Place the potato in the oven and roast at 350 degrees Fahrenheit until the potato is soft to the touch.

- Cut the potato in half and scoop out the inside of the potato. Pass the potato through a tamis.

- Gather the potato into a pile sprinkle ½ of the flour on top of the potato along with the salt and pepper. Make a little well in the potato pile and place the yolk in the center.
- Using a bowl scraper chop the potato and flour together. When you have chopped the ingredients together as much as you can, sprinkle the rest of the flour onto the potato and gently knead the flour into the potato until all of the flour is incorporated.
- Take your ball of potato "dough" and roll it out into a long thin log and cut it into ½-inch pieces.
- Bring small pot of water with a pinch of salt to a boil.
- Put all of the gnocchi into the boiling water at once. They will sink to the bottom of the pot. After a few moments the gnocchi will rise back up to the top.
- When the gnocchi have come to the top of the water they have finished cooking. Scoop them out with a slotted spoon, place on a baking sheet and drizzle with a little olive oil. Allow to cool.

Vadouvan Butter Sauce:

- Place canola oil in a large sauté on high heat.
- Add the shallots and cook until for a few moments (no color).
- Deglaze the pan with white wine.
- Reduce the wine *au sec* (until almost dry).
- Next add the vegetable stock, butter, and Vadouvan then reduce the heat to medium and reduce the liquid until the liquid creates a glaze.
- At this point add the gnocchi and cook until they are hot.
- Be careful not to reduce the sauce too much as that it breaks. If the sauce does break and become separated add a tiny bit of water until it comes back together.

Vegetables:

- Place a large sauté pan on high heat and add the canola oil.
- When the oil is hot add the mushrooms and sauté until they have a little color and are cooked through.
- Once the Mushrooms are cooked deglaze the pan with wine and cook *au sec* (until almost dry).

- Then add the vegetable stock, butter, chives, preserved lemon, asparagus and butter. Reduce to a shiny gaze and season to taste with sherry vinegar and salt.

NOTE

For dietary purposes, may reduce butter by half.

> **Nutrition Facts (per serving)**
> Calories: **583** • Calories from fat: **46%** • Fat: **30g**
> Saturated fat: **13g** • Cholesterol: **240.5mg** • Carbohydrates: **26g**
> Protein: **46g** • Sodium: **1,568mg** • Fiber: **3g**

Massachusetts

•

Abe & Louie's,
Boston, MA, and Boca Raton, FL

2200 West Glades Road, Boca Raton, FL 33431 • (561) 447-0024
793 Boylston Street, Boston, MA 02116 • (617) 536-6300
www.abeandlouies.com

Abe & Louie's is considered one of the top prime steakhouses in Boston, as well as in beautiful Palm Beach County, Florida. Known for great steaks, excellent seafood, an extensive menu of incredible soups, salads, starters, sides, and specials, outstanding service, and an extensive wine list, Abe & Louie's is a favorite choice for lunch and dinner.

Recipe courtesy of Abe and Louie's and Head Chef Gary Mitchell.

. . . .

Roasted Beet, Poached Pear, and Goat Cheese Salad

Salad/Entrée • Serves 6

INGREDIENTS

12 ounces red beets

12 ounces golden beets

1 pear

½ cup white wine

6 ounces Vermont goat cheese

freshly cracked black pepper, to roll
   goat cheese in (optional)

3 Tbsp. minced fresh herbs (tarragon,
   parsley, and chives)

1½ tsp. olive oil

1½ tsp. fresh lemon juice

Sea salt, to taste

2 cups mâche (mixed greens or
   spring mix)

4 ounces Pomegranate Vinaigrette

INSTRUCTIONS

- Place the beets in a shallow pan with a cup of water and roast for about 2 hours at 300 degrees Fahrenheit.

- Check to be sure they are cooked through. The beets should be soft but not mushy. Cut beets into ¼-inch slices (a mandoline is ideal for slicing).

- Cut pear in half and core before cooking. Cook pear in a shallow pan with ½ cup white wine for about 15 minutes at 300 degrees Fahrenheit until soft.

- Cut goat cheese in ½-inch slices and roll the outside edge only in pepper.

Assembly:

- On each of 6 plates, arrange beets and pears in alternating slices around the plate: first a red beet, then a golden beet, and then the pear; you should use 4 slices of each.

- In the middle of the plate place the peppered goat cheese and top this with the mâche that has been drizzled with a little bit of olive oil, lemon juice, and sea salt.

- Drizzle the pomegranate vinaigrette over the beets and pears only.

NOTE

This is an excellent, beautiful salad that can easily go well with some grilled or pan-seared fish, shrimp cocktail, lobster tail, or sliced steak, such as Filet Mignon, to make a truly satisfying meal.

Nutrition Facts (per serving) for the Salad, without the dressing.
Calories: **197** • Calories from fat: **54%** • Fat: **12g**
Saturated fat: **7g** • Cholesterol: **30mg** • Carbohydrates: **13g**
Protein: **11g** • Sodium: **196mg** • Fiber: **3g**

. . . .

Pomegranate Vinaigrette[34]

INGREDIENTS

½ cup Abe and Louie's dressing
  (see below)

½ cup pomegranate juice
½ cup olive oil

---

34 Yields 2 cups.

INSTRUCTIONS

Place Abe and Louie's dressing and the pomegranate juice in a mixer and turn on to medium-high; drizzle in the olive oil slowly, being careful not to pour oil too fast.

NOTE

This dressing contains 42 calories per one Tbsp. serving. Therefore, the beet, pear, and goat cheese salad, with one Tbsp. of dressing, contains 242 calories per serving.

. . . .

Abe and Louie's Dressing

Quantities adjusted for home use to yield approximately 2 cups, or 32 servings, of 1 Tbsp. per serving.

INGREDIENTS

1 cup canola oil	2 Tbsp. grated Parmesan
⅓ cup olive oil	pinch salt
⅓ cup good red wine vinegar	pinch white pepper
1 Tbsp. Dijon mustard	juice from 1 lemon

INSTRUCTIONS

• Place all ingredients in a mixer except the oils and the cheese.

• On medium-high speed slowly add the oils until incorporated, turn down to low speed, and add the cheese.

• Place in a container and refrigerate until needed for service.

Nutrition Facts (per serving) for Pomegranate Vinaigrette (1 Tbsp.):
Calories: **85** • Calories from fat: **100%** • Fat: **10g**
Saturated fat: **1g** • Cholesterol: **1mg** • Carbohydrates: **1g**
Protein: **0g** • Sodium: **13mg** • Fiber: **0g**

. . . .

Beef and Mushroom Barley Soup

Soup/Entrée • Phases Two–Four • Serves 8

INGREDIENTS

4 ounces salted butter

1 ½ pounds good-quality stew beef, diced small

½ pound carrots, diced small

1 Spanish onion, diced small

¼ pound celery, diced small

½ pound sliced white mushrooms

4 Tbsp. beef base

¾ gallon good-quality beef stock or broth

¼ Tbsp. thyme leaves

4 bay leaves

pinch salt and black pepper

¾ pound barley pearls

INSTRUCTIONS

• Place butter in a stock pan and melt on low heat. When butter is melted, turn up the heat to medium-high and place beef in the pan.

• Cook the beef until almost done and then add the carrots, onions, celery and mushrooms and cook until vegetables are tender.

• Pour all the beef base and beef stock into the pan and stir to incorporate; add the seasonings and the barley and turn up the heat until soup boils, then turn down to a simmer.

• Simmer about 40 minutes until the barley is cooked.

• Adjust seasoning if necessary.

Nutrition Facts (per serving)
Calories: **498** • Calories from fat: **40%** • Fat: **22g**
Saturated fat: **11g** • Cholesterol: **102mg** • Carbohydrates: **37g**
Protein: **35g** • Sodium: **1582mg** • Fiber: **7g**

Wheatleigh, Lenox

Hawthorne Rd., Lenox, MA 01240 • (413) 637-0610 • www.wheatleigh.com

Wheatleigh was built in 1893 by Henry H. Cook as a wedding present for his daughter (quite a generous father), Georgie, who married Carlos de Heredia, a Spanish Count. Cook was a New York financier, banker, railroad magnate and real estate tycoon. He was a descendant of Captain Thomas Cook, founder of Portsmouth, R.I., and the son of Constant Cook, who helped build the Erie Railroad. Reportedly, Cook built Wheatleigh as a "summer cottage" for his daughter because she had brought a title into the family. Wheatleigh was designed by the prominent Boston architectural firm of Peabody and Stearns in the style of a sixteenth century Florentine palazzo. Many of the materials and over 150 artisans were brought from Italy to accomplish the intricate carvings. Frederick Law Olmsted, the landscape architect who designed New York's Central Park, was responsible for creating "Wheatleigh Park" on the land surrounding the palazzo. During the "Gilded Age" Wheatleigh was the site of many grand parties and musical events. Today, this ultra-luxurious hideaway features the ultimate in accommodations, flawless service, and some of the best cuisine in the country, by Chef Jeffrey Thompson. Dining at Wheatleigh one can expect the freshest regional, and seasonal cuisine with global influences, exquisitely presented and paired with an outstanding wine list, and flawlessly served by a gracious European trained staff.

Recipe courtesy of Wheatleigh and Chef Jeffrey Thompson.

. . . .

Butternut Squash Soup with Chestnut and White Truffle

Soup • Phases Two–Four • Serves 4

INGREDIENTS

2 pounds peeled and chopped butternut squash	2 quarts water
1 shallot, sliced	2 Tbsp. canola oil
½ cup orange juice	1 Bay Leaf
1 sprig rosemary	¼ orange peel
	2 ounces white wine

¼ cup dark brown sugar (optional)

salt and pepper to taste

4 chestnuts

1 Tbsp. olive oil to sauté chestnuts

handful of chives for garnish

truffle oil to drizzle (optional)

several shavings of white truffle
(see Note)

INSTRUCTIONS

Squash:

- In a large pot, sweat the squash in 2 Tbsp. canola oil with the shallot, orange peel, rosemary and Bay Leaf.
- When squash is softened add the brown sugar and cook for one minute.
- Deglaze with the white wine and reduce.
- Add the juice and water and season with salt and pepper.
- Cook until the squash is tender.
- Remove from heat and purée soup in the blender and strain through a *chinois* or sieve.

Garnish:

- For the garnish, crack several chestnuts, removing the shell, sautée the chestnuts in olive oil for several minutes, and seasoning and chives.

Assembly:

- Spoon soup into bowls, place the chestnut in the center of the soup, drizzle with a drop of white truffle oil and shave fresh white truffle on the top.

NOTE

White truffles from Italy are a prized and expensive delicacy, and typically sell for well over $100 an ounce. For this recipe, a one-ounce white truffle will more than suffice. There are special truffle shavers available at specialty markets and online, or you may use a mandoline. White truffles are typically available during the autumn in the United States at specialty markets, and online. Depending on availability, you may omit the white truffles, and substitute with black truffles, which are more widely available (and considerably less expensive).

Nutrition Facts (per serving)
Calories: **386** • Calories from fat: **41%** • Fat: **18g**
Saturated fat: **2g** • Cholesterol: **0mg** • Carbohydrates: **56.6g**
Protein: **3g** • Sodium: **54mg** • Fiber: **5g**

. . . .

Seared Tuna with Broccolini, Couscous, and Squash

Entrée • All Phases • Serves 4

INGREDIENTS

4 5-ounce portions of tuna

1½ cups cooked couscous[35]

1 bunch broccolini

1 each small delicate squash

1 Tbsp. thinly sliced chives

citrus *fleur de sel*[36], to season

4 Tbsp. lemon glaze (see below)

INSTRUCTIONS

Tuna:

• Rub each fillet with olive oil, salt and pepper and mark on the grill on both sides.

• Place fish on a tray and place in the oven to finish the cooking.

• Season with the *fleur de sel*.

Broccolini[37]*:*

• Clean and trim broccolini into florets with small stems.

• Blanch in boiling salted water, then shock in ice-water bath.

• When cooled, drain on a towel.

• Lightly warm in olive oil, season with fleur de sel and chives for serving with the tuna.

---

35 Also called *fregola sarda*—cook according to instructions on packaging.

36 Make it at home with fleur de sel, dried citrus zest, orange, lemon, lime, chives, and pink peppercorn.

37 Prepare Broccollini, Couscous, Squash, and Lemon Glaze in advance.

Couscous:

- In a pan place the couscous and a little water and olive oil to glaze. Finish with seasoning and chives.

Squash:

- Slice squash into rings and take out the seeds, toss in olive oil and grill, place in the oven to finish the cooking and then season with fleur de sel and chives.

Lemon Glaze:

- 1 each thyme sprig
- 1 each Bay Leaf
- 3 cloves garlic confit
- 1 shallot confit
- ½ cup honey
- ¾ cup grain mustard
- ¾ cup water
- 1 cup lemon juice
- salt and white pepper to taste

INSTRUCTIONS

- Place all items in a pot and simmer and reduce by half. Strain and continue to reduce to a glaze consistency. Season to taste.

Assembly:

- Place a spoon of the couscous in the delicate squash ring on the right side of the plate, place the fish on the left, arrange the broccolini with the slices of tuna. Spoon the glaze over the fish and around the plate.

NOTE

This would be suitable for Phase One without the couscous.

Nutrition Facts (per serving)
Calories: **696** • Calories from fat: **16%** • Fat: **12g**
Saturated fat: **2.5g** • Cholesterol: **44mg** • Carbohydrates: **95.5g**
Protein: **50g** • Sodium: **133mg** • Fiber: **6g**

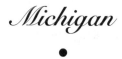

Michigan

•

Charley's Crab, Grand Rapids and Palm Beach, FL (See Florida)

See recipe for Chilled Gazpacho with Charley's Crab's Fat-Free Italian Vinaigrette Dressing at Charley's Crab in Palm Beach, Florida

•

Chateau Chantal

15900 Rue de Vin, Traverse City, Michigan 49686
231.223.4110 • www.chateauchantal.com

The beautiful Chateau Chantal winery and B&B sits on a commanding hill in the heart of the Old Mission Peninsula overlooking East & West Grand Traverse Bays near beautiful Traverse City. The Begin family, Robert, Nadine and daughter Marie-Chantal, opened their doors in 1993 upon the completion of a French style three room B&B, winery, and vineyard estates. By July 2003, the B&B's circle of friends has grown considerably and the family completed a 15,000-square foot expansion, which increased the total units available to eleven. Located on a sisxty-five-acre estate in one of the most scenic areas of the Great Lakes, the B&B provides a unique destination that combines vineyards and winery, a bed & breakfast, gourmet food, great local wine, fresh air, and great hospitality.

Chateau Chantal focuses on Michigan wines, producing Riesling, Chardonnay, Pinot Grigio, Pinot Noir, Cabernet Franc and other varietals. While Chateau Chantal was not incorporated until 1991, its history began in December 1983, when Robert and Nadine formed Begin Orchards and purchased 60 acres of cherry orchards on the estate property. Between 1984 and 1991, the Begins cleared much of this land, planted various grapes varieties and purchased additional land. In July 1990, Mr. Begin received a Special Use Permit from the Peninsula Township to operate the Chateau. If you are looking for an elegant place to stay in the heart of Traverse City's wine country, Chateau Chantal is the place. If you are looking to experience the best in Michigan wines, definitely call to schedule a tasting, and be sure to inquire about special events, dinners, and Jazz at sunset. Traverse City has an excellent locavore food scene, which draws from the local bounty of the land and Lake Michigan, as well as numerous wineries to enjoy. As Chateau Chantal is a winery, we have selected these two recipes for starters that pair nicely with a glass of wine and are perfect for entertaining!

Recipes courtesy of Marie-Chantal Dalese.

· ·

Baby Portabella Mushroom Caps with Caramelized Shallot & Fontina

Starter • All Phases • Serves 12

INGREDIENTS

48 Cremini mushroom caps
  (Baby Portabellos)

10 shallots
  4 Tbsp. olive oil for sauté
1 cup shredded Fontina cheese

INSTRUCTIONS

- Clean and de-stem mushrooms—do NOT use water.
- Par cook mushrooms in olive oil in a sauté pan—approximately 5 minutes. Remove from heat.
- Chop shallots. Sautée shallots in olive oil until golden brown.
- Place mushroom caps upside down on a sheet pan.
- Place a scoop of caramelized shallots in each cap and cover with shredded fontina.
- Bake in oven at 350 degrees Fahrenheit for 10 minutes or until cheese is melted.

NOTE

This is excellent with Chateau Chantal's Pinot Noir. This dish serves 12 with 4 mushroom caps per person.

Nutrition Facts (per serving)
Calories: **74** • Calories from fat: **52%** • Fat: **4g**
Saturated fat: **2g** • Cholesterol: **10mg** • Carbohydrates: **5.5g**
Protein: **6.5g** • Sodium: **77g** • Fiber: **0g**

· ·

Fruit, Avocado, and Goat Cheese Roll

Starter • All Phases • Serves 6

INGREDIENTS

1 avocado

½ pint strawberries

¼ watermelon

6 ounces mild goat cheese

1 cup Israeli couscous (dry yields)

3 sheets rice paper

INSTRUCTIONS

- Cook couscous.

- Slice all veggies and goat cheese.

- Place one thin layer of couscous on the bottom side of the paper leaving 1 inch from the edge.

- Next place fillers in this order: avocado, strawberry, goat cheese, watermelon.

- Tightly roll ingredients into the rice paper starting at the bottom and rolling towards the top.

- Slice fruit sushi into ¾-inch portions (24 total).

NOTE

This dish is excellent with Chateau Chantal's sparkling wine.

Nutrition Facts (per serving)
Calories: **298** • Calories from fat: **33%** • Fat: **11g**
Saturated fat: **5g** • Cholesterol: **13mg** • Carbohydrates: **42g**
Protein: **11g** • Sodium: **123mg** • Fiber: **5g**

•

Grand Traverse Resort and Spa, Aerie Restaurant

100 Grand Traverse Village Blvd., Acme, Michigan 49610

(231) 534-6000 • www.grandtraverseresort.com

Grand Traverse Resort and Spa is the ultimate year-round family-friendly destination, offering something for everyone just minutes from vibrant downtown Traverse City in the heart of beautiful northern Michigan! Choose from a variety of accommodations. At Grand Traverse Resort, enjoy championship golf on three great courses, indoor and outdoor pools, children's activities, spa, fitness, lakefront beach, and gourmet dining on the 16th floor of the main tower, overlooking Grand Traverse Bay. It is the perfect place to catch the sunset while enjoying locally and seasonally inspired cuisine, paired with a cocktail or wines from around the world, as well as a selection of the best local wines from the award-winning nearby Old Mission and Leelanau Peninsulas. Aerie has become a mecca for those who love bold, exciting flavors, unparalleled views, and attentive service. Aerie is an ideal spot for a special occasion, and makes any occasion special. The culinary team is dedicated to bringing the best of everything, from wherever they can source it, to create an inventive, exciting menu within a setting unlike any other Traverse City dining venue.

If you prefer beer, the Traverse City region has more than half a dozen microbreweries, whose brews are featured at Aerie. The resort features several other casual dining venues, offering something for everyone on the beautiful, park like grounds. Enjoy the very best of #PureMichigan hospitality at Grand Traverse Resort and Spa and excellent cuisine in an unforgettable setting. After a few days at the resort and exploring the best of Traverse City's incredible food, wine, and craft beer scene, you will come away feeling refreshed and anxious to book your next trip to Traverse City!

Recipe courtesy of J. Michael De Agostino, Public Relations Manager Grand Traverse Resort and Spa.

. . . .

Vegetable Terrine

Vegetable/Side • All Phases • Serves 4

INGREDIENTS

3 summer squash

4 turnips

1 rutabaga

3 yellow beets

5 ounces fresh basil

fresh Italian parsley to taste

lemon zest to taste

drizzle olive oil

salt and pepper to taste

INSTRUCTIONS

· Cut all vegetables to fit terrine mold.

· Layer the vegetables alternating each.

· Layer herbs between layers and salt and pepper all layers.

· Finish with olive oil drizzle over terrine.

· Bake at 325 degrees Fahrenheit for 1½ hours.

Nutrition Facts (per serving)
Calories: **147** • Calories from fat: **18%** • Fat: **3g**
Saturated fat: **0.4g** • Cholesterol: **0mg** • Carbohydrates: **28.5g**
Protein: **5g** • Sodium: **705mg** • Fiber: **9g**

Nevada

•

Café Martorano, Las Vegas

See recipe for Bucatini Amatriciana with Guanciale and Onions in Fort Lauderdale, FL.

New Jersey

•

Café Martorano, Atlantic City

See Bucatini Amatriciana with Guanciale and Onions in Fort Lauderdale, FL.

New York

•

Almond Restaurant

Almond Bridgehampton: One Ocean Road, Bridgehampton, NY 11937
(631) 537-5665 • www.almondrestaurant.com
Almond NYC: 12 East 22nd Street, New York, NY 10010
(212) 228-7557 • www.almondnyc.com

In 2001, Jason Weiner and Eric L emonides opened Almond, which quickly became the "un-Hamptons" restaurant the Hamptons needed, featuring fresh, straightforward, locally sourced, seasonally inspired French-American bistro cuisine. Almond is a favorite for locals, celebrities, tourists, and fellow restaurateurs and has garnered accolades from the *New York Times*, *Newsday*, and *Wine Spectator*. Jason began his culinary career in San Francisco, where he worked with Michael Mina. Eric Lemonides grew up in Brooklyn into a family of restaurant owners, where he learned the business as a child. He later moved to San Francisco, where he managed Piemonte Ovest. He returned to New York to oversee Della Femina in East Hampton and later F. Illi Ponte in Tribeca, as well as several of his own restaurants until teaming up with childhood friend Jason Weiner to open Almond. Almond proudly supports local growers and features them on their website.

. . . .

Monkfish Cioppino

Entrée • All Phases • Serves 4

INGREDIENTS

4 5-ounce monkfish fillets	1 tsp. minced jalapeño
2 Tbsp. olive oil	1 Bay Leaf
salt and pepper, to taste	1 ounce white wine
2 cups crushed canned tomatoes	12 mussels
2 tsp. chopped garlic	4 large shrimp (peeled and deveined)
2 tsp. sliced shallots	8 clams
¼ cup diced piquillo peppers	

½ pound cleaned squid (cleaned and cut into big pieces)

1 Tbsp. chopped parsley

4 basil leaves (torn)

8 grissini (imported Italian breadsticks, such as Real Torino or Alessi)

INSTRUCTIONS

- Pre-heat oven to 500 degrees Fahrenheit.
- Put a large ceramic casserole in your oven until it is extremely hot.
- Take it out of the oven and put it on your stovetop.
- Season the monkfish with salt and pepper.
- Put the olive oil in the casserole.
- Carefully add the monkfish and quickly put the casserole back in the oven.
- After 5 minutes take the casserole out of the oven and turn the fish over.
- Now add all the remaining ingredients **except** for the parsley, basil, and breadsticks.
- Quickly return the casserole to the oven for another 3–4 minutes, until the shellfish open up.
- Take the casserole out of the oven and now toss in the parsley and basil.
- Garnish with the breadsticks (2 per serving—optional).
- Put the whole casserole on a trivet and serve family-style.

Nutrition Facts (per serving)
Calories: **372** • Calories from fat: **30%** • Fat: **13g**
Saturated fat: **2g** • Cholesterol: **212mg** • Carbohydrates: **14g**
Protein: **48g** • Sodium: **451mg** • Fiber: **1g**

●

The American Hotel, Sag Harbor

49 Main Street, Sag Harbor, NY 11963 • (631) 725-3535 • www.theamericanhotel.com

The illustrious American Hotel, one of Sag Harbor's historic buildings, was built in 1846 in the height of the whaling era. The hotel is regarded by locals and visitors as one of the most charming, elegant, and professionally run establishments on Long Island's East End. Situated in the heart of charming, historic Sag Harbor, the Hotel has eight sumptuous guest rooms and an award-winning restaurant, which make guests feel right at home, as if they were staying with family. Staying and dining at the American is truly a pleasure. Everybody knows your name and anticipates your every need.

Recipes courtesy of Tom Allnoch and Chef Jonathan Parker.

. . . .

Seared Tuna a la Nage

Entrée • All Phases • Serves 1

INGREDIENTS

Tuna:

2 Tbsp. canola oil

7 ounces sushi-grade tuna

salt and pepper, to taste

1 Tbsp. mixed black and white
   sesame seeds

Salad:

1 ounce mixed field greens

1 Tbsp. julienned carrot

1 Tbsp. julienned daikon radish

1 Tbsp. sliced radishes

1 ounce enoki mushrooms

¼ English cucumber, sliced on bias

1 cup of Soy and Lemongrass Nage,
   heated (see below)

Lemongrass Nage:

10 ounces white wine

4 ounces mirin

1 ounce sliced ginger

zest of ½ lemon

1 quart water

¼ cup of low-sodium soy sauce

1 stalk lemongrass, chopped in
   food processor

1 pinch of bonito flakes

INSTRUCTIONS

Tuna:

- Heat a sauté pan until very hot. Add the oil.

- Season tuna on both sides with salt and pepper, press into sesame seeds, and sauté quickly on each side to desired doneness. Take tuna out of pan, rest for 2 minutes, and slice thinly.

- In a suitable bowl, place the mixed greens, and garnish around the greens with carrots, radishes, mushrooms, and cucumber.

- Place the tuna, fanned out, on top of Salad. Serve the Nage on the side to be poured at tableside.

Lemongrass Nage:

- Place the white wine, mirin, ginger, lemon zest, and water in a medium pot and bring to a boil. Simmer for 15 minutes.

- Add the soy sauce, lemongrass, and bonito flakes.

- Take off the heat and leave to infuse, covered, for 30 minutes more.

- Pass through a chinois.

- Refrigerate until needed.

NOTE

The Lemongrass Nage yields 4 servings.

Nutrition Facts (per serving) for the Tuna without any sauce:
Calories: **406** • Calories from fat: **45%** • Fat: **20g**
Saturated fat: **2g** • Cholesterol: **90mg** • Carbohydrates: **5g**
Protein: **48g** • Sodium: **88mg** • Fiber: **2g**

-

Nutrition Facts (per serving) for the Nage:
Calories: **75** • Calories from fat: **0%** • Fat: **0g**
Saturated fat: **0g** • Cholesterol: **0mg** • Carbohydrates: **10g**
Protein: **2g** • Sodium: **1,349mg** • Fiber: **0g**

· · · · · · · · · · · · · · ·

Bison Carpaccio

Starter/Entrée • All Phases • Serves 1

INGREDIENTS

3 ounces of bison filet, trimmed

1 Tbsp. olive oil

½ ounce of Parmesan shards

1 tsp. diced shallot

1 tsp. very finely sliced chives

½ cup of mixed field greens

½ ounce of vinaigrette of your choice
   (see Note)

salt and pepper, to taste

INSTRUCTIONS

· Freeze bison as it facilitates cutting.

· Slice paper thin and lay overlapping slices directly on an appetizer plate.

· Drizzle with olive oil and scatter the Parmesan, shallots, and chives over the bison.

· Toss the greens with the vinaigrette of your choice, and season, to taste.

· Stack the greens in the center of the carpaccio and serve.

NOTE

This can be shared among several diners as an appetizer. This can also be made with beef Filet Mignon. For the vinaigrette, we will use 1 tablespoon extra-virgin olive oil and 2 tablespoons red wine vinegar for the calorie computation. In earlier Phases, this could be shared as a starter or be considered an entrée.

Nutrition Facts (per serving)
Calories: **450** • Calories from fat: **70%** • Fat: **36g**
Saturated fat: **8g** • Cholesterol: **83mg** • Carbohydrates: **4g**
Protein: **29g** • Sodium: **431mg** • Fiber: **0g**

●

Angelo's of Mulberry Street, New York, NY

See recipe for Zucchini Flowers at Tramonti in Delray Beach, FL.

•

Barbetta, New York, NY

321 West 46th Street, New York, NY 10036

(212) 246-9171 • www.barbettarestaurant.com

New York's renowned Barbetta, located in the theater district, is the oldest restaurant in New York City to be owned and operated by its founding family. Barbetta celebrated its 100th anniversary in 2006, and is also the oldest Italian restaurant in New York! The exquisite restaurant, with its lovely outdoor patio and beautiful eighteenth-century antiques, features exceptional northern Italian cuisine, with an emphasis on the Piemonte region of northwest Italy. The Maioglio family is from Torino, and Barbetta was the first restaurant in New York to feature authentic Piedmontese dishes, such as tartufi bianchi, or the famed white truffles from Alba, or *Bagna Cauda*, and numerous other delicacies. Owned and operated by Laura Maioglio, Barbetta's menu features many classic dishes along with the year they were first introduced in the restaurant. Barbetta has received countless awards throughout the years, and was featured in *Wine Spectator* in the April 2002 issue, the only restaurant to receive an entire page in their story "Where to Eat."

Recipes courtesy of Laura Maioglio, Barbetta.

. . . .

Roasted Fresh Peppers alla Bagna Cauda (1962)

Appetizer/Side • All Phases • Serves 6

This is a classic *Piemontese* dish from Italy's northwestern-most region, Piemonte.

INGREDIENTS

8 fillets of anchovies (may use up to 12) and water to soak

¾ cup olive oil for Bagna Cauda (anchovies and garlic)

2 to 4 cloves of garlic (use from 2 to 4, according to taste)

2 ounces of olive oil (to brush over peppers)

3 large red bell peppers

3 large orange bell peppers

3 large yellow bell peppers

2 heads oak leaf lettuce

INSTRUCTIONS

- Soak anchovies in water to reduce salt. Strain, pat anchovies dry, and chop.

- Cut garlic cloves into very thin slivers (adding more cloves will intensify the garlic taste of the Bagna Cauda).

- Pour ¾ cup olive oil into a heavy frying pan. Add anchovies and garlic and place over a low heat. Cook, stirring occasionally, for about 20–30 minutes. The Bagna Cauda is done when the anchovies and garlic have disintegrated. Set aside.

- Cut each pepper in half, remove the white ribs and all the seeds. Brush the peppers with the 2 ounces of olive oil and place in a baking pan, exterior skin side up.

- Place under high heat broiler for 5–7 minutes. Remove from baking pan and place in another pan and cover with plastic wrap. Allow to cool.

- When peppers are cool enough to handle, remove the skin.

Assembly:

- To serve, place 3 pieces of peppers interior side up (one of each color) on a large dinner plate.

- Spoon 2 Tbsp. of the Bagna Cauda into each half pepper.

- Prepare 6 dinner plates in all. Serve at room temperature. At Barbetta, they insert leaves of oak leaf lettuce between each slice of pepper.

Nutrition Facts (per serving) for the Nage:
Calories: **337** • Calories from fat: **77%** • Fat: **29g**
Saturated fat: **4g** • Cholesterol: **4.5mg** • Carbohydrates: **19g**
Protein: **5g** • Sodium: **203mg** • Fiber: **3g**

•

Ben's Kosher Deli,
Manhattan, Bayside, Carle Place, Greenvale, Scarsdale, and Woodbury, NY, and Boca Raton, FL

Ben's Delicatessen
9942 Clint Moore Road, Greenvale, New York 11548 • (561) 470-9963
140 Wheatley Plaza, Boca Raton, FL 33496 • (516) 621-3340
www.bensdeli.com
Also with locations in Bayside, Carle Place, Manhattan, Scarsdale, and Woodbury, NY.

"Ronnie" Dragoon founded the incredibly popular Ben's Delicatessen in 1972, which he considers to have been a calling, inspired by his Eastern European heritage. Ben's has been my long-time favorite for Jewish deli food, since I grew up on Long Island. Ben's operates a Kosher kitchen under rabbinical supervision. According to Ronnie, Ben's "cures their own corned beef" and their chicken soup "cures everything else!" I always enjoyed their chicken matzo ball soup (Jewish penicillin) whether I was under the weather or well! Fortunately, Ronnie listened to the flock of New York snowbirds and snowflakes and took his popular restaurant concept to New York South (Boca Raton), so I no longer have to get on a plane for my fix!

Recipe courtesy of Ronald M. Dragoon.

. . . .
Ben's Israeli Salad

Salad/Entrée • All Phases • Serves 4

INGREDIENTS

¼ cup olive oil
¼ cup freshly squeezed lemon juice
¼ cup white vinegar (10 percent acidity)

1 Tbsp. freshly chopped cilantro
1½ tsp. salt

1¼ pounds cucumber, halved lengthwise, seeded, and chopped fine

1 pound finely chopped tomatoes

¾ pound finely chopped celery

½ pound finely chopped celery

½ cup finely chopped scallions

¼ cup of fresh parsley sprigs

INSTRUCTIONS

- In a large bowl, combine the olive oil, lemon juice, vinegar, cilantro, and salt.

- Add to bowl the cucumber, tomatoes, and other vegetables and toss to coat. Cover and refrigerate.

NOTE

I often enjoy this salad with a bowl of Matzoh Ball Soup, or Ben's famous Chicken in a Pot or Roasted Chicken, or with some sliced Jewish deli meat on the side as a meal at Ben's. At home, this is excellent with slices of grilled chicken breast, turkey, shrimp, or grilled/pan-seared seafood, like tuna or salmon and makes a very satisfying, healthy meal.

Nutrition Facts (per serving)
Calories: **109** • Calories from fat: **82%** • Fat: **9g**
Saturated fat: **1g** • Cholesterol: **0mg** • Carbohydrates: **7g**
Protein: **1g** • Sodium: **33mg** • Fiber: **2g**

•

Dario's, Rockville Centre

13 North Village Avenue, Rockville Centre, NY 11570 • (516) 255-0535

Dario's has been regarded as one of the top Italian restaurants in Nassau County for years, owing much of its success to the family's hands-on approach, the freshest ingredients, and an accommodating staff ready to go the extra mile to please.

Recipes courtesy of Dario's.

. . . .

Mussels Fra Diavola

Entrée • All Phases • Serves 2

INGREDIENTS

2 dozen fresh PEI (Prince Edward Island) mussels

2 Tbsp. extra-virgin olive oil, for sauté

2 cloves fresh garlic, sliced very thin

salt and pepper, to taste

red chili flakes, to taste

1 cup dry white wine

1 cup tomato sauce

2 Tbsp. minced fresh Italian parsley

INSTRUCTIONS

- Rinse the mussels under cold water and let stand in a bowl of water for several minutes to remove any grit.
- Heat a stockpot with oil over medium-high heat.
- Lightly brown the garlic.
- Add mussels and reduce heat to medium. Add the salt and pepper, chili flakes, white wine, tomato sauce, and parsley.
- Cover the pot and allow to cook for several minutes.
- When the mussels open, they are done!

NOTE

This is excellent as an entrée over *al dente* linguine. I suggest 3–4 ounces pasta per person (approximately 100 calories per ounce for the pasta) for Phases Two and beyond. Simply boil the linguine, toss with a little sauce, and top with the mussels. This preparation is also great with any or all of the following in addition to mussels: lobster tails, clams, calamari, or shrimp (just note that the cooking time of each type of seafood is different, so don't add them all at the same time). Try a combination for "frutti di mare." For the tomato sauce, use my recipe for *San Marzano Sauce*, or purchase a quality sauce like Rao's Marinara.

Nutrition Facts (per serving)
Calories: **387** • Calories from fat: **42%** • Fat: **18g**
Saturated fat: **3g** • Cholesterol: **54mg** • Carbohydrates: **25g**
Protein: **25g** • Sodium: **1,998mg** • Fiber: **2g**

•

Estia's Little Kitchen, Sag Harbor

1615 Sag Harbor-Bridgehampton Turnpike, Sag Harbor, NY 11963
(631) 725-1045 • www.eatshampton.com

Estia's, owned by chef Colin Ambrose, has been a Hamptons tradition dating back to 1991 when Colin purchased Estia's in Amagansett. In 1998, he opened the Sag Harbor location, transforming a sleepy coffee shop into a full-service restaurant. Chef Colin grew up on the East End, and grows his own fresh produce, something he is passionate about, having started a chef's garden co-op on Lorne Michael's Amagansett property. Estia's is a charming little restaurant that is slightly out of the way, serves wonderful breakfasts, and features local seafood and produce. The menu is influenced by the flavors of Mexico. Those in-the-know line up and wait for a table; regular Alec Baldwin has a dish named after him, "Big Al's Burrito," which contains egg whites and vegetables, and is served with fruit and home-made salsa—it has also become a favorite of regulars Alan Alda and his wife.

Recipe courtesy of Colin Ambrose.

. . . .

Whole-Grain Pancakes

Breakfast • Phases Two–Four (see Note) • Serves 5

INGREDIENTS

1 cup whole-wheat flour

¼ cup wheat germ

2 tsp. baking powder

1 tsp. salt

1 cup skim milk

2 large eggs

3 cups cooked steel-cut oatmeal
 (chilled)

2 Tbsp. canola oil (for griddle)

1 cup fresh blueberries (optional)

INSTRUCTIONS

• Combine all dry ingredients in a large bowl.

• Combine milk and eggs in a separate bowl and whisk together.

- Add the chilled oatmeal.

- Mix all ingredients together in a large bowl.

- Heat a griddle over medium heat with non-stick cooking spray. (The restaurant suggests oil or butter; if you use, spread just enough to coat the griddle.)

- Place one pancake on griddle to test cooking time and paying attention to the clock. These pancakes take more time than your average white flour pancakes. Then proceed to griddle remaining pancakes.

NOTE

I suggest a drizzle (maximum 1 Tbsp.) of maple syrup and a sprinkle of cinnamon to garnish. Regular maple syrup contains 52 calories per Tbsp., and should be avoided in Phase One. Sugar-free (Log Cabin) contains 35 calories.

If using berries, sprinkle them over pancakes while on the griddle. There are 83 calories in 1 cup of blueberries. Blueberries are an excellent source of vitamins and are considered one of the best antioxidants. Fresh strawberry slices to garnish, optional (There are 49 calories in a cup of strawberries.

Nutrition Facts (per serving)
Calories: **413** • Calories from fat: **26%** • Fat: **12g**
Saturated fat: **2g** • Cholesterol: **86mg** • Carbohydrates: **62g**
Protein: **16g** • Sodium: **308mg** • Fiber: **9g**

•

The Frisky Oyster, Greenport

27 Front Street, Greenport, NY 11944 • (631) 477-4265 • www.thefriskyoyster.com

Chef and Owner Robert Beaver, a Richmond, Virginia native, began his culinary career in Washington, DC. Working as a chef, he found the rush of a busy night in the kitchen captivating. He graduated from and went back to complete a fellowship at the Culinary Institute of America in Hyde Park, NY. He then headed back to Virginia, where he was awarded a position at the renowned Inn at Little Washington. "Robby," as Chef Beaver is often called, honed his skills under culinary master Patrick O'Connell. He developed relationships with local farmers and enhanced his craft utilizing the seasonal bounty and freshest ingredients possible. Being introduced to "farm-to-table" cooking, sustainable farming, and fishing led Robby to Long Island's North Fork, where in 2008 he accepted the Chef position at The Frisky Oyster, and in 2010, when the opportunity presented itself, jumped at the chance to become the new owner of the extremely popular restaurant. Robby's cuisine features the freshest local, seasonal produce and top-quality, locally caught and harvested seafood, as well as sustainable and organic products.

Recipe courtesy of Chef Robert Beaver.

. . . .

Montauk Tuna with Cilantro Walnut Pesto, Mushrooms, Hearts of Palm, and Bok Choy

Entrée • All Phases (see Note) • Serves 6 (see Note)

INGREDIENTS

Tuna:

3 pounds Montauk or fresh Sashimi Grade Tuna Fillet

sea salt and freshly ground black pepper to taste

Pesto:

2 cups fresh cilantro

½ cup toasted walnuts

1 Tbsp. chipotle peppers

5 cloves fresh garlic

½ cup extra-virgin olive oil

sea salt and pepper to taste

Additional ingredients:

4 cups mushrooms of your choice

1 cup hearts of palm

1 head fresh baby bok choy

4 cups vegetable stock

sea salt and pepper to taste

INSTRUCTIONS

• Season fish and grill to preferred degree (recommended rare).

• Place all pesto ingredients in a food processor and run until smooth.

- Place the mushrooms, hearts of palm, and bok choy in a sauté pan, season with salt and pepper, and heat over a high flame adding stock to keep moist.

Assembly:

- Place a large spoonful of pesto on each plate (use less in Phase One).
- Top with the vegetables.
- Slice the tuna and place on top of the vegetables.

NOTE

For weight-loss purposes, you may want to limit your Tuna portion to 4–6 ounces per person, and for Phase One either 4 ounces or less.

Nutrition Facts (per serving)
Calories: **675** • Calories from fat: **56%** • Fat: **42g**
Saturated fat: **6.6g** • Cholesterol: **70mg** • Carbohydrates: **8.5g**
Protein: **67.4g** • Sodium: **429mg** • Fiber: **3.7g**

●

Gabriel Kreuther, New York, NY

41 W. 42nd St., New York, NY 10036 • (212) 257 5826 • www.gabrielkreuther.com

Looking onto Bryant Park in the heart of Midtown Manhattan, chef Gabriel Kreuther's eponymous restaurant offers a comfortably luxurious, Alsatian-inspired dining experience infused with the best of New York. During the first decade of his career, Chef Gabriel worked at Michelin-starred kitchens throughout Germany, France and Switzerland before bringing his talent to the States. Gabriel began at La Caravelle & Restaurant Jean-Georges and then as Executive Chef at Atelier in The Ritz-Carlton and The Modern for nearly a decade, where he received numerous accolades. Chef Kreuther is a long-time member & mentor for the prestigious Bocuse d'Or USA Culinary Council and received a 2009 James Beard Foundation award for "Best Chef: New York City."

In June 2015, Gabriel opened his own restaurant, Gabriel Kreuther, which combines his classic French training and Alsatian heritage with his love of New

York City. Gabriel Kreuther has received the AAA 5 Diamond Award, a Michelin Star, and was recently named on the list of "The 9 best new restaurants in The World, 2016" by *Robb Report*.

. . . .

Baked Black Sea Bass, Fennel Seeds–Coriander Broth, Green Tomato Marmalade

Entrée • Phases Two–Four • Serves 4

INGREDIENTS

Green Tomato Marmalade:

1 pound green tomatoes, washed and cored

5 ounces sugar (see Note)

3 Tbsp. lemon juice

Spice mix:

2 Tbsp. fennel seeds

2 Tbsp. black peppercorn

6 Tbsp. coriander seeds

Bass preparation & garnish:

4 6-ounce black sea bass fillets, skin off

5–6 ounces each 4 scallions, cleaned and cut on the bias into 6–8 pieces each

1 Tbsp. of blanched lemon zest

4 Bay Leaves

4 pieces of blanched baby fennel (keeping the fennel ferns on the side for garnish)

½ cup of dry white wine or vermouth

1½ cups of fish stock or vegetable broth

salt and pepper

Cayenne pepper

4 medium glazed shallots or a dozen pearl onions, blanched

4 Tbsp. fresh butter (see Note)

8 small fingerling potatoes, cooked, peeled, and then sliced into coins (see Note)

Juice of 2 lemons

INSTRUCTIONS

Green Tomato Marmalade:

- Dice the tomatoes into ½-inch cubes.

- Mix all the ingredients together in a plastic or glass container, cover a lid or plastic wrap and then let rest 24 hours in the refrigerator.

- The next day put the tomato mix into a small stock pot and bring it to a light boil.

- Reduce the heat and let simmer for about 2½–3 hours, stirring occasionally.

- When it is cooked, let the whole thing cool down.

- Lastly, pack it away into a marmalade or mason jar and reserve in the refrigerator until further use. This will keep in the refrigerator just like any marmalade.

Spice mix:

- Mix all spices well together and grind them in either a spice grinder or a coffee grinder.

- Grind until you obtain a rough consistency of a powder, not too fine.

- Reserve in a closed container until needed.

Bass preparation & garnish:

- Take a deep casserole dish and butter it out so that the fish won't stick in the pan later on.

- Take each bass fillet and season it with salt, pepper, and a good amount of the spice mix on both sides.

- Place the bay leaves into the dish and add in the seasoned bass fillet, making sure that under each fillet you have a Bay Leaf.

- Next add into the casserole the sliced scallions, the baby fennel, the shallots, and the potato slices. Pour the dry white wine or vermouth which ever you prefer over the ingredients and add on top of it the fish stock.

- Cover the casserole slightly with a piece of aluminum foil and bake in the oven at 375–400 degrees Fahrenheit for about 6 minutes.

- Take the dish out from the oven and turn each fillet over with a spatula and put the dish back into the oven for another 6–8 minutes. You can check the doneness with a cake taster or a knife. It should go through the fish with a very slight resistance, making sure to not overcook the fish because it will carry over while you are working on the next step.

- When the sea bass is cooked, separate the fish onto a different platter and cover with the foil. Keep it warm.

- Place the vegetables into a small pot to keep them hot as well. Pour the cooking liquid into a sauce pot and bring it to a running boil on a burner and then reduce it by 25 percent. When reduced, take the butter and add it in with either a whisk of a stick blender (preferably a stick blender). Blend it until nice and frothy; season to taste with cayenne and salt. Taste some broth with a spoon to see if you need to add in some more spice mix. This is the time to get the broth to your liking. Lastly, finish it with the lemon juice to bring the broth to a nice balance between the spices and the acidity.

- Take 4 soup bowls and split the vegetables evenly, do not serve the Bay Leaves.

- Then take the black bass fillet and add it on top of the vegetables on each plate.

- Finish the dish with the well-seasoned fennel coriander broth nice and frothy, add on top the lemon zests. The dish is ready to be served.

- At the table each person can then finish the dish by topping it with a large tablespoon of green tomato marmalade.

NOTE

You may wish to reduce butter, sugar, and potatoes for dietary purposes even in Phases Two and on. For nutritional analysis, we used white wine and vegetable broth were used in this recipe.

Nutrition Facts (per serving) for Marmalade:
Calories: **66** • Calories from fat: **0.04%** • Fat: **0.3g**
Saturated fat: **0g** • Cholesterol: **0mg** • Carbohydrates: **17g**
Protein: **1g** • Sodium: **8mg** • Fiber: **1g**

Nutrition Facts (per serving) for Fish:
Calories: **485** • Calories from fat: **32%** • Fat: **17g**
Saturated fat: **8g** • Cholesterol: **121mg** • Carbohydrates: **36g**
Protein: **44g** • Sodium: **2,299mg** • Fiber: **7g**

•

The Golden Pear Café,
Southampton, Bridgehampton, East Hampton, and Sag Harbor

99 Main Street, Southampton, NY 11968 • (631) 283-8900 • www.goldenpearcafe.com
Bridgehampton: 2426 Montauk Highway • (631) 537-1100
East Hampton: 34 Newtown Lane • (631) 329-1600
Sag Harbor: 111 Main Street • (631) 725-2270

Since 1987, owner Keith Davis has been serving up delicious breakfasts, lunches, gourmet coffees, baked goods, healthy salads, wraps, and more at his popular mini-chain of East End cafés that are extremely popular with the Hampton's crowd, and are a tradition for great food and great people-watching in a relaxed, charming setting. Whenever I am "out east," a daily stop at the Golden Pear for something—even a cup of coffee—is mandatory! The Golden Pear has locations in Southampton, Sag Harbor, Bridgehampton, and East Hampton. Keith Davis stated, "I am delighted and inspired by Fred Bollaci's vision of educating the world about enjoying a healthy, gourmet lifestyle." Also, Keith recently launched his already famous Keith's Nervous Breakdown Ultra Premium Cocktail Mixes, starting with his cranberry-pomegranate Margarita Mix, followed by his Rum Punch. Inspired by the pink margarita he had after missing a three-foot putt in a competitive round of golf, the rest is history! Keith's drink mixes are all-natural, and organic, sweetened with organic agave nectar as opposed to high fructose corn syrup. If you are going to drink, I suggest doing it the right way by having a #NervousBreakdown! www.nervousbreakdown.com

Recipes courtesy of Keith Davis.

. . . .
Grilled Fresh Wild Salmon Salad

Entrée • All Phases • Serves 4

INGREDIENTS

Dressing:

4 Tbsp. extra-virgin olive oil

2 Tbsp. fresh lemon juice

2 tsp. Dijon mustard

2 Tbsp. fresh chopped dill

pinch of kosher salt   pinch of black pepper

Salad:

1 pound fresh wild salmon fillet   1 cup fresh grilled asparagus
4 Tbsp. extra-virgin olive oil   4 cups Bibb lettuce
pinch of kosher salt   fresh dill, for garnish
pinch of black pepper   4 lemon wedges, for garnish
1 cup (1 large stalk) fresh
    chopped celery

INSTRUCTIONS

- Pre-heat grill to medium-high setting.
- Brush salmon fillet with olive oil.
- Sprinkle both sides with salt and pepper.
- Grill salmon 4–5 minutes on each side.
- Remove salmon from grill and put in refrigerator to cool.
- Wash and trim asparagus spears.
- Toss asparagus in olive oil, salt and pepper.
- Grill asparagus for 2–3 minutes.
- Remove asparagus from grill and set aside to cool.
- When cool, chop asparagus on angle into 1-inch pieces.
- Wash celery stalk and chop on angle; set aside.
- In large salad bowl combine the celery and asparagus.
- Remove salmon from refrigerator and break into small pieces into the salad bowl.
- In a small bowl whisk together the dressing ingredients and pour over the salad.
- Toss together gently to complete.
- Serve over Bibb lettuce garnished with fresh dill and lemon wedge.

Nutrition Facts (per serving)
Calories: **196** • Calories from fat: **92%** • Fat: **20g**
Saturated fat: **3g** • Cholesterol: **0mg** • Carbohydrates: **4g**
Protein: **1g** • Sodium: **152mg** • Fiber: **1g**

. . . .

Citrus Veggie Tuna Salad

Entrée • All Phases • Serves 6

INGREDIENTS

Dressing:

½ cup canola oil

juice from 1 lemon

juice from ½ lime

2 Tbsp. fresh chopped parsley

1 Tbsp. fresh chopped thyme

1 tsp. fresh chopped oregano

1 Tbsp. coarse grain mustard

1 tsp. kosher salt

freshly ground black peppers

Salad:

2 (10-ounce) fresh tuna steaks (may substitute with 2 6-ounce cans white tuna pieces)

¼ cup canola oil to brush on tuna steaks

½ cup diced celery (1 stalk)

½ cup diced carrots (½ medium)

1 cup diced zucchini (1 small)

1 cup diced, peeled, and seeded cucumber (1 small)

1 cup diced yellow squash (1 small)

2 heads of Boston Bibb lettuce

1 cup cherry tomatoes

INSTRUCTIONS

- Pre-heat your grill on high setting.

- Brush the tuna steaks with canola oil, and salt and pepper both sides.

- Grill for 4 minutes on each side, remove, place on a plate, and put in the refrigerator to cool completely.

- When cool, remove from refrigerator; break into pieces into large bowl.

- If you are using the canned tuna, strain all water and spoon tuna into large bowl.

- Prep all vegetables, except lettuce and tomatoes, and add to tuna; fold together using a spatula.

- In a separate bowl, whisk together all dressing ingredients (oil, citrus, mustard, and fresh herbs).

- Pour over tuna salad and fold together.

- Add more salt, pepper, and fresh lemon juice according to your liking.

- In a large serving bowl or platter place Bibb lettuce leaves on bottom and sides to cover.
- Spoon tuna salad over the Bibb lettuce.
- Arrange tomatoes around the edge of the bowl or platter.

NOTE

You can also assemble this salad on individual salad plates.

Nutrition Facts (per serving)
Calories: **303** • Calories from fat: **69%** • Fat: **29g**
Saturated fat: **3g** • Cholesterol: **43mg** • Carbohydrates: **8g**
Protein: **24g** • Sodium: **675g** • Fiber: **3g**

. . . .

Garden Vegetable Egg White Omelet

All Phases • Serves 1

INGREDIENTS

4 egg whites

2 tsp. unsalted butter

¼ cup of seeded, diced plum tomato

¼ cup of diced zucchini

¼ cup of diced yellow squash

6 small broccoli florets

1 tsp. fresh chopped scallion

2 Tbsp. fresh chopped Italian parsley

salt and black pepper, to taste

canola oil-based cooking spray to
    coat pan (substitute for 2 tsp.
    sweet butter)

INSTRUCTIONS

- Pre-heat your broiler on high setting and move a rack close to the broiler.
- Prepare all vegetables and set aside.
- Separate the egg whites from the egg yolks and set aside in a bowl.
- Heat 1 teaspoon of butter in a non-stick sauté pan.
- Add the vegetables and sauté over medium-high heat for about 2 minutes until *al dente*.
- Add the herbs and salt and pepper and mix together.
- Remove the vegetables and set aside in a small bowl.

- Wipe the pan clean.
- Heat the other teaspoon of butter in the non-stick pan.
- Let the pan get fairly hot and pour the egg whites into the pan.
- Using a spatula, gently lift the edges of the omelet and shape omelet into a circle. Cook for 1 minute.
- To cook the egg whites further, place the pan under the broiler for 30 seconds.
- Remove the pan from the broiler and spoon the vegetables over the omelet.
- Place the omelet pan under the broiler for another 30 seconds.
- Gently slide the omelet out of the pan folding the omelet in half to complete.

NOTE

Substitute diced asparagus or diced green peppers for the broccoli. About 1 ounce of low-fat Swiss cheese also may be added. Low-fat Swiss ranges from 48–70 calories per one-ounce slice, and averages 100 calories for regular. In calculating calories, use about 2 1-second sprays of Pam olive oil cooking spray, which is 9 calories per spray.

Nutrition Facts (per serving)
Calories: **159** • Calories from fat: **3%** • Fat: **3g**
Saturated fat: **0g** • Cholesterol: **0mg** • Carbohydrates: **17g**
Protein: **19g** • Sodium: **630mg** • Fiber: **6g**

●

La Bussola, Glen Cove

40 School Street, Glen Cove, NY 11542 • (516) 671-2100 • www.labussolaristorante.com

La Bussola's tradition of serving excellent Neapolitan-style cuisine can be traced back to sunny Napoli, when Italian immigrant Pasquale Lubrano came to America in 1957 and began working in the restaurant industry. In 1980, he fulfilled a lifelong dream by opening his own restaurant, La Bussola (the compass) in Glen Cove to rave reviews. The business grew and the family expanded to Huntington and Mineola, with each of Pasquale's four sons joining in the family business. Today Tony, John, and Carlo each manage a restaurant, and Chef Marco oversees the kitchens for all locations. La Bussola has built and maintained a stellar reputation by procuring nothing but the best ingredients (hand-selecting the fish at the Fulton Fish Market) and going "above and beyond" to treat their customers like part of the *famiglia*, to continue the legacy established by Pasquale. "We are honored that Fred has chosen us to be part of his healthy gourmet living family. We have always made it a priority to provide our clientele with healthy gourmet options and we are proud to be a part of Fred's success," Chef Marco said.

Recipe courtesy of Marco and Carlo Lubrano.

· ·
La Bussola's "Combination Salad"

Side Salad or Entrée • All Phase • Serves 2

INGREDIENTS

Salad:

1 cup arugula

1 Belgian endive, sliced

1 head radicchio, sliced

1 cup roasted red peppers

½ cucumber, sliced

1 large ripe tomato, sliced

½ medium red onion, sliced

½ cup mixed black and green imported olives

La Bussola's Vinaigrette:

2 Tbsp. extra-virgin olive oil

2 Tbsp. balsamic vinegar

1 clove fresh garlic, crushed

pinch of dried oregano

pinch of salt and pepper

INSTRUCTIONS

Mix or shake the dressing ingredients to emulsify. Place salad ingredients in a large bowl, toss with dressing, and serve on chilled salad plates.

NOTE

This salad is excellent to accompany grilled chicken or seafood, like La Bussola's famous Grilled Branzino, or as an accompaniment to a small plate of pasta (Phases Two–Four). To make it an entrée, consider serving it with the addition of grilled, pan-seared, or poached seafood on top.

Nutrition Facts (per serving) for the Salad with dressing:
Calories: **272** • Calories from fat: **59%** • Fat: **18g**
Saturated fat: **3g** • Cholesterol: **0mg** • Carbohydrates: **27g**
Protein: **6g** • Sodium: **443mg** • Fiber: **13g**

. . . .

Pork Chop Scarpariello

Entrée • PhasesTwo–Four (see Note) • Serves 2

INGREDIENTS

2 10-ounce bone-in pork chops

all-purpose flour for dredging

4 Tbsp. extra-virgin olive oil for sauté

2 cloves garlic, sliced

2 cherry peppers, sliced

½ cup white wine

1 cup chicken broth

salt and pepper, to taste

1 Tbsp. fresh Italian parsley, minced

juice of 1 lemon

INSTRUCTIONS

- Pre-heat skillet on high.

- Dredge pork chops in flour, shake off excess.

- Add olive oil to skillet and sauté pork chop until brown on both sides.

- Add sliced garlic and cherry peppers.

- When garlic is golden brown, add the white wine, chicken broth, and salt and pepper.

- Lower heat to medium, cover, and cook for approximately 8 minutes.

- Before serving, add parsley and lemon juice.

NOTE

This is also good served with the addition of sliced, grilled Italian sausage or chicken sausage. This preparation works nicely with chicken as well. At home or in the restaurant, I recommend sharing this dish, as 10 ounces of meat is a lot. A 5-ounce portion (smaller pork chop, or cutting in half) at home would go nicely with La Bussola's salad and/or vegetables.

Nutrition Facts (per serving)
Calories: **529** • Calories from fat: **53%** • Fat: **31g**
Saturated fat: **6g** • Cholesterol: **109mg** • Carbohydrates: **19g**
Protein: **38g** • Sodium: **774mg** • Fiber: **1g**

•

La Ginestra, Glen Cove

50 Forest Avenue, Glen Cove, NY 11542 • (516) 674-2244 • www.laginestrarestaurant.com

For nearly thirty years, La Ginestra (the broom) has been one of the top Italian restaurants on Long Island, serving delicious, authentic, rustic Southern Italian and Sicilian specialties. A personal childhood favorite when I was growing up in Glen Cove, La Ginestra remains a perennial favorite. Among my favorite dishes there were always their grilled vegetables and Portobello mushrooms, along with grilled shrimp and calamari. La Ginestra's veal, seafood, and pasta dishes are also delicious. Chef/Owner Enzo Alessandro said, "There are no shortcuts to excellent cooking. We are dedicated to consistently meeting our clients' needs which is why we have such a loyal customer like Fred and wish him much success."

Recipes courtesy of Enzo Alessandro, La Ginestra.

Grigliata di Verdure e Gamberi (*Mixed Grill of Vegetables and Shrimp*)

Starter or Entrée • All Phases • Serves 4

INGREDIENTS

3 Tbsp. olive oil for coating vegetables
2 cloves minced garlic

12 slices green zucchini, cut ¼-inch thick

12 slices yellow zucchini, cut
¼-inch thick
12 slices baby eggplant, cut
¼-inch thick
12 scallions (white part only)
4 small artichokes, outer leaves
removed, cut in half

4 small Portobello mushrooms,
gills removed
12 slices each of red and yellow
bell peppers
salt and pepper, to taste

INSTRUCTIONS

- Mix oil and garlic in a bowl.
- Use a brush to coat each of the vegetables with oil/garlic mixture.
- Pre-heat grill.
- Grill items until tender, turn frequently to avoid a burned taste.
- Grill the artichokes and Portobello mushrooms first, as they take longer to cook.
- Add salt and pepper, to taste, as vegetables cook.

Nutrition Facts (per serving)
Calories: **159** • Calories from fat: **59%** • Fat: **11g**
Saturated fat: **1g** • Cholesterol: **10mg** • Carbohydrates: **15g**
Protein: **5g** • Sodium: **110mg** • Fiber: **6g**

. . . .

Marinated Jumbo Shrimp

INGREDIENTS

Shrimp:
20 U-12 shrimp (12 per pound), peeled
and deveined

Marinade:
3 cloves garlic
6 ounces extra-virgin olive oil
25 mint leaves
juice of ½ lemon

1 ripe Roma tomato, skin and
seeds removed
salt and pepper, to taste

INSTRUCTIONS

- Combine all ingredients except shrimp in a food processor.
- Process for 1 minute and transfer to a bowl.
- Add shrimp and marinate for 1 hour.
- Pre-heat grill. Grill shrimp for 2 minutes on each side.

NOTE

This dish is typically served as a starter for the table at La Ginestra, with the addition of a small home-made fresh mozzarella, as well as calamari, which are marinated and grilled along with the shrimp. Burrata is a good substitution. Fresh mozzarella and burrata are widely available at specialty markets as well many grocery stores. You can do this with other types of seafood as well, such as prawns, scallops, and lobster tails. The marinade and grilling will work with larger fillets of fresh fish, such as swordfish and halibut. This is nice served with a mixed salad of your choice. For example, tricolore of arugula, radicchio, and endive, tossed with olive oil, lemon, and/or balsamic.

Nutrition Facts (per serving)
Calories: **144** • Calories from fat: **68%** • Fat: **11g**
Saturated fat: **2g** • Cholesterol: **53mg** • Carbohydrates: **4g**
Protein: **8g** • Sodium: **105mg** • Fiber: **1g**

●

La Grenouille, New York, NY

3 East 52 Street, New York, NY 10022 • (212) 752-1495 • www.la-grenouille.com

For over fifty years, La Grenouille has been known for some of the finest French cuisine in New York City, prepared with precision and graciously served. Anyone who has had the pleasure of dining in their lovely, elegant townhouse can attest that the floral arrangements are also *magnifique*!

Recipe courtesy of Wade at La Grenouille.

. . . .

Grilled Chicken Paillard with Summer Vegetables and Aged Balsamic Vinegar

Entrée • All Phases • Serves 4

INGREDIENTS

4 boneless, skinless chicken breasts
(approximately 6 ounces each)
salt and pepper, to taste
4 Tbsp. extra-virgin olive oil
1 tsp. fresh thyme leaves
1 fennel bulb, trimmed, quartered, and
sliced thinly

12 cherry tomatoes, halved
1 zucchini, quartered, seeds removed,
thinly sliced
4 Tbsp. aged balsamic vinegar
4 cups wild arugula

INSTRUCTIONS

- Place chicken breast on a cutting board, cover loosely with several sheets of plastic wrap or parchment paper, and pound gently with a meat mallet until breast is of desired thickness.

- Season the chicken with salt and pepper, lightly coat with olive oil, and sprinkle the thyme leaves on the chicken.

- Place the chicken breasts on a hot grill, and cook about 1 ½ or 2 minutes on each side, or until chicken is cooked thoroughly. Set aside.

- In a hot sauté pan, add some olive oil, then the fennel.

- Season the fennel and zucchini with salt and pepper, cook for 1 minute.

- Add the tomatoes and remove the pan from the heat.

- Place each chicken breast on a plate.

- Arrange the vegetable mix over the chicken.

- Lightly dress the arugula with olive oil and place on top of the chicken and vegetables.

- Drizzle each dish with the aged balsamic vinegar and additional drizzle of olive oil.

Nutrition Facts (per serving)
Calories: **202** • Calories from fat: **63%** • Fat: **14g**
Saturated fat: **2g** • Cholesterol: **21mg** • Carbohydrates: **10g**
Protein: **10g** • Sodium: **201mg** • Fiber: **4g**

•

Matteo's,
Huntington & Roslyn (See Florida)

See recipe for Matteo's Shrimp alla Wendy and Burned String Beans in Boca Raton and Hallandale, Florida.

•

Mirabelle Restaurant at The Three Village Inn

150 Main Street, Stony Brook, NY 11790 • (631) 584-5999 • www.threevillageinn.com

Chef Guy Reuge, who was born in the heart of France's Loire Valley, has been recognized for years as one of the most celebrated *cuisiniers* on Long Island. Chef Reuge, who was chef-owner of the incredibly successful, critically-acclaimed Mirabelle in St. James, which has been considered one of Long Island's top restaurants and favorite places for a special occasion has brought his exceptional cuisine to nearby Stony Brook, where he joined Lessing's Three Village Inn and where he operates two restaurants: the four-star Restaurant Mirabelle and the Mirabelle Tavern. Reuge is the author of the cookbook *Le Petit Mirabelle*, and in 2010, he was honored as a James Beard Award semifinalist for "Best Chef in the Northeast."

Recipes courtesy of Chef Guy Reuge.

. . . .

Escabeche of Red Snapper

Entrée • Phases Two–Four • Serves 6

INGREDIENTS

½ cup extra-virgin olive oil

6 6-ounce red snapper fillets

3 large onions, sliced

1½ Tbsp. minced fresh coriander

1½ tsp. coriander seeds

1½ tsp. saffron threads

1½ Tbsp. green peppercorns

zest of 2 oranges

1 tsp. minced garlic

2 red bell peppers, cored, seeded, and sliced

2 orange bell peppers, cored, seeded, and sliced

2 yellow bell peppers, cored, seeded, and sliced

2 green bell peppers, cored, seeded, and sliced

¾ cup dry white wine

juice of 1 orange

juice of 1 lemon

6 plum tomatoes, peeled, seeded, and cubed

salt and pepper, to taste

½ pound mussels, scrubbed well and steamed, for garnish (optional)

INSTRUCTIONS

- In a large skillet, heat 3 tablespoons of the oil over moderately high heat until it is hot, add the fillets, skin side down, and cook them for 4 minutes, or until the skin is very crisp.

- Turn the fillets and cook them for 2 minutes more.

- In another large skillet cook the onion in the remaining oil over moderately high heat, stirring, for 2 minutes.

- Add the fresh coriander, coriander seeds, saffron, green peppercorns, orange zest, garlic, and bell peppers and cook the mixture, stirring occasionally, for 7 minutes.

- Add the wine and the orange and lemon juice and tomatoes and cook the mixture with the salt and pepper.

- Transfer the fish to a large glass or ceramic dish, cover it with the vegetable mixture and chill it, covered, overnight.

- Before serving, let the fish stand in a cool place for 1½ hours.

- Garnish each serving with 2 of the steamed mussels, if desired.

NOTE

For calorie analysis, the mussels were included. Mussels are approximately 7 calories each.

> **Nutrition Facts (per serving)**
> Calories: **520** • Calories from fat: **39%** • Fat: **23g**
> Saturated fat: **3g** • Cholesterol: **82mg** • Carbohydrates: **31g**
> Protein: **50g** • Sodium: **540mg** • Fiber: **7g**

•

Noah's, Greenport

136 Front Street, Greenport, NY 11944 • (631) 477-6720 • www.chefnoahs.com

Executive Chef Noah Schwartz, a Long Island native and graduate of New England Culinary Institute, began his culinary career in Sonoma, California. While working as a chef in Sonoma, he met his wife, Sunita. A restaurateur herself, Sunita always had a passion for wine, having studied under one of the best winemakers in the region. The wine list reflects Sunita's extensive knowledge of wine, and features many top Long Island wines. After they wed, the couple relocated to Long Island's North Fork, an increasingly important wine region, known also for excellent local bounty of produce and seafood to open their own restaurant. Noah's is located in the heart of Greenport, a picturesque seafaring town, and offers outdoor seating during summer months. Since opening in 2010, Noah's has received numerous accolades. Chef Noah has been lauded by Best Chefs America in both 2012 and 2013. Known for its trademark seafood inspired small plates featuring locally sourced ingredients, a raw bar with fresh oysters shucked to order, as well as an extensive wine list that features one of the largest selections of local wines, Noah's is not to be missed!

Recipes courtesy of Chef Noah Schwartz

. . . .

Noah's Fluke Crudo

Starter/Entrée • All Phases • Serves 4

INGREDIENTS

1 lb. freshest local fluke fillet	1 Tbsp. wasabi powder
1 watermelon radish	1 lime juiced
1 ripe avocado	1 tsp. Yuzu juice

sea salt, to taste

INSTRUCTIONS

- Trim fluke of any bones and slice on a 45-degree angle as thinly as possible.
- Peel and slice watermelon radish thinly on a mandoline or with a very sharp knife.
- Clean avocado of skin and pit and purée with wasabi, lime juice, and yuzu juice.
- Season with sea salt.

Assembly:

- Spread a thin layer of avocado purée on 4 plates.
- Layer alternating slices of fluke and radishes on top of the purée.
- Sprinkle with sea salt and finish with a squeeze of fresh lime juice.

NOTE

This dish serves 4 as an excellent, light appetizer or snack. To make it an entrée, I would double the portion per person. The success of this dish, like in all seafood dishes, begins with the freshest, preferably locally sourced seafood. Wherever you live, be sure to find the freshest and best! You can substitute whatever is available locally and prepare it in the same manner; Snapper, Tuna, Salmon, Flounder, and Scallops all work very well in this recipe.

Nutrition Facts (per serving)
Calories: **248** • Calories from fat: **18%** • Fat: **12g**
Saturated fat: **2.5g** • Cholesterol: **77mg** • Carbohydrates: **7g**
Protein: **28.5g** • Sodium: **162mg** • Fiber: **4g**

. . . .

Noah's Local Seafood Bouillabaisse with Saffron Fennel Broth

Entrée • All Phases (see Note) • Serves 4

INGREDIENTS

1 large yellow onion, julienned

2 bulbs fennel, julienned

3 cloves garlic, sliced thinly

16 ounce fish stock or clam juice

1 cup white wine

1 pinch saffron

1 Tbsp. Harissa or chili paste

4 large sea scallops

8 medium-sized shrimp (peeled and deveined)

8 ounces salmon cut into 2 ounce pieces

8 ounces striped bass or halibut, cut into 2-ounce pieces

2 pounds mussels, cleaned and de-bearded

2 pounds clams

2 Tbsp. butter (omit for Phase One)

4 plum tomatoes (halved, roasted, peeled)

3 Tbsp. olive oil

salt and pepper, to taste

INSTRUCTIONS

Broth:

- In a large pot, sauté the onions and fennel over low heat until almost tender,

- stirring occasionally.

- Add the garlic, saffron, and white wine, allow wine to burn off, about 1 minute. Stir to incorporate.

- Add the stock and bring to a simmer for 5 minutes.

- Add chili paste.

Bouillabaisse:

- In a large pot, heat up olive oil.

- Sear the fish, scallops, and shrimp over medium-high heat, on one side only.

- When the fish has a nice golden color, add the broth and mussels, bring back to a simmer.

- When the mussels open, season to taste with salt and pepper, and stir in cold butter (optional) to finish.

NOTE

Noah recommends serving this hot with grilled baguette slices, or over your favorite pasta (for Phases 2 and up).

In the chili paste, you may want to add additional saffron based on desired color and flavor.

For Phase One, omit the butter. There are 102 calories in a tablespoon of butter, thus 204 calories would be removed from the entire recipe. For all Phases, I suggest reducing the portion size—prepare the above quantities for 8 diners, or preparing half the quantity for 4 diners, and enjoy the Crudo recipe as a starter!

Nutrition Facts (per serving)
Calories: **751** • Calories from fat: **42%** • Fat: **27g**
Saturated fat: **7g** • Cholesterol: **208mg** • Carbohydrates: **58g**
Protein: **57g** • Sodium: **2,196mg** • Fiber: **3.5g**

•

The Plaza Café

61 Hill Street, Southampton, NY 11968 • (631) 283-9323 • www.plazacafe.us

The Plaza Café offers some of the finest seafood in the Hamptons, where chef and owner Douglas Gulija uses the freshest ingredients to create culinary magic in a cozy, elegant setting in tony Southampton village. The Plaza Café has been one of the top restaurants in the Hamptons since opening in 1997.

Recipe courtesy of Douglas Gulija.

. . . .

Pan-Roasted King Salmon with Friseé, Roasted Shallots, Haricot Verts, Red Bliss, and Mustard Seed Vinaigrette

Entrée • All Phases (see Note) • Serves 4

INGREDIENTS

Salmon:

6 red bliss potatoes, boiled (reduced from 12 for weight-loss purposes, omit for Phase One)

Mustard Seed Vinaigrette (see below)

2 heads frisée, white part only

4 roasted shallots

20 haricots verts, blanched

1 bunch chives, minced

4 king salmon fillets, 7 ounces each

4 Tbsp. canola oil, seasoned with salt and pepper, to taste (for coating salmon)

1 cup white wine

4 chive spears

salt and pepper, to taste

Mustard Seed Vinaigrette:

2 Tbsp. olive oil

3 Tbsp. mixed olive and canola oil

1 Tbsp. minced shallots

pinch of cayenne pepper

pinch of white pepper

pinch of salt

2 Tbsp. red wine vinegar

2 tsp. Dijon mustard

INSTRUCTIONS

Salmon:

• Smash red bliss potatoes in a bowl and drizzle with mustard seed vinaigrette.

• Add friseé and shallots.

• Warm salad mixture over a low flame until potatoes are warm and frisée is wilted.

• Add haricots verts and chives.

• Add more vinaigrette if needed.

• Adjust seasoning with salt and pepper and keep warm while salmon is cooking.

• Place salmon on half sheet pan, brush with seasoned oil, and season with salt and pepper.

- Add enough wine to cover bottom of pan.
- Broil salmon until desired doneness (approximately 7–8 minutes for medium-rare, 9–10 minutes for medium).
- Gently flip salmon over to clean fat from fish.
- Portion warm salad mixture in center of serving plate.
- Top with salmon and drizzle plate with remaining mustard seed vinaigrette.
- Garnish with fresh chive spears.

Vinaigrette:

- Combine all ingredients, except the oils. Slowly add oils to emulsify by whisking/shaking. Set aside.

NOTE

Omit potatoes in Phase One—omitting the potato saves approximately 180 calories per serving; with 12 small red bliss potatoes, there are 880 calories total per serving. Also, I would suggest a smaller portion for home preparation, such as 4–6 ounces of salmon per person. The mustard seed vinaigrette is adapted for home use.

Nutrition Facts (per serving)
Calories: **700** • Calories from fat: **37%** • Fat: **30g**
Saturated fat: **4g** • Cholesterol: **109mg** • Carbohydrates: **73g**
Protein: **53g** • Sodium: **221mg** • Fiber: **0g**

•

Red Bar/Brasserie, Southampton

210 Hampton Road, Southampton, NY 11968

(631) 283-0704 • www.redbarbrasserie.com

Red Bar/Brasserie, a Southampton favorite, has the look of a sophisticated Hamptons house with creamy walls, hardwood floors, large potted palms, wainscoting, and French doors overlooking the garden. In the evening, the ambience is warm, the restaurant glowing from soft lighting and candlelight. Excellent food and friendly staff make Red Bar a winner.

Recipe courtesy of Red Bar/Brasserie.

. . . .

Grilled Prawns with Romesco Sauce

Entrée • All Phases • Serves 4

INGREDIENTS

¼ cup olive oil

1 Tbsp. chopped almonds

1 Tbsp. chopped hazelnuts

1 cup torn-up stale bread (optional)

1 Tbsp. chopped garlic

2 jarred piquillo peppers

1 medium tomato, seeded and cubed

1 Tbsp. Spanish sherry vinegar

2 tsp. smoked paprika

pinch of cayenne pepper

salt to taste

2 pounds jumbo prawns with heads on, peeled and deveined

INSTRUCTIONS

Romesco:

• Heat the oil in a skillet over medium heat.

• Add the nuts and the bread and cook for about 5–6 minutes until the bread becomes toasted.

• Add the garlic and continue cooking 2–3 more minutes.

• When the garlic begins to brown slightly, add the peppers and tomatoes.

• Cook until the tomatoes have completely softened.

• Transfer the mix to a food processor and add the vinegar, paprika, and cayenne.

• Pulse to form a pesto-like consistency.

• Season with salt, to taste.

Prawns:

• Toss the prawns with a little olive oil and salt.

• Grill over medium heat for 3–4 minutes on each side until cooked and opaque.

- Spoon a small bed of the Romesco on the center of each plate and arrange the prawns over the Romesco.
- Serve with lemon wedge.

NOTE

The bread is roughly 80 calories per slice, so if omitting, there would be roughly 405 calories per serving. Omit bread for Phase One. If prawns are not available, you may use shrimp or lobster tail. This preparation is nice with other grilled seafood as well.

Nutrition Facts (per serving)
Calories: **425** • Calories from fat: **44%** • Fat: **21g**
Saturated fat: **3g** • Cholesterol: **345mg** • Carbohydrates: **8g**
Protein: **48g** • Sodium: **426mg** • Fiber: **1g**

•

1770 House, East Hampton

143 Main Street, East Hampton, NY 11937 • (631) 324-1770 • www.1770house.com

The 1770 house, one of Long Island's top restaurants is also a lovely bed and breakfast, featuring six luxuriously appointed guest rooms, a private carriage house, and a staff that caters to guests' every need. The inn was originally built as the home of William Fithian in 1663, and in 1770 was converted into an inn, beginning "an enduring reputation for warmth and welcome." The award-winning 1770 House restaurant features refined contemporary American cuisine and an outstanding wine list. Also, check out sister restaurants in town, including Cittanuova (also featured in this book), East Hampton Point, and The Grill. This recipe was featured on the Food Network's *Barefoot Contessa* with East Hampton's own Ina Garten.

Recipe courtesy of Chef Kevin Penner, 1770 House.

· · · · · · · · · · · · · · · · · · ·

1770 House Meatloaf

Entrée • Phases Two–Four • Serves 8

INGREDIENTS

1 pound ground veal (preferably naturally raised)1 pound ground pork (preferably naturally raised Berkshire)

1 pound ground beef (preferably naturally raised)

1 Tbsp. chopped, fresh chives, plus 1 tsp. for the sauce

1 Tbsp. chopped, fresh thyme leaves, plus 1 tsp. for the sauce

1 Tbsp. chopped, fresh Italian parsley, plus 1 tsp. for the sauce

3 large eggs (preferably organic)

1⅓ cups finely ground panko

⅔ cup whole milk (preferably hormone and antibiotic free)

1 Tbsp. kosher salt

1½ tsp. freshly ground black pepper

2 Tbsp. olive oil, to coat pan

2 stalks of celery, finely diced

1 large Spanish onion, finely diced

2 cups chicken or beef stock

10 cloves roasted garlic

1 Tbsp. butter, at room temperature (reduced from 3 Tbsp. for home/weight-loss preparation)

INSTRUCTIONS

· Pre-heat the oven to 350 degrees Fahrenheit.

· Place the veal, pork, beef, chives, thyme, parsley, eggs, Panko, milk, salt and pepper in a large mixing bowl.

· Heat a medium sauté pan over medium-high heat and film it with extra-virgin olive oil.

· When the oil is hot, add the celery and onion to the pan and cook, stirring, until softened.

· Remove the celery and onion from the pan and let cool.

· When the mixture is cool, add it to the mixing bowl with the other meat loaf ingredients.

· Using clean hands, mix the ingredients until well combined and everything is evenly distributed.

· Place a piece of parchment paper on a sheet pan (it should have sides at least 1½ inches high to prevent grease runoff from the pan).

· Place the meat on the sheet pan and pat it and punch it down to remove any air pockets.

- Shape the meat into a loaf (about 14½ inches long by 5 inches wide by 2 inches high).
  - Place the sheet pan in the oven and bake 40–50 minutes or until a meat thermometer indicates an internal temperature of 155–160 degrees Fahrenheit.
  - Remove the meatloaf from the oven and let it rest for 10 minutes.
  - Meanwhile, for the sauce, combine the chicken or beef stock, roasted garlic, and butter over medium-high heat and simmer for about 10–15 minutes, or until lightly thickened.
  - Add 1 teaspoon of each of the chopped chives, thyme, and parsley to the sauce. Slice the meatloaf into serving portions and spoon the hot sauce over the meatloaf and serve.

NOTE

With modifications, this recipe is for Phases Two–Four, because of the butter content. You may substitute reduced-fat milk for weight-loss purposes.

Nutrition Facts (per serving)
Calories: **402** • Calories from fat: **38%** • Fat: **17g**
Saturated fat: **6g** • Cholesterol: **191mg** • Carbohydrates: **18g**
Protein: **42g** • Sodium: **1,224mg**

•

75 Main, Southampton

75 Main Street, Southampton, NY 11968 • (631) 283-7575 • www.75main.com

One of the hottest, hippest restaurants in the Hamptons, 75 Main is the place to see and be seen in Southampton. The restaurant's motto is "when in the Hamptons, do as the Hamptons does...live to love, and love to live!" Owner Zach Erdem has created a sensational spot, with a stylish and graceful café-like feel, where one can dine among celebrities, including guests like Madonna, Alec Baldwin, Bono, Christie Brinkley, and more, and is frequently mentioned in *The New York Post's* "Page Six." In addition to some of the best food on the

East End, 75 Main transforms into the hottest night spot in the Hamptons with featured bands and a euphoric atmosphere, with plenty of Louis XIII, Cristal, and signature cocktails. Zach also owns the Hamptons hotspots KOZU and AM Southampton.

. . . .

The "Spa Burger"

Entrée • All Phases • Serves 4

INGREDIENTS

Burgers:

2 pounds ground chicken cutlet

1 Tbsp. diced red pepper

1 Tbsp. diced Bermuda onion

1 Tbsp. diced chives

1 tsp. pink peppercorns

1 Tbsp. each of finely chopped fresh Italian parsley, sage, rosemary, and thyme.

Garnish (per serving):

1 slice ripe tomato

3 slices cucumber

1 tsp. Grey Poupon Dijon mustard

optional whole-grain brioche bun (not included for calorie count)

INSTRUCTIONS

Combine the burger ingredients thoroughly and cook on a medium-hot grill, being careful not to char the burgers, as that will bitter the herbs. Assemble plate with garnishes alongside the burger.

NOTE

You may try this with turkey as well as with traditional ground beef or lamb, for a very tasty alternative.

Nutrition Facts (per serving)
Calories: **233** • Calories from fat: **11%** • Fat: **3g**
Saturated fat: **1g** • Cholesterol: **137mg** • Carbohydrates: **2g**
Protein: **55g** • Sodium: **212mg** • Fiber: **1g**

. . . .

The "Chop-Chop" Salad

Salad/Entrée • All Phases • Serves 1

The "Chop-Chop" Salad combines the classic café salad with a contemporary twist that puts sweet, salty, and savory flavors into a harmonious whole.

INGREDIENTS

1 head green leaf lettuce (julienne cut), or mixture of curly red leaf and green leaf lettuce

1 Tbsp. diced roasted red pepper

1 Tbsp. diced Bermuda red onion

1 Tbsp. dried cranberries

1 Tbsp. candied walnuts

1 Tbsp. crumbled gorgonzola

2 Tbsp. white balsamic vinaigrette (whisk together 1 Tbsp. white balsamic vinegar, 1 Tbsp. extra-virgin olive oil, and salt and pepper to taste)

INSTRUCTION

Combine all the ingredients, except the gorgonzola, with the vinaigrette, toss gently, and place in a stylish bowl. Sprinkle gorgonzola on top and serve.

NOTE

This salad is great with the addition of grilled chicken, salmon, seared tuna, shrimp, or lobster meat as an entrée.

Nutrition Facts (per serving)
Calories: **245** • Calories from fat: **68%** • Fat: **19g**
Saturated fat: **3g** • Cholesterol: **4mg** • Carbohydrates: **16g**
Protein: **5g** • Sodium: **242mg** • Fiber: **3g**

Starr Boggs, Westhampton Beach

---

6 Parlato Drive, Westhampton Beach, NY 11978
(631) 288-3500 • www.starrboggsrestaurant.com

Starr Boggs began his career as a chef and restaurateur on eastern Long Island three decades ago at the Inn at Quogue. Starr grew up on a farm on the eastern shore of Virginia, where his family raised most everything they ate. Starr found himself at home on eastern Long Island, whose climate and availability of fresh, local produce and seafood is similar to Virginia's coast. At Starr Boggs, you can enjoy gourmet dining in a historic home that has been beautifully renovated, with lovely gardens and outdoor seating areas. Starr Boggs has a wonderful wine list with many local selections. The famous mahogany bar is known for some of the best people-watching in the Hamptons.

Recipe courtesy of Starr Boggs.

. . . .

Grilled Harissa–Marinated Calamari Appetizer

Appetizer • All Phases • Serves 6

INGREDIENTS

Calamari:

1 ½ pounds calamari, cleaned (both tentacles and tubes)

3 cups mesclun

1 red pepper, roasted

1 medium red onion, grilled

1 orange, segmented

1 medium head of fennel, shaved

Marinade:

½ cup harissa paste

1 cup olive oil

2 Tbsp. Cholula Hot Sauce

1 Tbsp. fresh basil, pureed

INSTRUCTIONS

Calamari:

• Marinate calamari in harissa marinade for ½ hour prior to grilling.

- Grill should be heated to medium-high heat.
  - Grill calamari 2 minutes per side. Should be slightly charred and firm. Take care to not overcook!
  - Distribute mesclun greens on each of 6 plates.
  - Toss calamari with remaining red pepper, onion, orange, and fennel. Place calamari mixture over greens.
  - Serve immediately.

Marinade:

- In a small bowl, blend together all marinade ingredients until well combined. Set aside for serving.

NOTE

There are 73 calories per Tbsp. of harissa paste and 119 calories per Tbsp. of olive oil. There are 0 calories in Cholula, and a cup of basil leaves contains 1 calorie (so essentially none). Assuming the marinade would add approximately 1 Tbsp. of oil and 1 teaspoon of harissa to each serving, the total calories added would be approximately 146, for a total of 289 calories per serving. In addition to calamari, this marinade works well with other seafood; try it with chunks of swordfish, chicken, or steak with bell peppers and onions on skewers for some very tasty shish kabobs.

> **Nutrition Facts (per serving) without the marinade:**
> Calories: **143** • Calories from fat: **11%** • Fat: **13g**
> Saturated fat: **0g** • Cholesterol: **265mg** • Carbohydrates: **7g**
> Protein: **19g** • Sodium: **67mg** • Fiber: **3g**

●

Stone Creek Inn, East Quogue

405 Montauk Highway, East Quogue, NY 11942
(631) 653-6770 • www.stonecreekinn.com

The beautiful Stone Creek Inn has graced East Quogue since 1996 when celebrated chef, Christian Mir from Southwest France, and his wife, Elaine DiGiacomo, purchased and renovated the historic property, creating one of the premiere dining destinations in the Hamptons, with excellent, modern French cuisine in an elegant setting. Stone Creek Inn features fresh, local, seasonal menus and an award-winning wine list, which includes many wonderful selections from the East End.

Recipe courtesy of Chef Christian Mir.

. . . .

Chilled Zucchini Soup with Lobster Tail and Avocado

Soup/Starter • All Phases • Serves 4

INGREDIENTS

½ small onion, chopped
1 clove garlic, crushed
2 Tbsp. olive oil
1 pound zucchini, chopped into
   large dice
1 quart chicken stock/broth (or water)
salt and pepper, to taste

10 fresh basil leaves
drizzle of good-quality olive oil
4 8-ounce fresh lobster tails, steamed
   or boiled (optional, see Note)
4 slices ripe Haas avocado to garnish
   each bowl (optional)

INSTRUCTIONS

Soup:

- In a heavy bottom casserole, cook onions and garlic in olive oil for 5 minutes, or until translucent.
- Add chopped zucchini and chicken stock.
- Bring to a boil and cook until zucchini are just cooked (about 5–7 minutes).
- Add salt and pepper, to taste.
- Transfer contents to an ice bath until warm.
- Add small amount to blender and blend at high speed for 1 minute.
- Transfer back to ice bath until cooled.
- Continue until all the soup is blended.
- Soup must be cool before storing in the refrigerator.

- Garnish Soup with fresh lobster and avocado.
  - Finish with drizzle of good-quality extra-virgin olive oil and a sprig of fresh basil.

  ### Ice Bath:

  - Place ice in a bowl or bucket.
  - Find another smaller bowl or bucket that fits inside the first.
  - Place the soup in the second container and place it inside the first to chill. This will keep the soup a bright green color.
  - Add only a small amount to blender, as hot liquid will quickly overflow and can be dangerous.

NOTE

There are 27 calories per ounce of lobster meat. An 8-ounce lobster "tail" yields approximately 4 ounces of meat.

Nutrition Facts (per serving)
Calories: **206** • Calories from fat: **40%** • Fat: **9g**
Saturated fat: **1g** • Cholesterol: **108mg** • Carbohydrates: **7g**
Protein: **23g** • Sodium: **1,082mg** • Fiber: **2g**

Vermont

•

The Perfect Wife Restaurant and Tavern, Manchester Center

2594 Depot St., Manchester Center, VT 05255 • (802) 362-2817 • www.perfectwife.com

Chef and Owner Amy Chamberlain enjoyed cooking since childhood. An enterprising young woman, Amy and her friend baked chocolate chip cookies one summer and set up a stand, making $11.00 a week! This not only kept them out of trouble, it helped Amy define her passion for the culinary arts and the entrepreneurial direction her life would take. She went on to attend and graduate from New England Culinary Institute and worked for a number of top chefs in New England and in Aspen, Colorado. Three of the largest influences on her style were Mark Gaier and Clark Frasier of Arrow's in Ogunquit, Maine, and Alex Kim, for whom she was sous-chef at Syzygy in Aspen, Colorado. In 1996, Amy's dream of opening her own place, The Perfect Wife Restaurant and Tavern, became a reality. She considers her style of cuisine "freestyle" as she likes to start with classics and "twist them just a bit." The menu changes to reflect the seasons and the market for fresh, local ingredients. Amy is a member of the Vermont Fresh Network and a firm supporter of local agriculture and locally produced foods. In 2015, Fred appeared on GNAT-TV in Vermont as a guest on Amy's show, *"Life of the Party,"* where he showcased his famous healthy preparation for Italian-American Meatballs and New England Cod Livornese to the delight of a live studio audience.

Recipe courtesy of Chef Amy Chamberlain.

. . . .

The Perfect Wife's Famous Howling Wolf Vegan Special

Entrée • Phases Three–Four • Serves 8 (see Note)

INGREDIENTS

Yellow Curry Satay:

1 large yellow onion, diced

4 Tbsp. chopped garlic

2 Tbsp. good-quality curry powder
   (look for Madras brand in a gold tin)

1 Tbsp. ground cumin

2 tsp. dried basil

2 tsp. dried oregano

½ cup mango chutney

1 can coconut milk

5 cups canned diced tomatoes

1 cup canned tomato purée

Sun-dried Cherry Chutney:

1 cup dried cherries

½ cup golden raisins

2 tsp. chopped shallots

2 tsp. green peppercorns

½ cup sherry (Harvey's Bristol Cream,
   etc.)

¼ cup port wine

1 Tbsp. red wine vinegar

Sweet Potato Hash:

6 sweet potatoes

1 large yellow onion

2 Tbsp. chopped garlic

salt and pepper to taste

2 Tbsp. olive oil

pinch of nutmeg

INSTRUCTIONS

Yellow Curry Satay:

• Sweat the onions and garlic until soft. Add spices and toast them a little. Add chutney and coconut milk. Simmer until combined nicely. Add tomato products. Simmer for one hour on medium-low heat. Season to taste with salt and pepper.

Sun-dried Cherry Chutney:

• Combine everything in pot and cover by 1 inch of water. Simmer over low heat till fruit is very plump, about 20 minutes.

Sweet Potato Hash:

• Dice 6 sweet potatoes and 1 onion. Toss with chopped garlic, salt, pepper, olive oil and a little bit of nutmeg. Put in roasting pan and cover. Bake at 325 degrees Fahrenheit for about 45 minutes or until tender.

Assembly:

• First, cook the rice according to directions on the package. Next combine all these items with your favorite steamed, grilled, or roasted vegetables (the restaurant serves with steamed vegetables).

NOTE

There are several components, which should be made in advance and come together in this unique and tasty dish, including Yellow Curry Satay, Sun-dried Cherry Chutney, and Sweet Potato Hash. These should be prepared along with 2 ounces of rice per person (cook according to directions on package) per person, and several cups per person of steamed vegetables of your choice, such as broccoli, cauliflower, carrots, zucchini, and squash, and plated, as shown. For nutritional analysis, we assumed 2 cups of broccoli and 2 cups of carrots were used. In addition, I suggest using brown rice instead of white, and recommend making this recipe at home, as shown, for 8 people. At the restaurant, the recipe is for 4.

Nutrition Facts (per serving)
Calories: **656** • Calories from fat: **17%** • Fat: **12g**
Saturated fat: **7g** • Cholesterol: **0mg** • Carbohydrates: **131g**
Protein: **10g** • Sodium: **131mg** • Fiber: **11g**

Nationwide

•

Ocean Prime

Nationwide locations, including: Beverly Hills, Boston, Dallas, Denver, Detroit, Indianapolis, Naples, New York City, Orlando, Philadelphia, Phoenix, Tampa, and Washington, D.C.

www.ocean-prime.com

Ocean Prime is an award-winning restaurant concept from the Cameron Mitchell Group of Ohio, which combines a prime steakhouse with great seafood, to create "the modern American supper club." With a great selection of food, a comfortable modern atmosphere, award-winning wine list, and locations nationwide, Ocean Prime is sure to please.

Recipe courtesy of Tracey Smith, Marketing Manager, Ocean Prime.

. . . .

Tangerine Tuna

Entrée • All Phases • Serves 4

INGREDIENTS

4 8-ounce portions yellowfin tuna

2 Tbsp. extra-virgin olive oil, for sautée

kosher salt, to taste

freshly cracked black pepper, to taste

12 ounces baby spinach, rinsed and
  picked through

4 ounces baby arugula, rinsed
  (optional)

½ cup tangerine or orange segments

¼ cup radishes

¼ cup julienned red onion

Juice of 2 lemons

2 Tbsp. extra-virgin olive oil,
  for dressing

2 ounces low-sodium soy sauce

2 Tbsp. honey

1 tsp. wasabi powder (optional)

2 Tbsp. extra-virgin olive oil, for drizzle
  (optional)

INSTRUCTIONS

- Begin by heating 2 Tbsp. of oil in a medium sautée pan over medium heat.
- Season tuna with salt and pepper and sear on both sides to desired degree.
- While tuna is cooking, combine spinach and arugula, tangerines, radishes, red onion, 2 Tbsp. olive oil, and juice from the lemon.
- Mix well and season with salt and black pepper as necessary.
- Divide salad evenly onto 4 dinner plates.
- Slice cooked tuna and fan out over top of salad.
- Mix soy sauce, honey, and wasabi powder in a small bowl.
- Using a spoon, drizzle the soy mixture over top of each dish.
- Sprinkle a little kosher or sea salt over the tuna slices, if desired.

NOTE

The restaurant finishes the dish with an optional drizzle of olive oil, which we have omitted for weight-loss purposes. In addition, tuna, and this type of preparation, are both low enough in calories to possibly allow as large as an 8-ounce portion (featured above) when prepared this way, depending on your calorie budget and Phase. This is both satisfying and light, a favorite at Ocean Prime.

Nutrition Facts (per serving) for the Tangerine Tuna:
Calories: **437** • Calories from fat: **32%** • Fat: **16g**
Saturated fat: **2g** • Cholesterol: **102mg** • Carbohydrates: **18g**
Protein: **55g** • Sodium: **671mg** • Fiber: **2g**

Truluck's (locations in California, Florida, and Texas)

Nationwide locations include Mizner Park, Boca Raton, Ft. Lauderdale, Miami, and Naples, FL, La Jolla, CA, and Austin, Dallas, and Houston, TX.
www.trulucks.com

Truluck's is renowned for excellent seafood, snazzy décor, and top-notch service. Truluck's owns its own fisheries and procures their stone crab fresh daily in season from the Isle of Capri, near Naples, Florida.

Recipes courtesy of Truluck's Head Chef Brian Wubbena.

. . . .

Chimichurri Sauce

All Phases (an excellent accompaniment to grilled, roasted, or pan-seared meat and seafood) • Yields about 1 cup (16 1-Tbsp. servings)

INGREDIENTS

2 Fresno chili peppers, grilled, deseeded, and finely chopped

¼ cup finely chopped fresh basil

¼ cup finely chopped fresh Italian parsley

¼ cup finely chopped cilantro

1 Tbsp. finely chopped fresh rosemary

1 Tbsp. finely chopped fresh thyme

2 Tbsp. fresh garlic, crushed, ends removed

1½ Tbsp. extra-virgin olive oil

1½ tsp. argan oil

1½ Tbsp. canola oil

juice of 1 lemon

½ cup rice wine vinegar

1 tsp. freshly ground black pepper (finely ground)

2 tsp. sea salt

INSTRUCTIONS

• In a large mixing bowl, combine all the ingredients.

• Transfer to an airtight container to store up to 5 days in the refrigerator, or use this sauce over grilled, baked, broiled, or pan-seared seafood, such as grouper, flounder, sole, snapper, halibut, swordfish, tuna steak, shrimp, sea bass, and similar fish.

Nutrition Facts (per serving)
Calories: **106** • Calories from fat: **86%** • Fat: **10g**
Saturated fat: **1g** • Cholesterol: **0mg** • Carbohydrates: **4g**
Protein: **1g** • Sodium: **780mg** • Fiber: **1g**

. . . .

Truluck's Cioppino—San Francisco—style Seafood Broth

All Phases • Serves 6 as broth base

INGREDIENTS

1 Tbsp. extra-virgin olive oil

2 ounces fresh garlic, chopped, ends removed

2 ounces dry white wine

1 quart shrimp or seafood stock

8 ounces Italian peeled tomatoes

2 Tbsp. chopped fresh basil, chopped

2 Tbsp. chopped fresh thyme

2 Tbsp. chopped fresh oregano, chopped

1 Tbsp. anchovies, chopped

2 tsp. sea salt

2 tsp. freshly ground black pepper

lemon juice, to taste (optional)

INSTRUCTIONS

• In a large pot, heat olive oil and sauté garlic until fragrant.

• Add white wine, shrimp or seafood stock, and tomatoes.

• Crush tomatoes while adding to break apart.

• Simmer for 45 minutes on low heat, then add herbs, anchovies, and salt and pepper.

• Simmer an additional 30 minutes on low to medium heat.

• This is best prepared a day in advance and left to chill in the refrigerator overnight for the flavors to marry.

• Serve with a variety and/or combination of seafood.

• To serve, heat up the broth first.

• To add seafood: rinse seafood and then cook the seafood directly in the hot broth until done. Note: Most of the above items only take several minutes to cook.

• Adjust the flavor with salt and lemon juice, to taste and serve.

NOTE

Truluck's suggests clams, mussels, white fish (such as snapper, grouper, flounder, or halibut), shrimp, calamari, crab, and lobster tail all work well with this broth.

Combine this dish with your favorite seafood. An 8-ounce lobster tail contains approximately 4 ounces of lobster meat when removed from the shell. Lobster meat is 27 calories per ounce. Thus, for 4 ounces of lobster meat with a portion of the Cioppino broth, the total is 188 calories. Shrimp and squid contain 30 calories per ounce; clams and mussels average 7 calories each.

Nutrition Facts (per serving)
Calories: **80** • Calories from fat: **52%** • Fat: **4g**
Saturated fat: **1g** • Cholesterol: **6mg** • Carbohydrates: **3g**
Protein: **5g** • Sodium: **1256mg** • Fiber: **1g**

Hall of Fame

The following restaurants are personal favorites, whose owners were generous enough to share their recipes, though have since retired.

•

Da Silvano (Silvano Marchetto), New York, NY

Silvano Marchetto, native of Tuscany, opened his namesake Da Silvano on May 1, 1975, combining favorites from both Tuscany and Silvano's native Rimini, on the Adriatic coast, with an American "rock and roll" vibe to make his restaurant "downtown cool" in Greenwich Village. Da Silvano went on to become one of the most successful restaurants in New York history, spanning over 40 years.

Recipe courtesy of Silvano Marchetto.

. . . .

Spiedino di Pesce Riminese (Seafood Skewers with Squid, Swordfish, and Shrimp—Inspired by Rimini)

Entrée • All Phases • Serves 8

INGREDIENTS

Skewers:

1 red pepper, stem, seeds, and ribs removed and cut into 1-inch pieces

1 yellow pepper, stem, seeds and ribs removed and cut into 1-inch pieces

3 Tbsp. olive oil, plus more for oiling the grill grate (or cast-iron pan if preparing inside)

1⅓ cups panata (seasoned breading; see below)

1 pound cleaned squid, cut into 1-inch rings

1 pound swordfish, cut into 1-inch cubes

1 pound large shrimp, peeled, deveined, and cut into 1-inch pieces

16 wooden skewers (8 inches long), soaked in cold water

2 cups salad greens

2 lemons, cut in 4 wedges

Panata:

½ cup plain breadcrumbs

½ tsp. minced garlic

6 Tbsp. minced Italian parsley

pinch of crushed red pepper

INSTRUCTIONS

- Place all the ingredients on a cutting board and chop together until thoroughly incorporated (or use a small Cuisinart if you prefer), place into a bowl. This mixture can be stored in an airtight container in the refrigerator up to 3 days.

- Prepare a fire in an outdoor grill and let it burn until covered with white ash. You can heat a cast-iron pan and do this inside as well—be sure the pan is very hot.

- Place the red and yellow pepper pieces in a small stainless steel or ceramic bowl and drizzle with olive oil. Toss and reserve.

- Spread out the panata mixture on a clean, dry surface. Press the squid, swordfish, and shrimp pieces in the panata and coat on all sides.

- Prepare the skewers by placing alternating pieces of seafood and peppers: 1 piece of red or yellow pepper after every 3 pieces of seafood, on each skewer.

- When the grill or pan is ready, oil the grate. Place the skewers on the grill, cooking for 1–2 minutes on each of the 4 sides. Keep a close watch so they do not burn.

- Place ½ cup salad greens on each of 8 plates and place 2 skewers atop each salad. Serve immediately, with a lemon wedge.

Nutrition Facts (per serving)
Calories: **265** • Calories from fat: **32%** • Fat: **10g**
Saturated fat: **2g** • Cholesterol: **241mg** • Carbohydrates: **10g**
Protein: **33g** • Sodium: **213mg** • Fiber: **1g**

Renzo's of Boca (Renzo Sciortino), Boca Raton, FL

Sicilian native Renzo Sciortino oversaw one of the most popular Italian restaurants in Boca Raton for over 20 years after operating restaurants on Long Island. His hands-on attention to detail made him legendary in the area.

Recipe courtesy of Renzo Sciortino.

. . . .

Renzo's Yellowtail Snapper Oreganato

Entrée • All Phases (see Note) • Serves 2

INGREDIENTS

2 Tbsp. extra-virgin olive oil

1 pound yellowtail snapper
  (2 8-ounce fillets)

¼ cup plain breadcrumbs

2 cloves garlic, chopped

juice of ½ lemon

½ cup dry white wine

1 Tbsp. fresh oregano, chopped

pinch fresh Italian parsley, chopped

dry oregano, salt, and pepper, to taste

INSTRUCTIONS

- Pre-heat oven to 350 degrees Fahrenheit.

- Add olive oil to an ovenproof sauté pan or casserole dish.

- Add the yellowtail fillet to the pan, sprinkle breadcrumbs over the top, add garlic, lemon juice, white wine, fresh oregano, parsley, and dry oregano, salt, and pepper, to taste.

- Bake in pre-heated oven for about 10 minutes, or until the fish is flaky to the fork.

NOTE

This recipe is also great with sea bass, flounder, sole, grouper, halibut, and similar fish. For weight-loss purposes, consider a smaller portion (4–6 ounces). This is suitable for Phase One if you have a half portion with vegetables and/or salad, Phase One does not allow bread, but the breadcrumbs here are negligible, and they are finished in the oven, rather than fried, which is better for you.

Nutrition Facts (per serving)
Calories: **500** • Calories from fat: **32%** • Fat: **18g**
Saturated fat: **3g** • Cholesterol: **107mg** • Carbohydrates: **16g**
Protein: **62g** • Sodium: **671mg** • Fiber: **1g**

•

San Domenico/SD26/The Rainbow Room (Tony May), New York, NY

New York's legendary restaurateur Tony May can be credited as one of the pioneers who introduced the art of authentic Italian cuisine to the United States, first operating the Rainbow Room, and then the legendary San Domenico on Central Park South, followed by SD26. It was at San Domenico where I first savored *tartufi bianchi* (white truffles), Uovo in Raviolo (Ravioli filled with spinach, ricotta, and an egg yolk), and rabbit with my dad back in the 1980's.

Recipe courtesy of Tony May & Marisa May-Metalli.

Vignarola Spring Vegetable Soup

Soup/Entrée • All Phases • Serves 4

INGREDIENTS

½ cup extra-virgin olive oil
½ cup dry white wine
4 ounces chopped onion
4 baby artichokes, cleaned, trimmed,
  with the dark outer green leaves
  discarded; cut into quarters
2 ounces asparagus spears, cut
  in diamonds

1 ounce scallions, cut in diamonds
4 ounces fresh fava beans, shelled
  and peeled
2 ounces fresh English peas, shelled
sea salt, to taste
freshly ground black pepper, to taste
1 ounce (per person) pecorino Romano
  shavings (optional)

INSTRUCTIONS

• In a pot, bring the oil and white wine to a simmer.

- Add the onions and artichokes.

- Simmer gently until both begin to soften.

- Return the mixture to a boil and add the asparagus and the scallions.

- Let cook for 3 minutes, then add the fava beans and peas.

- Season mixture with sea salt and pepper, to taste, and let cook for 10 more minutes—not longer. Stir occasionally. Vegetables should retain their bright green colors.

- Spoon the "Vignarola" into 4 warmed, individual soup bowls and then sprinkle the pecorino Romano cheese shavings on top.

NOTE

The nutrition facts include 1-ounce pecorino per serving; 1 ounce of pecorino Romano contains 110 calories.

Nutrition Facts (per serving)
Calories: **432** • Calories from fat: **72%** • Fat: **35g**
Saturated fat: **9g** • Cholesterol: **25mg** • Carbohydrates: **15g**
Protein: **15g** • Sodium: **853mg** • Fiber: **3g**

Italy

Hotel Santa Caterina

S.S. Amalfitana, 9, 84011 Amalfi (Salerno), Italy

+39 089 871012 • www.hotelsantacaterina.it

The stunningly beautiful Hotel Santa Caterina, *my favorite hotel in the world*, is perched on a bluff draped with bougainvillea and terraces of lovingly tended olive groves and fruit orchards, surrounded by the unforgettable blue Mediterranean Sea and sky in the heart of the Amalfi Coast. The main hotel is a beautifully restored late nineteenth century liberty style villa, and features the very best in regional Italian and Continental cuisine, with an emphasis on fresh, local seafood, produce, and cheeses, a wonderful spa, and beautifully appointed guest rooms overlooking the sea. Come experience the very best in Italian luxury and hospitality at what will surely become your favorite destination for enjoying *La Dolce Vita* in Italy too!

· ·

San Pietro (John Dory) and Artichoke Roll with Asparagus Bundles and Potatoes

Entrée • All Phases • Serves 4

INGREDIENTS

4–6-ounce fillets of San Pietro fish
(see Note)

2 artichokes, peeled and sliced
(see Note)

2 ounces leeks, chopped

2 ounces extra-virgin olive oil

3 tsp. grated Parmesan cheese

8 ounces chopped potatoes (see Note)

1 ounce capers (salt packed or in brine)

1 ounce Taggiasca olives

4 ounces 'del pendolo' cherry tomatoes
(see Note)

4 ounces red peppers

1 clove garlic

INSTRUCTIONS

- Sauté the artichokes and leeks in a little olive oil until softened. For convenience, you may substitute with peeled, canned or jarred baby artichoke hearts. Rinse, especially if they are marinated to remove added flavors that could detract from the delicate flavor of the fish.
- Flatten the fillets of San Pietro between 2 sheets of cling film, season with salt and pepper, place the artichokes, previously pan cooked with the leeks, on top.
- Sprinkle the fish with Parmesan cheese and roll.
- Bake the chopped potatoes in the oven until lightly golden. (Omit potatoes for Phase One, or substitute with sweet potato.)
- Create 4 bundles of asparagus, tie with slithers of red pepper, and blanch in a pan with some water. Remove when cooked to *al dente*, and place in an ice bath for about 10 seconds to help retain green color. Set aside.
- Cut the San Pietro rolls into 12 slices and cook in a non-stick pan with a little oil for roughly 2 minutes on each side, until lightly browned. Set aside.
- Rinse the capers. Chop the garlic, olives, and tomatoes.
- Brown the capers, olives, garlic, and chopped tomatoes in a little oil and simmer for several minutes until ingredients are well amalgamated.
- Place the fish and vegetables on 4 plates and garnish with the sauce obtained.

NOTE

John Dory is favored among international chefs for its beautiful fillets, and lives in coastal waters of Europe, Africa, Asia, and the Australia-New Zealand. Although it is not commonly imported into the U.S. due to availability and cost, if you are traveling abroad and see it featured, it is worth having. You may occasionally see it at a higher-end restaurant in the States. A good substitute is Dover sole or Sole.

The "del pendolo" tomatoes are a prized variety of tomato cultivated in the rich volcanic soil surrounding Mt. Vesuvius near Naples. Substitute with the best quality imported San Marzano canned tomatoes from the same area of Italy. For weight-loss purposes, omit potatoes in Phase One.

Nutrition Facts (per serving)
Calories: **379** • Calories from fat: **41%** • Fat: **1617g**
Saturated fat: **2g** • Cholesterol: **121mg** • Carbohydrates: **11g**
Protein: **45g** • Sodium: **488mg** • Fiber: **5g**

•

Toscana Saporita Cooking School

Via Pietra a Padule al Sasso 5102, Massaciuccoli Lucca (LU) Italia
+39 335 8129442 • info@toscanasaporita.com • www.toscanasaporita.com

As someone particularly fond of authentic Italian cooking, having had the pleasure to attend Toscana Saporita twice so far, I can safely say it is the greatest hands-on culinary experience one can have in Italy! If attending cooking school in Italy is on your bucket list, this is *THE* place. Chef and Owner/Managing Director of the renowned Toscana Saporita Cooking School near Lucca, Italy, Sandra Rosy Lotti is known throughout Italy for her cookbooks on Tuscan regional cuisine. She has also co-authored with her cousin Anne Bianchi, *Dolci Toscani,* the definitive compilation of Tuscan dessert recipes and is a contributing writer for *Intermezzo* Magazine. Sandra frequently contributes to Italy's most prestigious cooking magazines and conducts private cooking lessons when classes are not in season. A frequent visitor the United States, she frequently presents her authentic Tuscan cuisine at the James Beard Foundation House, The French Culinary Institute, La Cucina Italiana, Degustibus, Ocean Reef Club in Key Largo, and at Eataly locations. She took care of the menu for the Birra Moretti Launch in London and in NY. Sandra's vivacious personality, passion for what she does, and genuine love of people makes Toscana Saporita the perfect place for eager students to learn the art of Tuscan cooking.

Pasta Fatta in Casa: Basic Pasta

Entrée • Phases Two–Four • Serves 4

INGREDIENTS

1 cup unbleached, all-purpose flour   ¾ cup semolina flour

2 eggs

pinch of salt

1 Tbsp. extra-virgin olive oil

2 Tbsp. water

INSTRUCTIONS

- Heap the flour onto a flat work surface and create a well in the center. Add the eggs, salt, oil and water to the well.

- Using a fork, beat the egg mixture, incorporating increasing amounts of the flour wall until smooth dough has been created. Knead with floured hands for 5 minutes.

- Pinch off a lemon-sized piece and pass through the widest setting on a pasta machine. Dust lightly with flour, fold into thirds and pass through the machine 3 times more. Narrow the setting on the machine, dust the sheet lightly with flour and pass through the machine.

- Continue to pass through even more narrow settings until you have reached the desired thickness (generally 4–5 on the machine will do it).

NOTE

Different types of flour such as chestnut, chickpea, whole-wheat, oat, soy, rye can be added. Adjust the measurements according to the hardness of the flour. For example, when using whole-wheat, chickpea, farro, or chestnut flours (all fairly hard), use 1 cup all-purpose, ⅜ cup semolina, and ⅜ cup whole-wheat.

Nutrition Facts (per serving)
Calories: **279** • Calories from fat: **20%** • Fat: **6g**
Saturated fat: **1g** • Cholesterol: **93mg** • Carbohydrates: **45g**
Protein: **10g** • Sodium: **326mg** • Fiber: **2g**

. . . .

Insalata di Farro – Farro Salad

Starter/Entrée • All Phases • Serves 5

INGREDIENTS

½ pound farro

4 large ripe tomatoes, diced

6 fresh basil leaves, finely chopped

1 leek, white part only, cut into thin slivers (or finely diced red onion)

1 clove garlic, minced

¼ cup extra-virgin olive oil

Salt and freshly ground black pepper

2 Tbsp. pine nuts, toasted in the oven for about 5 minutes (optional)

½ cup Parmigiano-Reggiano, shaved

INSTRUCTIONS

- Rinse the farro carefully in cold water.
- Place the farro in a soup pot with enough water to cover by 4 inches and add salt.
- Cover and cook over moderate heat for 35 minutes or until tender.
- Drain thoroughly, rinse it in cold water to remove the starch, drain it again and transfer to a large bowl.
- Add the remaining ingredients and toss until well blended. Serve lukewarm or refrigerate and serve cold.

NOTE

Every pound of farro serves 10 people (medium portions) Every pound of farro needs to be cooked in about 2 quarts of water. Make sure it is covered by 4 inches of water when you cook it.

For another variation, try Octopus Farro Salad. Cook the octopus in cold salted water where you have diluted 1 cup of red vinegar and have added a couple of wine corks. Cover the pot with a lid. To cook the octopus perfectly, calculate 20 minutes after the water has started to boil per pound of octopus. Leave the octopus in the pot with its cooking water until it gets warm. Then slice it and add it to the cooked farro at 5. Add shaved Parmigiano-Reggiano, extra-virgin olive oil, salt and pepper and serve warm.

Nutrition Facts (per serving)
Calories: **355** • Calories from fat: **44%** • Fat: **17.5g**
Saturated fat: **3g** • Cholesterol: **6mg** • Carbohydrates: **40g**
Protein: **11g** • Sodium: **617.5g** • Fiber: **8g**

· ·

Branzino in Cartoccio– Sea Bass Marinated in Orange Juice & Cooked in Parchment with Vegetables

Entrée • All Phases • Serves 4

INGREDIENTS

Fish:

10 Tbsp. extra-virgin olive oil

1 leek, white part only, cleaned
   and diced

1 potato, peeled and thinly sliced

2 plum tomatoes, diced

1 fennel bulb, thinly sliced

2 small zucchini, cut into thin rounds

1 carrot, julienned

1 cup white wine

24 Gaeta olive, pitted (or Kalamata)

2 Tbsp. capers (salt packed or in brine,
   rinsed)

1 yellow pepper, thinly sliced

1 red pepper, thinly sliced

freshly chopped parsley, as much as
   you want

fresh thyme

4 thick sea bass fillets, totaling
   1 pound

Marinade:

2 blood oranges

½ cup extra-virgin olive oil

1 tsp. grated lemon zest

salt and pepper

freshly chopped parsley

INSTRUCTIONS

· Marinated fish fillets for 1 hour in orange juice, extra-virgin olive oil, lemon zest, salt, pepper and parsley.

· Heat the oil in a skillet and sauté the leek for 8 minutes over moderate heat, stirring constantly until soft.

· Add the potato, tomatoes, fennel, zucchini, peppers and carrot and wine and cook for 10 minutes, stirring frequently until the vegetables are almost cooked. Add the wine olives and capers and stir to blend.

· Dust with parsley.

· Pre-heat the oven to 350 degrees Fahrenheit.

· Cut 4 large, heart shaped pieces of parchment and divide the vegetables mixture among them, spooning it onto one side of each heart only.

- Top with the sea bass fillets, fold over the hearts and roll the edges to seal.

  - Bake for 15 minutes, then make a small slit in each of the parchment packages and bake for 3 more minutes.

  - Transfer the packages onto individual plates and serve immediately.

NOTE

For nutritional information, we assumed ¼ of the marinade ingredients would end up being consumed with the dish. In Phase One, omit the potatoes. The amount of orange juice is negligible since it is a marinade, it is allowed in Phase One.

Nutrition Facts (per serving)
Calories: **591** • Calories from fat: **48%** • Fat: **51g**
Saturated fat: **7g** • Cholesterol: **0mg** • Carbohydrates: **28g**
Protein: **4g** • Sodium: **576mg** • Fiber: **7g**

Chapter Nine
A Few of Fred's Favorite Healthy Gourmet Recipes

INDEX OF RECIPES

- Cedar Plank Grilled Salmon "Two Ways"—with Blood Orange Reduction and Honey Dijon (Entrée) (All Phases)
- Escarole & Cannellini Beans and "Neapolitan-Style" (Side Dish) (All Phases)
- Strawberries with Balsamic Vinegar and Black Pepper (Dessert) (All Phases)
- Casey's Baked Fruit (Dessert) (All Phases)

· ·

Smoked Salmon and Asparagus Frittata

Breakfast· All Phases · Serves 4

This combines the best of Jewish and Italian—taking smoked Nova Salmon, tomato, and onion (the essence of a Nova platter) and adding the ingredients to a frittata, a baked Italian omelet flavored with fresh grated cheese. The asparagus adds more flavor and color, though you can easily use broccoli, spinach, escarole, mushrooms, or roasted peppers in any combination. Anything you might put into an omelet would work in a frittata. If you don't feel like baking, cut the ingredients in half and make an omelet instead. I love combining eggs with another protein and vegetables, and a little cheese, to hit three food groups in a healthy balance. Eggs are very satisfying, and make great fuel to get you through the day. Protein is important, especially if you are building muscle. If you have cholesterol issues, talk to your doctor, and consider Egg Beaters, or all egg whites.

This can be refrigerated and served chilled as a snack. It tastes like a quiche without the pastry. You can add any combination of ingredients you like in a frittata. They are a great way to use up leftovers and are excellent for breakfast, lunch, or dinner. I like mine with some Cholula hot sauce (0 calories) on the side!

INGREDIENTS

1 cup asparagus, blanched, bottoms removed, cut on bias

2 sprays non-stick cooking spray

3 large eggs

3 egg whites

2 Tbsp. skim milk

1 Tbsp. freshly grated Parmigiano-Reggiano

1 Tbsp. grated pecorino Romano

freshly ground black pepper, to taste

4 ounces smoked Nova Salmon, thinly sliced and cut into bite-sized strips

1 red or yellow onion, chopped

1 ripe tomato, chopped

4 ounces goat cheese, crumbled

2 Tbsp. fresh chopped dill or fennel fronds, for garnish

INSTRUCTIONS

- Pre-heat the oven to 400 degree Fahrenheit.

- Bring a medium pot of salted water to a boil. Blanch the asparagus for about 2 minutes. Drain and immediately shock in an ice-water-bath. Remove, pat dry with paper towels, cut into 1-inch diagonal pieces.

- Whisk eggs, grated cheese, and freshly ground black pepper.

- Heat a 12-inch, non-stick, ovenproof skillet, coated with cooking spray over medium heat. Add onions and sauté until softened, about 3 minutes. Add the diced tomato and simmer another minute.

- Add the smoked salmon and cook for 1–2 minutes, depending how cooked you like it.

- Reduce heat to low and pour the egg mixture over the onions and tomato.

- Add the asparagus.

- Cover and cook until the bottom and sides are firm and lightly golden brown.

- Uncover and bake for about 10 minutes. Remove from the oven and sprinkle the goat cheese over the top. Bake an additional 2 minutes. Remove and let rest for 5 minutes.

- To remove the frittata from the pan, run a rubber spatula around the edges. Gently slide frittata from the skillet to a large plate or serving dish. Slice frittata into wedges, garnish with dill or fennel, and serve.

> **Nutrition Facts (per serving)**
> Calories: **230** • Calories from fat: **49%** • Fat: **13g** • Saturated fat: **6g**
> Cholesterol: **181mg** • Carbohydrates: **8g** • Protein: **21g** • Sodium: **984mg**

. . . .

French Toast With "Sprouted Bread"

Breakfast • All Phases • Serves 2

INGREDIENTS

2 egg whites, beaten
¼ cup skim milk
1 Tbsp. honey
1 tsp. vanilla extract

pinch cinnamon
pinch freshly ground nutmeg
pinch salt

2 slices Ezekiel 4:9 brand sprouted
   bread, defrosted if frozen

2 sprays non-stick cooking spray
Fresh fruit and/or berries, for topping

INSTRUCTIONS

- Whisk together egg whites, milk, honey, cinnamon, salt and vanilla extract in a bowl.
- Soak the sprouted bread slices in the mixture for a minute on each side.
- Spray a large skillet or griddle with non-stick cooking spray and heat on medium.
- Brown the soaked bread on each side for 2–3 minutes.
- Serve topped with fresh fruit! Strawberries, blueberries, raspberries, or peaches are excellent with this. You can heat the fruit in a saucepan, it is really delicious!

NOTE

You may substitute agave nectar for the honey. Agave nectar contains 60 calories per Tbsp., honey contains 64.

Nutrition Facts (per serving)
Calories: **154** • Calories from fat: **15%** • Fat: **3g** • Saturated fat: **1g**
Cholesterol: **3mg** • Carbohydrates: **24g** • Protein: **8g** • Sodium: **334mg**

. . . .

Fred's Chicken Vegetable Soup

Soup/Entrée • All Phases • Serves 6

Chicken Vegetable Soup is a healthy, hearty comfort food. Why go out or open a can for salty soup with hardly any satisfying chicken when you can make a delicious, easy meal with leftovers in no time!

INGREDIENTS

1 4-pound chicken (fresh, free-range, and organic, if possible)
sea salt and freshly ground pepper, to taste
12 cups water

1 large yellow onion
4 cloves garlic, whole or sliced (optional)
3 large carrots, sliced (or baby carrots cut-up)

3 celery stalks, chopped

1 Bay Leaf

1 bunch fresh Italian parsley, finely chopped, to garnish

1 tsp. per person grated Parmigiano-Reggiano, or Pecorino Romano as garnish

INSTRUCTIONS

- Remove the giblets bag from inside the chicken. Wash and dry the chicken with paper towels, inside and out.
- Sprinkle sea salt and freshly ground black pepper over the chicken.
- Bring the water to a boil over medium-high heat in a 12-quart stockpot.
- Add the chicken, onion, garlic, vegetables, and Bay Leaf.
- Reduce heat to medium-low and let simmer for an hour and a half with the lid on the pot, partially lifted.
- Skim and remove fat from the top as the soup cooks.
- Carefully remove the hot chicken onto a platter. Let it stand a few minutes. Remove skin and discard, pull off the loose meat, chop some into bite-sized pieces, set aside bones, wings, and larger pieces, which can be served separately on a platter.
- Add the chopped-up chicken back to the pot. The soup is ready to be served.
- To prepare optional pasta, boil it separately until *al dente*.
- Serve the soup in bowls, adding optional pasta. Garnish with fresh Italian parsley, freshly grated cheese, and pepper to taste. *Salute!*

NOTE

If you refrigerate the soup before eating it, any fat will harden on the surface and will be easy to remove. The calorie count is for 6 servings of the soup, including the entire meat only (no skin) yield from a 4-pound chicken and one teaspoon of grated cheese per person. If you are in Phases Two–Four, you may include up to 4 ounces of pasta (egg noodles or tortellini are excellent with this) per person.

Nutrition Facts (per serving)
Calories: **458** • Calories from fat: **63%** • Fat: **32g** • Saturated fat: **9g**
Cholesterol: **145mg** • Carbohydrates: **6g** • Protein: **35g** • Sodium: **236mg**

. . . .
Auntie Jo's Lentil Soup

Soup • All Phases • Serves 8

No visit to Auntie Jo's around lunchtime was complete without a bowl of her healthy lentil soup. Auntie Jo lived to the ripe old age of ninety-four, eating a healthy Mediterranean diet and walking everywhere, as her parents had done back in Sicily. In fact, she never got a driver's license! It was her lifestyle of eating a healthy mix of foods and doing a lot of walking that helped her live such a long and happy life.

INGREDIENTS

Lentil Soup:

2 Tbsp. extra-virgin olive oil

1 large yellow onion, finely chopped

2 cups carrots, finely chopped

1 cup celery with leaves, finely chopped

2 cloves garlic, smashed

1 Bay Leaf

salt and freshly ground black pepper, to taste

1 pound lentils

1 cup canned San Marzano tomatoes, hand-crushed with the juice

pinch of dried Sicilian oregano (or regular oregano)

6 cups hot water

2 cups chicken broth (optional, otherwise add more water)

2 cups chopped Spinach or Swiss chard

Garnish:

½ cup fresh Italian parsley, finely chopped

1 tsp. grated Parmigiano-Reggiano or Pecorino Romano, per serving

red chili flakes (optional)

INSTRUCTIONS

• Soak lentils in hot water for 20 minutes beforehand, as they will cook faster and easier.

• In a twelve-quart stockpot, heat the oil over medium heat.

• When the oil is hot, add the onion, garlic, carrots, celery, and Bay Leaf, and cook until the vegetables are soft.

• Add the lentils, crushed tomatoes, chopped kale or Swiss chard, water, and broth.

• Add the salt, pepper, oregano, and optional chili flakes.

- Bring to a rolling boil, then reduce the heat to medium-low, cover, and allow to simmer for at least an hour, stirring occasionally.

NOTE

You will want to taste the lentils to make sure they are done. I like them a little *al dente*, though this soup is also good slow and long-cooked for several hours. It will be rich and thicker, more like a stew. In Phases Two–Four, you may add a couple links of Italian sausage (omit in Phase One due to calories). An average link of Italian sausage contains roughly 250 calories. Remove the meat from the casing and brown it with the vegetables.

Nutrition Facts (per serving)
Calories: **234** • Calories from fat: **19%** • Fat: **5g** • Saturated fat: **1g**
Cholesterol: **3mg** • Carbohydrates: **34g** • Protein: **16g** • Sodium: **225mg**

. . . .

Fred's Turkey Chili

Soup/Entrée • All Phases • Serves 8

INGREDIENTS

Lentil Soup:

2 Tbsp. extra-virgin olive oil

1 pound ground turkey

1 cup yellow onion, finely chopped

1 Tbsp. minced fresh garlic

1 cup celery, finely chopped

1 cup carrots, finely chopped

2 Tbsp. tomato paste

1 cup chicken stock or broth

½ cup dry white wine

2 cups crushed tomatoes

2 cups red kidney beans, drained and rinsed

1 Bay Leaf

1 Tbsp. chili powder

½ tsp. paprika

½ tsp. dried oregano

½ tsp. ground cayenne pepper

1 tsp. cumin

1 tsp. coriander

pinch red chili flakes, to taste

salt and freshly ground black pepper, to taste

chopped hot pepper of your choice (habanero works well) (optional)

Garnish:

chopped red onion (3 calories per Tbsp.)

1 tsp. Breakstone's Reduced Fat Sour Cream (10 calories per tsp.)

Cholula hot sauce (Zero calories)

INSTRUCTIONS

- In a twelve-quart stockpot, heat the oil over medium heat.
- Cook the turkey in the pot until it is evenly brown.
- Stir in the onion, garlic, veggies, seasonings and Bay Leaf. Cook until vegetables are tender.
- Add the white wine to deglaze the pan.
- Add the tomato paste, and let it brown for a minute with the meat and vegetables.
- Add the crushed tomatoes, beans, seasonings, and stock.
- Bring to a boil. Reduce heat to low heat, cover and simmer for one hour.
- Uncover and simmer another 30 minutes to thicken.

NOTE

To make this dish a turkey or veggie chili, you may want to add the following:

- 1 red bell pepper, seeds removed, chopped
- 1 green bell pepper, seeds removed, chopped
- 1 zucchini, diced
- 1 cup canned corn or fresh corn sliced from a cob (optional)

Nutrition Facts (per serving)

Calories285 • Calories from fat: **15%** • Fat: **5g** • Saturated fat: **1g** • Cholesterol: **25mg** • Carbohydrates: **37g** • Protein: **23g** • Sodium: **140mg**

. . . .

Fred's Famous San Fratello Salad

Salad/Entrée • All Phases • Serves 6

I named my famous salad after San Fratello, the picturesque town in Sicily overlooking the sea, where the Bollaci family is from. The flavors and colors remind me of the beauty of our native Sicily. I have been making this salad for dinner guests for years. For purposes of this weight-loss book, I am using the quantities I included during my weight loss. Of course, they may be adjusted. The combination of flavors and colors make this very satisfying salad a winner!

INGREDIENTS

Salad:

2 cups baby arugula

2 cups mixed baby greens of your choice

1 head radicchio, chopped

1 Belgian endive, chopped

1 cup roasted peppers (such as Mancini brand, or you may roast your own in the oven or on the grill)

2 large, ripe tomatoes, large dice (or 2 cups cherry tomatoes)

½ cup imported Italian olives with pits

1 red onion, thinly sliced into ½-inch pieces

2 ripe Haas avocados, sliced into chunks

1 cup fresh basil leaves, torn or cut into chiffonade

1 ounce crumbled gorgonzola, or blue cheese, per person (may use shaved Parmesan, goat cheese, or feta if you prefer)

freshly ground black pepper, to taste

Lemon vinaigrette:

½ cup fresh lemon juice

3 Tbsp. extra-virgin olive oil

2 cloves garlic, minced (optional)

pinch dried oregano

sea salt, to taste

INSTRUCTIONS

- Rinse, dry, and combine vegetables, except for the avocado in a large salad bowl, or in individual bowls.
- Add the cheese, sliced avocado, and dressing to the top.
- Serve with freshly ground black pepper, to taste.

NOTE

To control the portion size, place the cheese individually on each plate. Alternately, to make the cheese flavor permeate the entire salad, place salad ingredients in a large bowl, dress it, add the cheese, and chop the salad with a handheld salad cutting tool. For balsamic vinaigrette, either substitute Balsamic vinegar for the lemon juice, or simply add ½ cup balsamic vinegar along with the lemon juice. The combination is wonderful. In addition, instead of the dressing the salad ahead of time, at the table add a drizzle of extra-virgin olive oil and a little balsamic vinegar or a squeeze of lemon. It is easy and good as well.

Nutrition Facts (per serving)
Calories: **337** • Calories from fat: **68%** • Fat: **27g** • Saturated fat: **8g**
Cholesterol: **21mg** • Carbohydrates: **20g** • Protein: **11g** • Sodium: **512mg**

. . . .

Auntie Jo's Famous Heart-Healthy Salad

Salad • All Phases • Serves 4

This is my adaptation of the salad my Great Aunt Josephine prepared and enjoyed every day! She lived to the age of 94, and was a big proponent of healthy lifestyle and nutrition. Apple cider vinegar is loaded with health benefits. In fact, this light and refreshing salad can easily be assembled in minutes and is very low-calorie! You may substitute red wine vinegar, balsamic, or lemon juice, in the dressing if you prefer. Add any vegetables you have on hand, or make into a salad. It's fun to be creative in putting together different colors, flavors, and textures. Any salad can easily be enhanced into a meal by adding a piece of grilled chicken breast, grilled salmon, or grilled shrimp.

INGREDIENTS

Salad:
1 head iceberg lettuce, chopped
1 head radicchio, chopped
2 tomatoes, chopped
2 cup carrots, rough chopped

1 stalk celery with and leaves, rough chopped
1 red onion, chopped
1 cup fresh Italian parsley, chopped

Dressing:
2 Tbsp. extra-virgin olive oil
½ cup apple cider vinegar
1 tsp. dried oregano

finely ground sea salt and freshly ground black pepper, to taste

INSTRUCTIONS

- Rinse, dry, and chop up ingredients.
- Combine dressing ingredients in a separate bowl.
- Combine veggies in a salad bowl with dressing and toss.
- Serve immediately.

. . . .

Calamari Amalfitana—Amalfi Style Calamari Salad

Sala • All Phases • Serves 6

This light, healthy, delicious chilled calamari salad is in the style of the Amalfi Coast, was inspired by Donatello Italian Restaurant which serves a lovely version of this.

INGREDIENTS

Calamari:

2 pounds tender, baby squid[38], cleaned and cut into ¼-inch rings, tentacles cut in half

4 Tbsp. extra-virgin olive oil

4 cloves garlic, minced

4 lemons, juiced

sea salt and freshly ground black pepper, to taste

Garnish:

2 additional lemons, sliced

½ cup fresh Italian parsley[39]

¼ cup imported Italian olives

1 tomato, cored and sliced vertically into segments, or 1 cup cherry tomatoes

1 head radicchio, chopped and added to the calamari salad, or individual leaves on the side to garnish

INSTRUCTIONS

• Boil the calamari (if it is not previously cooked) for 2 minutes. Drop the calamari into an ice bath, drain it, and pat dry with paper towels. Set it aside.

• Mix the olive oil, minced garlic, lemon juice, and salt and pepper, to taste.

---

38 Let your fishmonger clean the squid for you to make life easier.

39 Finely mince all but 4 sprigs, garnish each dish with one whole sprig in addition to the minced parsley.

- Toss with the calamari, plate, garnish with additional lemon, parsley, radicchio, tomato, and olives.

NOTE

The chopped veggies listed as garnish can also be added to the salad rather than being used as garnish. This recipe works beautifully with steamed shrimp, sliced lobster tail, as well as your choice of clams, mussels, scallops, and scungilli. To make a *"Frutti di Mare"* salad, you may wish to add any of the above items, plus optional cup each of chopped celery, carrots, and possibly cannellini beans. Be sure to serve chilled.

Nutrition Facts (per serving)
Calories: **253** • Calories from fat: **43%** • Fat: **12g** • Saturated fat: **2g**
Cholesterol: **353mg** • Carbohydrates: **12g** • Protein: **24g** • Sodium: **195mg**

· · · · · · · · · · ·

Tabbouleh

Salad • All Phases • Serves 4

This is a favorite from the Middle East. It includes finely chopped parsley, onion, tomato, and cracked bulgur wheat, with lots of lemon and a drizzle of extra-virgin olive oil. Tabbouleh is great with roasted or lemon-chicken, with pita bread, or in a wrap with grilled chicken or turkey, sliced from the frame. As a substitute for the bulgur, you may also want to try quinoa, couscous, or farro.

INGREDIENTS

4 cups packed of fresh Italian parsley,
   finely chopped (approximately
   4 cups)
1 large red or yellow onion,
   finely chopped
3 large ripe tomatoes, finely chopped
½ cup fresh mint, finely chopped
1 cup bulgur (cracked wheat)
1 cup boiling hot water (to soften
   the bulgur)
¾ cup fresh lemon juice
¼ cup extra-virgin olive oil

salt and freshly ground black pepper,
   to taste

INSTRUCTIONS

- Prepare the bulgur in a bowl. In the bowl, mix it with the hot water and a drop of oil. Cover and let stand for 15 minutes. Drain through a sieve. Squeeze the moisture out by hand.

- Finely chop the vegetables.

- Combine the vegetables with the bulgur.

- Squeeze the lemons into a bowl, add the olive oil, salt, and pepper to taste and mix.

- Pour over the salad and mix. Serve with additional freshly ground pepper.

Nutrition Facts (per serving)
Calories: **320** • Calories from fat: **41%** • Fat: **15g** • Saturated fat: **2g**
Cholesterol: **0mg** • Carbohydrates: **46g** • Protein: **8g** • Sodium: **95mg**

. . . .

Fred's Boca Cobb Salad with Lemon Pepper Vinaigrette

Salad/Entrée • All Phases Serves • 4 as an entrée

This delicious and satisfying salad is actually a meal in itself and was inspired by a dish at Addison Reserve Country Club.

INGREDIENTS

Cobb Salad:

4 cups mixed baby greens

8 jumbo shrimp, grilled

8 ounces jumbo lump crabmeat

1 cup hearts of palm, sliced

1 Haas avocado, diced

2 cups grape tomatoes

1 cup mandarin oranges

4 ounces crumbled goat cheese

4 Tbsp. toasted almonds

4 large hard-boiled eggs, peeled, sliced

8 charred scallions

2 Tbsp. Lemon Pepper Vinaigrette
 (per serving)

Fred's Lemon Pepper Vinaigrette:

½ cup fresh lemon juice

zest of ½ lemon

2 Tbsp. extra-virgin olive oil

1 shallot, finely minced

1 Tbsp. freshly ground black pepper

finely ground sea salt, to taste

INSTRUCTIONS

Cobb Salad:

- Grill the shrimp until just cooked, set aside.

- Also grill scallions until just lightly charred, set aside.

- Hard boil the eggs, set aside to cool.

- Make the vinaigrette.

- Rinse, dry, slice, and dice salad ingredients.

- Assemble the ingredients on 4 chilled salad plates, starting with the greens and veggies and construct your salad, finishing with the oranges, crumbled goat cheese, toasted almonds, and sliced egg.

- Place the grilled shrimp and lump crabmeat on top of each salad.

- Dress and serve immediately.

Fred's Lemon Pepper Vinaigrette:

- Vigorously whisk or shake ingredients in a jar immediately prior to serving.

Nutrition Facts (per serving)
Calories: **537** • Calories from fat: **55%** • Fat: **34g** • Saturated fat: **8g**
Cholesterol: **131mg** • Carbohydrates: **22g** • Protein: **40g** • Sodium: **734mg**

. . . .

Fred's Light Honey Mustard and Honey Dijon Dressing or Sauce

Dressing/Sauce • All Phases • Serves 4

INGREDIENTS

¾ cup Hellman's Light Mayonnaise

4 Tbsp. honey

1 Tbsp. yellow mustard (or Dijon mustard for Honey Dijon)

1 tsp. apple cider vinegar

1 pinch cayenne pepper

INSTRUCTIONS

Whisk ingredients together and serve chilled as a salad dressing, sauce or dip.

Nutrition Facts (per serving)
Calories: **89** • Calories from fat: **57%** • Fat: **6g** • Saturated fat: **1g**
Cholesterol: **0mg** • Carbohydrates: **10g** • Protein: **0g** • Sodium: **132mg**

. . . .

Tzatziki—Greek Yogurt & Cucumber Dip

Dip/Snack • All Phases • Serves 4

This is a great dip to serve with crudités of raw vegetables.

INGREDIENTS

1 English cucumber, peeled, seeded, and diced (see Note)
1 cup plain low-fat Greek yogurt
3 cloves garlic, peeled
½ lemon, juiced

sea salt and pepper, to taste
1 tsp. extra-virgin olive oil
1 tsp. chopped fresh mint leaves or fresh dill

INSTRUCTIONS

• Process ingredients in a food processor until well amalgamated.

• Place in a bowl, cover with plastic wrap, and chill for at least one hour before serving.

NOTE

English cucumbers are better in dips because they have fewer seeds and a lower water content. If using regular cucumbers, slice vertically and remove as many of the seeds as possible.

Nutrition Facts (per serving)
Calories: **64** • Calories from fat: **38%** • Fat: **3g** • Saturated fat: **1g**
Cholesterol: **9mg** • Carbohydrates: **5g** • Protein: **6g** • Sodium: **327mg**

· ·

Baba Ghanoush—Middle Eastern Roasted Eggplant Dip

Dip/Snack • All Phases (see Note) • Serves 4

This dip can be made with either roasted or baked eggplant. Serve at room temperature with grilled pita bread and/or veggies of your choice. For Phase One, serve only with raw vegetable crudités (carrots, celery, broccoli, cauliflower, tomatoes, radishes, etc.).

INGREDIENTS

Baba Ghanoush:

1 large or 2 medium eggplants (2 pounds)

¼ cup tahini (roasted sesame paste), additional to taste

3 garlic cloves, minced (more or less, depending how garlicky you want it)

¼ cup fresh lemon juice, additional to taste

1 pinch ground cumin

sea salt and freshly ground black pepper, to taste

sprinkle of cayenne pepper, to taste

Garnish:

1 Tbsp. extra-virgin olive oil to swirl in the dip at the end

2 Tbsp. chopped fresh Italian parsley

¼ cup imported black olives with pits (Kalamata and Gaeta are great)

INSTRUCTIONS

• You can either grill or bake the eggplant. To grill the eggplant, heat a grill to medium-hot. Prick the eggplant all around and grill it whole for 10–15 minutes, turning every couple minutes so the entire surface gets blistered and the juices start to come out. Transfer eggplant to a brown paper bag and fold the bag shut, allowing the eggplant to steam in its skin for 15–20 minutes.

• To bake the eggplant, pre-heat the oven to 350 degrees Fahrenheit. Prick eggplant all around and bake it whole on a baking sheet for 35–40 minutes, or until it is very soft.

• Allow the cooked eggplant to cool slightly, peel, and discard skin.

• Place eggplant flesh in a large bowl and mash it into a paste.

- Add the tahini, garlic, lemon juice, cumin, salt, and pepper, and mix and mash very well by hand. Taste and add additional lemon, tahini, cayenne, salt, or pepper if necessary.
- Transfer to a serving bowl. Create a well in the middle of the surface. Swirl the Tbsp. of olive oil in the middle, and surround with olives. Garnish with chopped parsley.

Nutrition Facts (per serving)
Calories: **273** • Calories from fat: **67%** • Fat: **22g** •Saturated fat: **3g**
Cholesterol: **0mg** • Carbohydrates: **18g** • Protein: **7g** • Sodium: **227mg**

. . . .

Fred's Fruit and Yogurt Smoothie

Snack • All Phases • Serves 1

INGREDIENTS

1 cup of mixed fruit of your choice
(strawberries, blueberries, banana, or
whatever you'd like!)

1 cup ice cubes
1 4-ounce container vanilla Dannon
Activia Light yogurt

INSTRUCTIONS

- Process ingredients in the blender until smooth.

NOTE

For a light variation, simply freeze a cup of your favorite fresh berries and process them in a blender. It comes out like "berry" ice.

Calorie analysis: total calories will vary depending on the fruit(s) used. There are 70 calories in Activia Light, which makes it an excellent, low-calorie snack or yogurt base for a smoothie. I also make this with plain low-fat Greek yogurt, which has an average of 130 calories per four-ounce container.

Calories in various fruits:

Banana (1 medium): 105
Blueberries (1 cup): 83
Strawberries (1 cup): 46
Raspberries (1 cup): 64

Fred's Lobster Lettuce Wraps

Snack/Entrée • All Phases • Serves 4

This is my light, lemony, low-calorie take on a lobster roll, using fresh Bibb lettuce instead of the traditional buttered hot dog bun. These make great hors d'oeuvres—elegant and easy finger food.

INGREDIENTS

1 pound of cooked lobster meat cut in bite-sized morsels (mixture of tail, claw, and knuckle) (see Note)

2 green onions, chopped

1 stalk celery with leaves, finely chopped

2 Tbsp. Hellmann's Light Mayonnaise

juice from 2 lemons or limes

dash of Tabasco

2 Tbsp. fresh chopped tarragon

sea salt and freshly ground black pepper, to taste

12 large butter lettuce leaves

INSTRUCTIONS

• Rinse and dry lettuce leaves. Set aside.

• Dice the lobster meat. If steaming your own, be sure the meat has cooled.

• Chop the onion and celery and place in a bowl.

• Add the lobster meat, mayonnaise, lime juice, Tabasco, tarragon, salt, and pepper. Gently mix to coat the lobster meat.

• Fill each lettuce leaf with an equal amount of the lobster mix.

• Plate and serve.

NOTE

A one-pound live lobster will yield roughly 3–4 ounces of meat. You can purchase and steam lobsters, or opt for lobster tails (an 8-ounce tail yields roughly 4 ounces of meat). If steaming your own lobsters, pick the meat from the carcass and you can freeze to use later for soup or broth. For convenience, you can purchase quality pre-cooked lobster meat at a good seafood or specialty market, or online direct from Maine.

Nutrition Facts (per serving)
Calories: **129** • Calories from fat: **21%** • Fat: **3g** • Saturated fat: **0g**
Cholesterol: **52mg** • Carbohydrates: **9g** • Protein: **16g** • Sodium: **493mg**

. . . .

Healthy Preparation for Fred's Famous Meatballs "Two Ways" Sicilian Style Three Meats with Raisins and Pignoli & Traditional Neapolitan–Style

Entrée • Yields approximately 15 meatballs
Sicilian Style is Phases Two–Four
Traditional Neapolitan-Style is all Phases

Sicilian Style

To reduce calories, I take my favorite recipe for three-meat Sicilian meatballs with golden raisins and toasted pine nuts, which are typically either fried or baked with oil and cook them directly in a pot of hot tomato sauce. They come out moist and delicious—the raisins plump up and give them an incredible flavor. My San Marzano Tomato Sauce recipe is below.

INGREDIENTS

2 Tbsp. golden raisins (optional)

¼ cup marsala wine to soak raisins (optional)

1 cup plain bread crumbs (store bought is fine)

¼ cup of skim milk

½ pound ground lean sirloin or round

½ pound ground veal

½ pound ground lean pork

4 large eggs

1 cup freshly grated Pecorino Romano cheese

1 cup fresh Italian parsley, finely chopped

2 cloves garlic, minced

2 Tbsp. pine nuts, lightly toasted (optional)

1 tsp. of chili flakes (optional)

1 tsp. salt

freshly ground black pepper, to taste

INSTRUCTIONS

- Soak raisins in marsala wine for half an hour (optional).

- To prepare the bread, remove the crusts, cut into small cubes, soak a couple of minutes in the milk.

- Mix the ingredients with a fork until well amalgamated.

- Roll the meatballs by hand, forming approximately 15 balls (you can adjust the size as you wish).

- Drop rolled meatballs into a large pot of hot simmering tomato sauce and let simmer for a minimum of 30 minutes on low heat, gently stirring occasionally so they don't stick.

NOTE

Both dishes are cooked directly in simmering San Marzano Tomato Sauce. The marsala has 47 calories per ounce. If you don't soak the raisins, the recipe will contain 188 less calories, or 13 calories less per serving. If you omit the raisins (33 calories per Tbsp. or 66 for the recipe), and pine nuts (75 calories per Tbsp. or 150 calories for the recipe), you will save a total of 404 calories or 27 per serving, so each meatball will contain 104 calories.

Traditional Neapolitan-Style Meatballs

INSTRUCTIONS

- Use the same quantities of the above ingredients, except use 1½ pounds lean ground sirloin (omit the pork and veal). Also omit the raisins, marsala, and pine nuts. Mix and roll the meatballs, cook in simmering sauce as above.

Nutrition Facts (per serving / meatball) *Sicilian Style*
Calories: **131** • Calories from fat: **42%** • Fat: **6g** • Saturated fat: **3g**
Cholesterol: **90mg** • Carbohydrates: **3g** • Protein: **14g** • Sodium: **357mg**

-

Nutrition Facts (per serving) for fried/baked meatballs without raisins or pine nuts. *Traditional Neapolitan-Style*
Calories: **97** • Calories from fat: **36%** • Fat: **7g** • Saturated fat: **3g**
Cholesterol: **90mg** • Carbohydrates: **2g** • Protein: **14g** • Sodium: **321mg**

· ·

Fred's San Marzano Tomato Sauce

All Phases • Yields 12 cups

This is a staple in my family. It combines simple, quality ingredients, including San Marzano tomatoes imported from Italy, and fresh basil. Naturally, this is great over pasta (Phases Two–Four), and is the base for poaching my meatballs. It can serve as a base for other sauces and recipes. Refrigerate the sauce for up to a week or freeze it for up to several months.

INGREDIENTS

2 Tbsp. extra-virgin olive oil

1 yellow onion, minced

1 clove garlic, minced

4 28-ounce cans San Marzano
tomatoes, hand-crushed

1 cup water

2 cups fresh basil leaves (packed), torn

sea salt and freshly ground black
pepper, to taste

INSTRUCTIONS

• Heat oil in a large stockpot.

• When the oil is hot, add the onion and garlic, and sauté until light golden brown (do not burn the garlic).

• Add the hand-crushed tomatoes with the juice from the cans. Put ¼ cup water in each can, swish it around to gather up all the last of the tomato goodness, and add it to the sauce (1 cup water total).

• Add the fresh basil, salt and pepper, to taste. Serve immediately or let it simmer.

NOTE

One cup of tomato sauce is sufficient for a 4-ounce serving of pasta. Most pasta contains 100 calories per ounce, so 4 ounces of pasta with 1 cup of my sauce is 481 calories. Add a Tbsp. of freshly grated Parmesan, which is 22 calories.

Nutrition Facts (per serving)
Calories: **81** • Calories from fat: **29%** • Fat: **3g** • Saturated fat: **0g** •
Cholesterol: **0mg** • Carbohydrates: **14g** Protein: **3g** • Sodium: **223mg**

. . . .

Fred's "Light Pasta Carbonara"

Entrée • Phases Two–Four • Serves 5

This typical Roman dish is traditionally made with diced, sautéed pancetta, egg yolks, and lots of black pepper and cheese. In America, it is frequently featured with the addition of heavy cream, making it like an Alfredo sauce with bacon and egg. Both versions are tasty, but very high in calories and fat. I have come up with a lighter version of this popular dish. Mine uses diced prosciutto, which is leaner than the traditional pancetta or bacon. I go the Italian way on this and skip the cream altogether, relying on the egg and a touch of pasta water to create the sauce. Since even a light Carbonara contains calories, I recommend a 3-ounce portion of pasta, perfectly assembled in a nest on a dish.

INGREDIENTS

sea salt, for the pasta water

1 pound pasta of your choice

1 Tbsp. extra-virgin olive oil, to coat the pan

½ yellow onion, finely chopped

1 clove garlic, finely minced

1 thick slice (approximately 2 ounces) imported prosciutto, diced

2 eggs (buy organic eggs if possible)

1 cup pasta cooking water, set aside

¼ cup Pecorino Romano, freshly grated

¼ cup Parmigiano-Reggiano cheese, freshly grated

an abundance of freshly ground black pepper, to taste

1 cup fresh Italian parsley, finely chopped, for garnish

INSTRUCTIONS

- Bring large pot of well-salted water to a boil. Cook pasta of your choice until it is *al dente*.

- While the pasta cooks, heat a skillet coated with a drizzle of olive oil.

- When the oil is hot, sauté the onion until it is translucent, add the garlic, continue to sauté on medium for about a minute. Do not burn the garlic.

- Add the cut-up prosciutto and sauté for 1–2 minutes. Remove the pan from the heat.

- Take a paper towel and blot up all extra grease.

- In a bowl, mix the eggs, cheese, and pepper, and set aside.

- Strain the pasta, reserving 1 cup of the pasta water.

- Add the pasta to the sauté pan with the prosciutto, garlic, and onion off the heat. Mix well.

- Add the egg-cheese-pepper mix.

- Add in a little pasta water at a time, continuing to stir. You will likely use several Tbsp. of the pasta water, not all of it. The strands of pasta should be lightly coated. If the sauce is too thick, add a little more pasta water. Just be sure to add a little at a time, you don't want the eggs to curdle. Garnish with parsley and serve.

Nutrition Facts (per serving)
Calories: **429** • Calories from fat: **21%** • Fat: **10g** • Saturated fat: **3g**
Cholesterol: **175mg** • Carbohydrates: **63g** • Protein: **20g** • Sodium: **286mg**

. . . .

Roasted Eggplant Parmigiana

Entrée • All Phases • Serves 4

In this satisfying dish, roasting the eggplant instead of sautéing greatly reduces the calories and results in an earthy, delicious flavor. This is essentially the traditional version in Italy, which uses *Parmigiano* rather than mozzarella. Mozzarella has approximately 100 calories per ounce (an average slice).

INGREDIENTS

2 Tbsp. extra-virgin olive oil, to coat baking pan

2 large eggplants

sea salt and freshly ground black pepper, to taste

2 cups San Marzano Tomato Sauce

¼ cup freshly grated Parmigiano-Reggiano or Pecorino Romano

8 ounces fresh mozzarella, thinly sliced (use only in Phases Two–Four)

1 cup fresh basil leaves cut into **chiffonade**, for garnish

INSTRUCTIONS

· Pre-heat the oven to 450 degrees Fahrenheit.

· Oil a baking sheet with olive oil.

· Slice eggplants into 1-inch-thick rounds. Lightly season each slice with salt and pepper, place on the lightly oiled sheet. Bake the eggplant for approximately 10–12 minutes, or until golden brown.

· Remove the eggplant from the oven. Remove the slices from the baking sheet and place them on a plate lined with paper towels to cool. Blot with additional paper towels to remove any excess oil.

· Reduce oven temperature to 350 degrees Fahrenheit.

· Place the eggplant slices in a baking dish, arranging them in 4 stacks.

· Sprinkle with grated cheese.

· Spoon sauce over each, then cover with a thin slice of fresh mozzarella.

- Bake uncovered until the cheese is melted and the tops are a light golden brown, about 20 minutes. Serve immediately garnished with chiffonade of basil.

Nutrition Facts (per serving)
Calories: **312** • Calories from fat: **52%** • Fat: **18g** • Saturated fat: **9g**
Cholesterol: **50mg** • Carbohydrates: **22g** • Protein: **18g** • Sodium: **1188mg**

. . . .

My Mother's Spanish Rice—with Brown Rice

Entrée • All Phases • Serves 6

This is a very satisfying favorite of mine. To make it healthier, I use brown rice. It tastes delicious. This dish demonstrates how a little bacon can flavor an entire sauce or dish. Cooking the bacon separately and blotting off the fat eliminates calories.

This dish is also excellent with shrimp in addition to or in place of the bacon. Use 3–4 large shrimp per person. Clean and devein them and toss them raw into the sauce when it is almost done. The shrimp will cook in only a few minutes. The same sauce is great with 3–4 ounces of pasta per person. Simply cook the pasta until *al dente* and toss in the pan with the sauce, adding a splash of pasta water while tossing over hot stove. Serve immediately.

If you like a little heat, you can add a pinch of red chili flakes.

INGREDIENTS

1 cup uncooked brown rice
2 strips bacon (Phases Two–Four), or may use an equivalent amount of diced ham
2 Tbsp. extra-virgin olive oil
1 large yellow onion, chopped
1 red bell pepper, seeds and stem removed, chopped
1 green bell pepper, seeds and stem removed, chopped
1 orange bell pepper, seeds and stem removed, chopped

1 yellow bell pepper, seeds and stem removed, chopped
1 cup white mushrooms, brushed clean, sliced
sea salt and freshly ground black pepper, to taste
2 cups San Marzano Tomato Sauce (see recipe in the Pastas and Sauces section)

INSTRUCTIONS

- Cook the rice according to the instructions on the package. Set aside.

- While the rice cooks, sauté the bacon in a small skillet until crispy. Set it aside to drain on paper towels.

- Heat the canola oil in a large sauté pan or Dutch oven over medium heat.

- Sweat the onion, peppers, and mushrooms until soft, add salt and pepper, to taste.

- Add the tomato sauce.

- Crumble the bacon into small pieces, and add to the sauce.

- Add the cooked rice.

- Simmer over medium-low heat for several minutes so flavors amalgamate.

NOTE

There are approximately 43 calories in a slice of bacon. Making this without the bacon results in 86 less calories total, or 14 calories less per serving.

Nutrition Facts (per serving)
Calories: **240** • Calories from fat: **26%** • Fat: **7g** •Saturated fat: **1g**
Cholesterol: **3mg** • Carbohydrates: **41g** • Protein: **6g** • Sodium: **390mg**

. . . .

Fred's Chicken Cacciatore "in the hunter's style"

Entrée • All Phases • Serves 6

INGREDIENTS

6 chicken thighs with skin[40], 6 chicken legs, with skin (can substitute or add breasts)

sea salt and freshly ground black pepper, to taste

2 Tbsp. extra-virgin olive oil or canola oil

4 cloves garlic, sliced

1 yellow onion, chopped

1 cup sliced white mushrooms

sprig rosemary

1 cup dry white wine

1 cup frozen peas

4 cups crushed imported San Marzano tomatoes or San Marzano Tomato Sauce

---

40 Cook with the skin on, but remove skin to eat.

½ cup fresh basil leaves

pinch dried Sicilian or regular oregano, to taste

½ cup fresh Italian parsley, finely chopped, to garnish.

INSTRUCTIONS

- Heat a large stock pot or Dutch oven over medium heat with the oil.

- When oil is hot, add the garlic, onion, rosemary, and mushrooms, and sautée for several minutes.

- Season the chicken with salt and pepper, and add pieces to the pot, several at a time to brown.

- Once they are browned to a light golden brown, remove and set aside, repeating until all pieces have been browned.

- Add the white wine to deglaze for several minutes.

- Add the tomatoes, basil, oregano, and peas, and return the chicken to the pot. Reduce heat to medium-low for 5 minutes, stirring gently.

- Reduce heat to low and allow to simmer for 30 minutes, gently stirring occasionally.

- Garnish with Italian parsley and serve.

Nutrition Facts (per serving)
Calories: **454** • Calories from fat: **29%** • Fat: **15g** • Saturated fat: **3g**
Cholesterol: **131mg** • Carbohydrates: **34g** • Protein: **40g** • Sodium: **1222mg**

Cedar Plank Grilled Salmon—"Two Ways"—with Blood Orange Reduction and Honey Dijon Salmon

Entrée • All Phases • Serves 4

Cooking salmon fillets directly on cedar planks over a hot fire gives the fish an extraordinary flavor. And it's fun to serve the salmon right on the plank. As the salmon cooks, check it frequently. If the planks catch fire, spray them with a light mist of water. You might need to move them to a cooler part of the grill. You can also cook the salmon right on the grill without the cedar plank.

INGREDIENTS

4 6-inch cedar planks

4 6-ounce wild salmon fillets, skin removed

sea salt and freshly ground black pepper, to taste.

INSTRUCTIONS

Grilling:

- Soak the cedar planks in warm salted water for at least an hour, drain.

- Remove skin from salmon. Rinse the salmon and pat dry with paper towels. Season with salt and pepper on both sides.

- See the instructions for 2 versions below: if you are making **Blood Orange Salmon**, grill the fish without coating or marinating. If you're making **Honey Dijon Salmon**, coat the salmon before grilling. If you're making **Asian Salmon**, marinate the fillets for 30 minutes before grilling.

- Pre-heat grill to medium.

- Place the planks on the grill.

- When the planks start to crackle and smoke, put one salmon fillet on each plank.

- Cover the grill and cook approximately 20 minutes, or until salmon flakes. The internal temperature should read 135 degrees Fahrenheit for medium-rare.

Blood Orange Reduction:

- While the salmon is grilling, heat 2 cups of strained blood orange juice in a saucepan and boil over medium heat for about 20 minutes, until it has reduced and thickened. Spoon the sauce over the salmon before serving.

Honey Dijon Salmon:

- Mix together 4 Tbsp. each coarse grain Dijon mustard and honey. Before grilling, rub the salmon fillets with mixture

- Before grilling, marinate the salmon in this mixture for 30 minutes.

Nutrition Facts (per serving)
Calories: **297** • Calories from fat: **33%** • Fat: **11g** • Saturated fat: **2g**
Cholesterol: **94mg** • Carbohydrates: **13g** • Protein: **35g** • Sodium: **115mg**

Nutrition Facts (per serving)
Calories: **316** • Calories from fat: **32%** • Fat: **11g** • Saturated fat: **2g** •
Cholesterol: **94mg** • Carbohydrates: **19g** • Protein: **34g** • Sodium: **289mg**

. . . .

Escarole & Cannellini Beans and Escarole Neapolitan-Style

Side Dish • All Phases • Serves 4 as a side dish

INGREDIENTS

1 large head of escarole

4 cloves garlic, thinly sliced

2 cups canned cannellini beans, rinsed

3 Tbsp. extra-virgin olive oil

½ cup chicken broth

pinch of sea salt and freshly ground black pepper

red chili flakes, to taste (optional)

INSTRUCTIONS

Escarole & Cannellini Beans:

• Rinse the escarole and remove and discard the bottom. Cut the leaves into bite-sized pieces.

• Heat the oil in a large skillet over medium heat.

• When the oil is hot, add the garlic and cook until lightly golden brown. Do not burn the garlic.

• Add the escarole, salt, pepper, chicken broth, and red chili flakes and cook until fork tender.

• Add the cannellini beans, toss for another minute, and serve.

Escarole Neapolitan-Style:

• To the above recipe, add 1 cup of tomato sauce or crushed tomatoes. You may also want to add up to ¼ cup toasted pine nuts, ¼ cup imported black olives with the pit (Gaeta or Kalamata), and ¼ cup golden raisins to the sautéed escarole in place of the beans. This is very Neapolitan and is also delicious.

Nutrition Facts (per serving)
Calories: **209** • Calories from fat: **44%** • Fat: **10g** • Saturated fat: **1g**
Cholesterol: **0mg** • Carbohydrates: **21g** • Protein: **9g** • Sodium: **277mg**

-

Nutrition Facts (per serving) for Neapolitan Escarole:
Calories: **243** • Calories from fat: **61%** • Fat: **17g** • Saturated fat: **2g**
Cholesterol: **0mg** • Carbohydrates: **23g** • Protein: **4g** • Sodium: **637mg**

· ·

Strawberries with Balsamic & Black Pepper

Dessert • All Phases • Serves 4

This is a surprisingly great combination and way to enhance strawberries, or a mixture of fresh berries. The balsamic vinegar soaks into the strawberries and enhances the flavor! Black pepper works very well with this, you may omit if you wish. Instead of marinating in balsamic vinegar, you can simply pour a little of an estate balsamic or balsamic glaze over the berries and enjoy immediately. In Phases 3 and 4, I also like to marinate my strawberries along with optional blueberries, blackberries, and raspberries for 30 minutes in a bowl with a couple ounces of Grand Marnier before serving, which makes an amazing dessert, and the small amount of Grand Marnier imparts wonderful flavor without a ton of calories.

INGREDIENTS

2 cups ripe strawberries, hulled
  and halved

¼ cup balsamic vinegar
freshly ground black pepper, to taste

INSTRUCTIONS

• Rinse, hull, and slice strawberries.

• Place in a bowl and pour in the balsamic vinegar, mix to coat the strawberries.

• Cover and let stand at room temperature for up to one hour to marinate.

• Garnish with optional freshly ground black pepper.

Nutrition Facts (per serving)
Calories: **160** • Calories from fat: **75%** • Fat: **14g** • Saturated fat: **2g**
Cholesterol: **0mg** • Carbohydrates: **10g** • Protein: **2g** • Sodium: **24mg**

· · · · · · · · · · · · · · · · · ·

Casey's Baked Fruit

Dessert • All Phases

This is perhaps the easiest, lowest calorie dessert that doesn't taste like a simple, low-calorie dessert! It works well with the fruit of your choice such as apples, pears, peaches, or nectarines.

INSTRUCTIONS

- Simply prick the fruit several times with a fork and place in a baking dish.
- Bake the fruit in a baking dish with a ½-inch of water surrounding them in a 350-degree pre-heated oven for 45 minutes, or until golden brown and soft.
- Sprinkle with cinnamon.
- Remove from oven and let stand for a few minutes.
- These can be served hot, at room temperature, or chilled, and are great with some frozen yogurt or low-fat whipped topping.

NOTE

Several golden raisins placed on top of each apple are excellent when baked with the apples.

Nutrition Facts (per serving)
Calories: **160** • Calories from fat: **75%** • Fat: **14g** • Saturated fat: **2g**
Cholesterol: **0mg** • Carbohydrates: **10g** • Protein: **2g** • Sodium: **24mg**

Appendix A
Top 12 Tips for Eating Out and Dining at Home

These simple tips should be part of your lifestyle throughout the first three Phases of losing weight. You will want to continue using them as you enjoy your new life in Phase Four.

1. **Simple advice for snacks:** light and low-fat Greek yogurt are great options, especially Dannon Activia Light and Light Greek yogurt. It is a good idea to keep lots of fresh fruit and vegetables on hand, so you can always have a healthy snack or throw together a salad. Some of the best items are seedless grapes, tomatoes, carrots, oranges, apples, peaches, nectarines, plums, bananas, strawberries, blueberries, raspberries, blackberries, grapes, pineapple, and grapefruit. Some fruits are high in sugar, so if you are diabetic, your doctor will likely restrict your intake of foods with a high glycemic index (high sugar content).

2. **Buy fruit already cut:** it is convenient to have fruit on hand that is already cut-up. I do this with a variety of melons. Having it ready to eat makes it a lot easier when you are in a rush. Make your life easier! If you are short on time, spend a little more for convenience—buy fruit already cut-up. I assure you, you will be more likely to eat it! Instead of having to peel carrots, buy the baby-cut carrots.

3. **Make sandwiches out of lettuce wraps instead of bread.** Save roughly 100 calories per slice of sandwich bread and use the large leaves from a head of iceberg lettuce to wrap the components of your sandwich. This also works as a substitute for a hamburger bun.

4. **Avoid regular mayonnaise, sour cream, whole milk, heavy cream.** Go for reduced-fat—in the case of mayonnaise, try Hellman's Light.

5. **Try sprouted bread in place of regular bread, try multi-grain bread or whole-wheat flour in place of white flour:** an excellent choice for French toast or toasted with a slice of cheese and some mustard, lettuce, tomato, and turkey.

6. **Buy lean and not-processed cold cuts:** it is a good idea to keep lean cold cuts, not the processed variety, on hand. Turkey sliced from the frame and roast beef are some good examples. Pre-packaged cold cuts (lunch meats) are not recommended.

7. **Grill or roast vegetables:** these can be brushed with a little olive oil and sprinkled with a touch of sea salt. Keep already roasted veggies on hand for an easy, healthy snack.

8. **Shrimp are your friend:** shrimp are an excellent source of protein and are 27 calories an ounce! A shrimp cocktail is an excellent, light snack!

9. **Eggs are excellent!** Eggs, egg whites, and Egg Beaters all make a healthy and easy meal or snack option. Try eating a hard-boiled egg as a snack—eggs are a great, satisfying breakfast that can be prepared a lot of healthy, delicious ways. A nifty trick is to make or order an omelet or frittata with half egg and half egg white. This provides the added flavor of egg, but is lower-calorie than if it were all egg. Include a variety of vegetables in your omelet or frittata—I often like to throw in leftover vegetables from the previous night's dinner, so nothing goes to waste.

10. **Don't skip breakfast:** while I'm personally not a fan of a large breakfast, except for the occasional Sunday brunch, it is essential to start your day out right with something for breakfast, even if it is as simple as some fruit, yogurt, or perhaps a couple eggs. Give your body the fuel it needs to get through the day and to be at peak performance—do not starve yourself. Statistics show that people who skip breakfast or who don't have a healthy, balanced, satisfying meal in the morning are more likely to overeat later in the day. Starving yourself in the morning actually works against efforts to lose weight by slowing down your metabolism. Think of your body and metabolism in terms of a furnace. You have to feed the furnace, preferably a little at a time, for it to burn more efficiently and consistently. My favorite breakfast choices include eggs, egg whites, smoked salmon with tomatoes and onions, or some fresh fruit, occasionally half of a bagel, a whole-wheat pancake (I like to add in fruit, like blueberries, bananas, strawberries, apples, etc.), or French toast made with sprouted or multi-grain bread. It is all about choices and balance. Reducing the amount of cheese in an omelet or frittata, or using reduced-fat cheese can save a lot of calories.

11. **Making amazing salads:** there are few things I enjoy more than a great salad. They are easy to put together and can be made with so many different choices of vegetables and other foods that it is nearly impossible to get bored. Vegetables and lettuces are low in calories and high in water content or volume, so you can consume a large bowl of salad (appropriately dressed, and so long as the other ingredients are healthy), which is a great way to satisfy yourself, especially early on, when you are accustomed to eating larger portions. Try always keeping a variety of ingredients for a good salad in the house: arugula, radicchio, crumbled blue cheese, gorgonzola, or feta, roasted peppers, avocado, hearts of palm, mandarin oranges, beets, and almonds, among others. To further enhance a salad and turn it into a full meal, add shrimp, grilled salmon, grilled chicken, seared tuna, slices of leftover steak, turkey, grilled or roasted vegetables, or hard-boiled eggs. For some healthy dressings, keep lemons, garlic, and good olive oil in the house, and keep vinegar options open by having quality balsamic and white balsamic as well as red wine, Champagne, and apple cider vinegar. If you crave the flavor of bacon or cheese in a salad, try a chopped salad. Put half a strip of bacon or turkey bacon or one ounce of crumbled cheese in with your veggies, add the dressing, and chop your salad, mixing it well! Every bite will have the flavor of bacon and cheese, but with a lot fewer calories than if you had added enough whole pieces of each item so that you'd have some in every bite.

12. **Buy a measuring scale and use it. Use your measuring cup and spoons.** Get in the habit of measuring every ingredient, especially when using things like oil, butter, and cheese, it makes it a lot easier to keep from adding too much fat or too many calories than if you were simply "guestimating."

Appendix B
Phase One Sample Breakfasts, Snacks, and Desserts

To get you started, I have included some sample breakfasts and desserts you may enjoy in Phase One (and forever), since I most frequently enjoyed them at home, and snacks can easily be taken with you to work.

PHASE ONE SAMPLE BREAKFASTS:

DAY 1:

- Egg White and Veggie Omelet
- 1 cup Irish steel-cut oatmeal, with cinnamon
- Coffee or tea with skim milk
- 6 ounces low-sodium V8 Vegetable Juice, Low Sodium

DAY 2:

- • 4 ounces Dannon Activia Light, Dannon Danactive, or low-fat Greek yogurt
- 1 cup mixed berries or fruit
- Coffee or tea with skim milk
- 6 ounces low-sodium V8 Vegetable Juice, Low Sodium

DAY 3:

- • ½ grapefruit
- *Egg White "Neo" Omelet—Nova, Eggs, and Onions*
- Coffee or tea with skim milk
- 6 ounces low-sodium V8 Vegetable Juice, Low Sodium

DAY 4:

- ½ cantaloupe
- ½ cup low-fat cottage cheese, drizzled with honey

- ½ cup mixed berries
- Coffee or tea with skim milk
- 6 ounces low-sodium V8 Vegetable Juice, Low Sodium

DAY 5:

- 4 ounces smoked salmon, sliced tomatoes, and onion
- 1 hard-boiled egg
- 1 cup mixed berries or fruit
- Coffee or tea with skim milk
- 6 ounces low-sodium V8 vegetable juice

ALL PHASES SNACK IDEAS:

You should typically enjoy 2 light snacks each day, the first snack around 10:30 a.m., between breakfast and lunch, and the second snack around 3:00 p.m., between lunch and dinner.)

- ½ grapefruit
- 1 cup seedless grapes
- 1 cup of mixed fruit or berries
- Fruit and yogurt smoothie
- Cup of soup, such as Chicken Vegetable, Minestrone, Lentil, or Roasted Butternut Squash
- Shrimp cocktail
- Tabbouleh
- Crudités of raw vegetables with ¼ cup Tzatziki—Greek Yogurt and Cucumber Dip
- 4 ounces Dannon Activia Light, Dannon Danactive, or low-fat Greek yogurt
- ½ cup prunes
- ½ cup canned peaches
- Apple, peach, nectarine, pear, etc.
- Sliced tomato, red onion, avocado, and fresh basil with a drizzle of extra-virgin olive oil and balsamic vinegar
- Tuna/salmon sashimi—3 pieces with 1 cup seaweed salad
- Banana
- Baked sweet potato

PHASE ONE DE SSERT IDEAS:

- Mixed berries and low-fat Greek yogurt or Dannon Activia Light
- Fresh berries and 1 cup frozen yogurt
- Home-made lemon or raspberry sorbetto (blend ice with the fruit and optional Splenda)
- Baked apple with cinnamon and optional low-fat whipped topping
- Baked peach
- Frozen yogurt (should be less than 100 calories for 4 ounces); avoid toppings

Resources

Calorie Counter and Exercise monitor: www.livestrong.com
Livestrong also has considerable online support and a huge community of users to assist one another.

Overeaters Anonymous: www.oa.org
OA utilizes the twelve steps and twelve traditions, adapted from Alcoholics Anonymous, to help overeaters find a spiritual solution to their overeating.

Codependents Anonymous (CoDA): www.coda.org
This program is a twelve-step group whose purpose is to help men and women develop healthy relationships.

Al-Anon: www.al-anon.alateen.org
This program is a twelve-step group designed for the families of alcoholics to share experience, strength, and hope. There are anonymous groups worldwide to help people deal with numerous addictions and their effects on family and friends.

Recipe analyzer/calorie estimators:
www.fitwatch.com/database/analyzer.php
http://recipes.sparkpeople.com/recipe-calculator.asp
www.caloriecount.about.com

Centers for Disease Control: www.cdc.gov

Web MD: www.webmd.com
This is a site that can be used for medical and health-related references.

Acknowledgements

I would like to acknowledge those whose support has been instrumental in helping me transform my life. There were times in my life, and especially during the year it took me to lose 150 pounds and during tough times that followed, when it seemed easier to give up, but each of your unique contributions have helped me persevere.

First, I would like to thank my godmother, Dr. Flavia Gusmano, and her husband, Dr. Daniel Galvin, for your support throughout the years and for encouraging me to try to lose weight "my way" rather than take any shortcuts. Thank you for making me the proud godfather to two amazing children, Daniel and Nicholas.

Thank you to my friend and cardiologist, Dr. Gene Myers, whose persistence and medical expertise helped make this all possible. Dr. Myers also referred me to Linda Sherr, my therapist, whose insight was key to helping resolve many years of unresolved emotional conflict that had contributed to, and resulted in, my obesity. Therapy has helped me to change my attitude and adopt a new, more positive outlook on life. Without a competent, compassionate doctor, and a qualified therapist, my weight loss certainly would not have happened so quickly. Thank you to Maureen Buchbinder for her expertise and help in ensuring that I was following a good, healthy food plan as I sought to diet my way.

Thank you to my friend Dick Smothers for being such an inspiration, my friend Suzi Karp for her words of support, my friend Elizabeth English Strickman for her encouragement and being a great walking buddy who helped me transition from simply walking to powerwalking. Thanks to my cousin Sandra and her husband, Kurt, for getting me into running, and inspiring me to give a half marathon and later a full marathon a shot. It is hard to imagine that, a few years earlier, I had a tough time walking.

Thank you to my friend and colleague, Deborah Burns for her vision in seeing a much bigger picture—an entire brand and persona in addition *The Restaurant Diet*, and for helping me to put my dream of living and sharing my international healthy gourmet lifestyle into action! Thank you to my friend Tracey Thomas, publisher of *Venu Magazine*, who offered me my first writing gig with a food and travel column. Thank you to Brian Thorne and Manny Santiago of Veritas Productions for your brilliant work in helping produce videos of me and my chef/restaurant partners, which has helped capture the visual essence of what the Fred Bollaci brand and philosophy is all about. Thank you to my agents, Doug Grad and Ellen Scordato who embraced *The Restaurant Diet* from day one and helped find my book a home. Thank you to my editor, Gary Krebs for your keen insight and advice in helping finalize this book into something better than I imagined! Thank you to Natasha Vera, my editor at Mango for your assistance and suggestions, and to cover designer Elina Diaz for your creative take in making a tape measure look like a long strand of *pappardelle* pasta!

There are many special people who have touched my life and helped me on my journey, too many to name, but you all know who you are. Good friends are hard to find. I am blessed to have so many special people in my life.

I firmly believe that God puts people in our lives for specific reasons, and I know I couldn't have transformed my life without a solid support system of family, friends, and professionals. Thank you all.

Lastly, I would like to thank and acknowledge all the wonderful chefs, restaurant owners, and their staff who have made *The Restaurant Diet* and its success possible. Special thanks to Chef Gabriel Kreuther, a phenomenal Michelin-Star New York chef who is quoted on the cover for your enthusiastic endorsement and for totally understanding and embracing my concept. Every restaurant owner and chef in here deserves my sincere gratitude and your patronage—you're not going to find a finer group of establishments, owners, and chefs anywhere. You all inspire me as a home cook and make what I do so enjoyable. A shout out to those establishments in the Boca Raton, Delray Beach, Palm Beach, and South Florida area, where I live and did a majority of my restaurant dieting, from the very beginning when I was over 300 pounds. You especially worked with and supported me during the most difficult part of my weight-loss journey, the transition from a gourmand who ate whatever I wanted into someone who learned to savor and appreciate great food, in moderation.

In fact, you may have noticed that the four phases of *The Restaurant Diet* actually spell "BOCA." Boca not only means "mouth" which is apropos since everything we eat comes through our mouths, but I have taken Boca one step further, a personal state of mind or mantra that stands for "Bold Ongoing Change in Attitude" that has been at the core of my weight loss and lifestyle transformation. One last note to you, my readers. Thank you for picking up and reading this book. I wish you all the success in the world and a life of health and happiness. Your future success is my success, and it would be most gratifying to know I helped inspire you. Please keep an open mind as you progress on your journey to a new and healthier you. To succeed, we must be bold. We must realize that the transformation is not quick; it takes time, dedication, and determination, and does not stop once the weight comes off—it is ongoing, forever! It all centers around attitude. A positive attitude can make all the difference in whether or not we succeed. No matter where you are starting from, be optimistic! Be kind to yourself. Look at the glass as half full rather than half empty, and look at your best days as being ahead of you. Forget all the times you may have failed and how much you dislike the thought of dieting. Start fresh, from a clean slate. Look at food as your friend, not something you have to fear. If you enjoy eating out, look at your favorite restaurants as potential partners in your success. You are their customer and they are there for you, you've just got to let them know. My hope is that *The Restaurant Diet* will help you find the strength and courage within yourself to embrace a new way of looking at weight loss, and open the door to the exciting new life you were always meant to live.

About the Author:
Fred Bollaci

Fred Bollaci is an attorney, entrepreneur, gourmand, world traveler, sommelier, and international healthy gourmet lifestyle, food, wine, travel, and fitness expert, who has enjoyed a gourmet lifestyle since childhood. After losing 150 pounds in twelve months in 2009–10, Fred has maintained his weight loss and has embraced a healthy version of gourmet living, which he writes about in his Golden Palate blog and shares on social media. Since losing the weight, Fred has helped motivate and inspire friends, family, and strangers with his positive, hopeful message. In 2014, Fred established his company, Fred Bollaci Enterprises, *the* definitive international healthy lifestyle brand and authority, and is dedicated to showing people across America and worldwide how to live a healthy, gourmet lifestyle. He has established excellent working relationships with hundreds of highly regarded restaurateurs, chefs, lodging destinations, and artisan producers, in both the United States and in Italy, establishments whose passionate owners, chefs, and staff are committed to providing guests with a high-quality experience, through healthy gourmet options. Fred has developed and trademarked both the Golden Palate Certificate of Excellence and the Platinum Palate Certificate of Excellence, two prestigious symbols of the very best in dining and hospitality. To date, Fred has awarded his prestigious Golden Palate Certificate of Excellence to over 750 establishments worldwide, and the coveted Platinum Palate Certificate of Excellence to over 100 exceptional establishments.

Fred is a practicing trusts and estates attorney in Florida, holds an MBA, and is a licensed real estate broker.

Fred offers consultations in-person, and via phone or Skype for anyone looking for motivation or assistance in losing weight and has been invited to speak to countless groups, sharing his valuable insight.

Fred is also a contributing writer and author of "The Golden Palate" Appetite Column in *Venu Magazine,* a prestigious contemporary culture publication based in the New York area with quarterly distribution in key markets nationwide, as well as an online digital issue. www.venumagazine.com

Fred currently resides in Delray Beach, Florida with his two dogs, a Cavalier King Charles Spaniel named Charlie, and a Zuchon (Teddy Bear) named Teddy. His passions include cooking, wine, dining out, travel, fitness, golf, photography, writing, gardening, and his dogs. For more information about Fred Bollaci, please visit Fred Bollaci Enterprises' website, www.fredbollacienterprises.com and subscribe to Fred's e-blast list to find out the latest and greatest places to dine and stay, delicious recipes, fabulous destinations, fitness tips, special events, breaking news, and more!